Introduction to Occupational Therapy
2nd Edition

Introduction to Occupational Therapy

2nd Edition

BARBARA SABONIS-CHAFEE, MS, OTR
FORMER SENIOR INSTRUCTOR
OCCUPATIONAL THERAPY DEPARTMENT
PALM BEACH COMMUNITY COLLEGE
LAKE WORTH, FLORIDA

SUSAN M. HUSSEY, MS, OTR
PROGRAM COORDINATOR AND INSTRUCTOR
OCCUPATIONAL THERAPY ASSISTANT PROGRAM
SACRAMENTO CITY COLLEGE
SACRAMENTO, CALIFORNIA

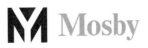 Mosby

St. Louis Baltimore Boston Carlsbad Chicago Minneapolis New York Philadelphia Portland
London Milan Sydney Tokyo Toronto

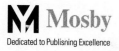
Dedicated to Publishing Excellence

PUBLISHER: John Schrefer
EXECUTIVE EDITOR: Martha Sasser
DEVELOPMENTAL EDITOR: Amy Christopher
PROJECT MANAGER: Gayle Morris
COVER DESIGNER: David Zielinski

Printed in the United States of America
Design, production, and composition: GraphCom Corporation
Printing and binding: RR Donnelley

Mosby–Year Book, Inc.
11830 Westline Industrial Drive
St. Louis, MO 63146

ISBN 0-8151-8251-1

99 00 01/9 8 7 6 5 4 3

Dedications

To the memory of my parents, Anna and Stanley Sabonis.

BSC

❖ ❖ ❖

To my mother, Lois, for her sense of values, pride in achievement, emphasis on advanced education, and frequent reminders to "take one day at a time."

SMH

Acknowledgments

This text would not have been possible without the contribution and support of several individuals. First of all, we would like to acknowledge all of the students and faculty who throughout each of our careers have provided feedback on our teaching and classroom resources. We would also like to thank AOTA for their willingness to provide various materials for this book. Finally, we would like to thank the staff at Mosby for all of their encouragement and assistance with this project. Martha Sasser, Amy Christopher, and Dana Peick have been an exceptional team with whom to work.

BSC and SMH

❖ ❖ ❖

My thanks to my son, Tom Sabonis-Chafee, for his assistance and to my daughters, Terry, Cathy, and Lisa, for their continued support. Although I am no longer actively teaching, I continue to be grateful for all that I have learned from my interaction with students—it is often said that teaching is the best possible learning experience.

BSC

❖ ❖ ❖

I would like to thank my friend and mentor, Albert Cook, for taking the time to review each chapter and provide much valued feedback, in spite of his own very hectic schedule. A rehabilitation engineer by training and an OT practitioner at heart, Al has a keen sense of knowledge on topics related to occupational therapy and health care. I want to also thank my friend, Maureen Paine, for her ongoing encouragement and support. Finally, many thanks go to my husband, Bruce, who filled many supportive roles during this project. I am so grateful for his patience, sense of humor, inspiration, and ability to adapt throughout my work on this project.

SMH

PREFACE

Introduction to Occupational Therapy, 2nd edition, is written for those entering study of the profession of occupational therapy. This text is especially written for those who intend to become practitioners at either the professional level (OTR) or the technical level (COTA) or for those who are exploring the profession to determine whether this is the field for them. *Introduction to Occupational Therapy* is written to give the reader a solid view of the important concerns and concepts of occupational therapy without burdening the student with information and details that he or she may not yet have the background to understand.

The text is divided into three sections. The first section introduces the reader to the field of occupational therapy, which includes a pictorial essay of the field, the history and philosophy of occupational therapy, occupational therapy personnel and educational requirements, the settings in which occupational therapy is practiced, professional ethics and regulations, and the national professional organization. Section Two focuses on the occupational therapy process and includes chapters on occupational performance, assessment, treatment planning and implementation, and the service management functions performed by the occupational therapy practitioner. Section Three takes into consideration the special skills that are needed by the individual practitioner in the field of occupational therapy, introducing medical terminology, development of therapeutic relationships, selection of therapeutic activities, and development of clinical reasoning.

This edition of *Introduction to Occupational Therapy* has been organized to make learning easy for the reader. Each chapter begins with a testimonial written by an OTR or a COTA about his or her experiences in occupational therapy. These personal accounts highlight the humanistic nature of our profession and relate theories and concepts to the real world of occupational therapy. Each chapter is introduced with learning objectives that outline the main points covered in that chapter; the learning objectives are followed by a list of key terms. These terms are typeset in boldface throughout the text. A summary at the end of each chapter provides a synopsis of the material covered. There are also suggested activities at the end of each chapter that provide ways to apply the information or concepts covered in the chapter.

To the teacher:

To make the best use of this text for occupational therapy students, it is suggested that it be used as the core text in conjunction with three other requirements:

❖ Self-paced medical terminology study
❖ Beginning field research (using suggested activities
❖ Individual and group classroom exercises

The student will not only form a coherent picture of occupational therapy and begin to develop problem-solving skills, he or she will also become an independent active learner.

Some of the suggested activities can be incorporated into class planning. One way to use the activities would be to expect each student to be involved in a term project, choosing one activity from those available. The end of the term review could be supplemented by each student presenting his or her project to the class.

TABLE OF CONTENTS

Section Two

THE PRACTICE OF OCCUPATIONAL THERAPY

Section Three

SPECIFIC SKILLS OF THE OCCUPATIONAL THERAPY PRACTITIONER

SECTION ONE OF <u>INTRODUCTION TO OCCUPATIONAL THERAPY</u> INTRODUCES THE FIELD OF OCCUPATIONAL THERAPY WITH A QUESTION-AND-ANSWER FORMAT THAT PROVIDES A BROAD OVERVIEW AND IS SUPPLEMENTED BY A PHOTOGRAPHIC ESSAY OF OCCUPATIONAL THERAPY IN APPLICATION. THE TERM "OCCUPATION," AS IT IS USED WITHIN THE PROFESSION, IS CLARIFIED.

THE RICH HISTORY OF OCCUPATIONAL THERAPY IS EXPLORED IN CHAPTER TWO, WHICH IS FOLLOWED BY AN EXAMINATION OF THE PHILOSOPHICAL BASE OF OCCUPATIONAL THERAPY IN CHAPTER THREE. THE CONTENTS OF CHAPTERS FOUR AND FIVE PROVIDE INFORMATION REGARDING OCCUPATIONAL THERAPY PERSONNEL, EDUCATIONAL REQUIREMENTS, AND VARIOUS EMPLOYMENT SETTINGS. CHAPTERS SIX AND SEVEN DEAL WITH THE ETHICS, STANDARDS, AND REGULATIONS THAT GUIDE THE PROFESSION. THE FINAL CHAPTER IN THIS SECTION, CHAPTER EIGHT, DESCRIBES THE ORGANIZATION, MISSION, AND ACTIVITIES OF THE NATIONAL ASSOCIATION THAT SUPPORTS THE PROFESSION.

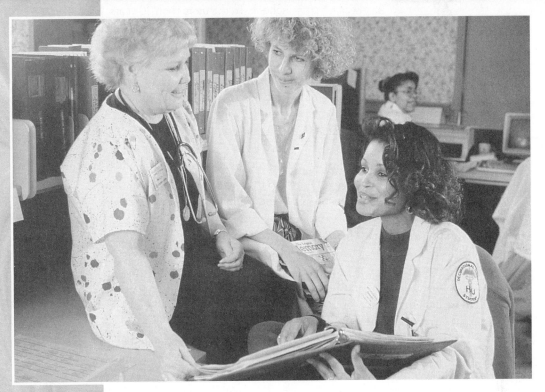

ONE

Occupational Therapy: The Profession

*f*or many years, I believed that I first became interested in occupational therapy when I worked as a research assistant in a psychiatric hospital. The occupational therapy clinic was a few doors from my office, and I had a first-hand view of the patients' responses to creating tie-dyed T-shirts and scented candles. Defeat and uneasiness were replaced by smiles and confidence, all in a matter of hours.

The activities reminded me of my childhood. My mother patiently taught me and my six younger sisters and brothers many different arts and crafts. More importantly, she let us loose in the "playroom" where we spent endless hours with glue, scissors, bits of wire, yarn, plastic lace, found objects, and scraps of paper from my father's office, making whatever we pleased. I learned needle crafts from my mother, and my grandmother taught me cross-stitch embroidery when I was 8 years of age. Throughout these formative years, a consistent theme was there—activities are fun and important; they can be life-long companions and sources of joy and self-esteem.

The link between my own childhood experiences of working through activities and the reactions of patients to occupational therapy grew stronger as I watched from my office. It wasn't long before I applied and was accepted into occupational therapy school. In the more than 20 years since I graduated, I never regretted my career decision and often look back with some amazement to the coincidences that led me to it. I love teaching people, especially those who fear they cannot learn or cannot do—because, of course, they *can* learn and *can* do. To me, it is the greatest pleasure to witness the "ah-hah!" look and the triumphant expression that comes with accomplishment in the face of fear.

It soon became obvious that my ties to occupational therapy predated my research assistant job. It wasn't until after I graduated from school and had been working several years and after one of my younger sisters also graduated from occupational therapy school that my mother revealed that she, too, had also been studying occupational therapy but left school to raise her family after meeting and marrying my father. Nowadays, when I think of the playroom of my childhood, I remember my mother—the almost–occupational therapist, quietly and secretly passing the message and mission to her children. ∎

Mary Beth Early, MS, OTR/L
Professor
Occupational Therapy Assistant Program
LaGuardia Community College
City University of New York
Long Island City, New York

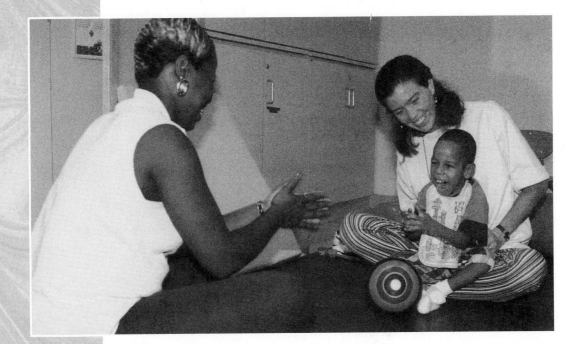

Introductory Questions

Objectives

After reading this chapter, the reader will be able to:
- ✤ Understand the basic terminology of occupational therapy
- ✤ Describe the nature and scope of the practice of occupational therapy
- ✤ Determine the personality traits that are suitable for a career in occupational therapy

Key terms

Occupation
Therapy
Goal
Activity
Independence
Function
Occupational therapy
Occupational therapy practitioner
Registered Occupational Therapist
Certified Occupational Therapy Assistant
Patient
Client
Media

As we consider occupational therapy, we will first look at the broad picture. We will scan—minus the detail—the field to give you an overview. We will begin with a series of questions that someone new to the profession may ask. You may already know some bits and pieces of the answers; in which case, compare your knowledge with new insights that may arise by looking at the overall picture.

WHAT IS OCCUPATIONAL THERAPY?

The American Occupational Therapy Association[1] (AOTA) has developed a definition for occupational therapy, which is intended for professional use (Box 1-1). For now, let us take a simplified approach to occupational therapy. Turning to *The Merriam-Webster's Collegiate Dictionary*®[3] for an understanding of six commonly used words, we find:

Occupation: Activity in which one engages
Therapy: Treatment of an illness or disability

Section I photo: American Occupational Therapy Association, , Bethesda, Md.

Chapter 1 photo: Case-Smith J, Allen AS, Pratt PN: *Occupational therapy for children*, ed 3, St Louis, 1996, Mosby.

Box 1-1

DEFINITION OF OCCUPATIONAL THERAPY

"...THE ART AND SCIENCE OF DIRECTING MAN'S PARTICIPATION IN SELECTED TASKS TO RESTORE, REINFORCE, AND ENHANCE PERFORMANCE, FACILITATE LEARNING OF THOSE SKILLS AND FUNCTIONS THAT ARE ESSENTIAL FOR ADAPTATION AND PRODUCTIVITY, DIMINISH OR CORRECT PATHOLOGY, AND TO PROMOTE AND MAINTAIN HEALTH. ITS FUNDAMENTAL CONCERN IS THE DEVELOPMENT AND MAINTENANCE OF CAPACITY THROUGHOUT THE LIFE SPAN, TO PERFORM WITH SATISFACTION TO SELF AND OTHERS, THOSE TASKS AND ROLES ESSENTIAL TO PRODUCTIVE LIVING AND TO THE MASTERY OF SELF AND ENVIRONMENT."[1]

Goal: End toward which effort is directed
Activity: State or condition of being active (participant)
Independence: State or condition of being independent (self-reliant)
Function: Action for which a person is fitted

These terms enable us to build a skeletal definition. **Occupational therapy** (OT) is a goal-directed activity that promotes independence in function. In Chapter 3 we explore the philosophy of OT in depth.

ARE THERE DIFFERENT LEVELS OF THE OCCUPATIONAL THERAPY PRACTITIONER?

An **occupational therapy practitioner** is commonly referred to as either a **Registered Occupational Therapist** (OTR) or a **Certified Occupational Therapy Assistant** (COTA), each a different level of practitioner. The OTR has more extensive education and training in both breadth and depth than the COTA, who works under the supervision of an OTR. Often the OTR is referred to as the "professional" level, and the COTA is referred to as the "technical" level of practice. Herein, OT practitioner refers to those within the field at either level. In Chapter 4 these two roles are discussed in greater depth.

WHAT DOES AN OCCUPATIONAL THERAPY PRACTITIONER DO?

There are many objectives that a therapy program seeks to accomplish, but all have the ultimate goal of increased independence in functioning of the client, or patient. The OT practitioner interacts with a client to assess and evaluate existing performance, set therapeutic goals, develop a plan, and implement treatment to enable the client to function better in his or her world. The OT practitioner must record progress and communicate treatment specifics to others (i.e., other professionals, families, agencies). However, it is important for the OT practitioner to establish personal rapport (a relationship of mutual trust) with the client, because the relationship itself has therapeutic value and plays a key role in the treatment partnership. The OT practitioner does not simply do something to or for the client; the OT practitioner guides the person to active participation in treatment.

WHY REFER TO BOTH "PATIENT" AND "CLIENT?"

In the field of OT, services are provided to people in many different settings. The term used to refer to those served varies depending on the setting. For example, in a hospital or rehabilitation setting we usually say **patient,** but in a mental health facility or training center we frequently use **client.** Some other terms—such as resident, participant, or consumer—may be dictated by the facility. For our purposes, *client* is inclusive.

IS THERE A TYPE OF PERSONALITY THAT IS BEST SUITED FOR A CAREER CHOICE IN OCCUPATIONAL THERAPY?

OT practitioners have many differing interests and expectations, but perhaps there is a common profile that describes those most likely to succeed in the field. The ideal practitioner genuinely likes people and relates to both individuals and small groups. As with any member of the health care professions, those interested in OT demonstrate the ability to handle their own personal problems and feelings before trying to help others. Occupational therapy is a lifelong profession, not a 9-to-5 job; therefore commitment and dedication are important. As in other professions, the OT practitioner is never *finished* with education but must always invest in growing with the field and continually maintaining competency. To support improved independent functioning, the OT practitioner empathizes with clients yet expects and demands effort from them. It has been said that a *strong constitution* helps because the OT practitioner is exposed to many medical problems in the field, from open wounds to degenerative disorders. Since OT practitioners must educate and instruct, an interest in teaching is also desirable. The personality trait most needed is flexibility; an OT practitioner needs to both teach *and* display the ability to adapt.

WHAT KINDS OF PROBLEMS OR DISABILITIES ARE ADDRESSED BY OCCUPATIONAL THERAPY?

The mandate of the profession is to develop life skills. The recipients of our therapy are those who have encountered problems that interfere with the ability to function in any stage of development. Potentially, we could be asked to solve problems for any functionally disabled person with the aim of increasing his or her independence. The scope of services includes physical, cognitive, and psychological and psychosocial disorders. Obviously, it is impossible to know everything, but with a focus on functional problem solving, the OT practitioner learns general principles that are applicable to nearly any dysfunction. Regardless of the setting, the OT practitioner is expected to be competent and make a contribution to the well-being of the client.

WHO ARE THE PEOPLE WHO ARE SERVED? IN WHAT KINDS OF SETTINGS ARE THESE SERVICES DELIVERED?

The range of OT services reaches from pediatrics (infants and children) to geriatrics (aged); from one time only consultations to short-term acute care to rehabilitation aimed at long-term adjustment. Occupational therapy personnel work in hospitals, clinics, schools, client's homes, community settings, or prisons. Recently, OT has expanded to include even more diverse services such as assistive technology, aquatics, animal-assisted therapy, ergonomics, and community integration. The OT practitioner works with clients who have a physical, cognitive, or psychological or psychosocial impairment. The impairment could be the result of an accident or injury, a disease, an emotional disorder, conflicts or stress, or from developmental delays or congenital anomalies (birth defects). The recipients of OT services are as diverse as the world itself.

OCCUPATIONAL THERAPY PRACTITIONERS WORK WITH WHAT TYPES OF CLIENTS?

A client could be a 1-pound newborn infant on a hospital neonatal unit, a preschool child in an early intervention program, or a child who has had cerebral palsy and has attended public school. An OT practitioner might work with an adolescent in a drug treatment center or a mentally retarded adult who has been trained to do productive work. A client could be someone paralyzed from a spinal cord injury after an automobile accident who needs to learn to adjust to living with a disability, or a homemaker who has had a stroke and must learn how to run her home and care for her family with one side of her body not functioning correctly. A client could be someone in a mental health clinic who needs to learn the simple skills of shopping, keeping a checkbook, and using public transportation—daily life tasks that most take for granted. An OT practitioner might have to make a splint for an outpatient with a hand injury or work with the geriatric population in a skilled nursing facility; an OT practitioner could work in a program that helps an individual train for a new job after an injury. Improving the independence of the person within the limits of his or her particular situation is the theme that unites these different circumstances. (See photographic essay at the end of this chapter.)

WHAT DOES AN OCCUPATIONAL THERAPY EDUCATIONAL PROGRAM COVER?

Because of the broad scope of the profession, the knowledge base for students in OT needs to represent several scientific areas including biological and behavioral sciences, sociology, anthropology, and medicine.[3] The student gains an understanding of the normal human development process and pathological processes that affect normal development and function. With these sciences as a foundation, the student learns the theory and processes related to OT. These educational programs focus on developing an attitude and awareness that enable the new professional to be sensitive to the various needs of those seeking treatment. OT education is aimed not only at specific skills, but it seeks to develop a way of thinking in the student. A generic problem-solving approach that relies on critical thinking is used. The student learns to evaluate function, analyze activities, and seek to increase the client's independence. This process is then applied to a wide range of dysfunction.

Although the acquisition of many specific skills occurs after entering a particular employment setting, some specific skill training is given for those techniques most widely used in the profession. Because the range of client needs is so far-reaching and the employment settings so diverse, it is not possible for students of OT to acquire all the skills with classroom training. Therefore a clinical training phase is an important aspect of all educational programs, at both the OTR and COTA levels. The student's clinical experiences provide the opportunity to integrate many elements of therapy. Students should, however, be prepared for the "I-didn't-learn-that" syndrome that every student experiences during clinical training. Upon completion of the clinical training phase, the student should be practicing at the entry level.

HOW ARE THE OCCUPATIONAL THERAPY CURRICULA DETERMINED? WHAT IS THE MAIN EMPHASIS?

Occupational therapy educational programs—the OTR (professional) and COTA (technical) levels—are accredited by the Accreditation Council for Occupational Therapy Education (ACOTE), which is a part of the AOTA. Programs are designed to conform to a series of guidelines called "essentials." The course of study features general theory, skills training, and the foundation for clinical reasoning. Occupational therapy education is designed *NOT* to give a set of unchanging answers but to teach the student problem-solving techniques and skills.

WHAT KINDS OF ACTIVITIES ARE USED BY THE OCCUPATIONAL THERAPY PRACTITIONER WHEN ADMINISTERING TREATMENT?

It is possible to use virtually anything that leads to functional improvement for the client. Ideally, the therapy session uses purposeful activity. A client who needs to develop fine motor skills may engage in an assembly task or puzzle building. If there is evidence of confusion, a simple sorting task may be in order. If there is a need to gain strength and endurance in hand movements, a macramé project or a woodworking project involving sanding may be selected. If there is a need for social interaction and gross motor improvement, a parachute activity may be chosen. If there is a need to improve visual discrimination, paper and pencil activities may be included in the treatment plan.

In each setting there may be activities that are frequently used, but they are never exclusive. The problem-solving process sets the parameters; the imagination of the OT practitioner sets the limits. Often a variety of specially designed equipment and activities are found in a setting, but OT also uses games, toys, dressing or self-care activities, work activities, art, crafts, computers, industrial activities, sports, music and dance, role-playing and theater crafts, gardening, homemaking activities, magic, clowning, pet care, and creative writing. If it meets the goals set in the client's treatment plan, it is a proper activity for OT.

The means employed are referred to as the **media** of therapy. OT practitioners turn trained and sensitive eyes to the assets (what the person does well), to the liabilities (what the person is unable to do well), to the interests of the client, to the needs and demands of the environment, and to the range of available options. The OT practitioner then uses the information gathered to build the person's program. Good problem solving requires that all relevant factors be considered. Therapists then reach into their imaginations to come up with activities that will best encourage improvement of functioning for the individual. This is not a field of recipe books and formulas. Occupational therapy requires an openness to life. "Whatever might help you, we will try," is the attitude good OT practitioners carry to media selection.

SUMMARY

These introductory questions show that the person pursuing a career in OT will not find a career with a set of ready-made answers; in this field one must be ready to seek solutions not yet known. Those looking for repetitive routines should not look to this profession.

An OT practitioner is a generalist in a world of specialists, that is, a generalist with a specific focus to find, by whatever means, the personal or technical adaptation that allows a client with an identifiable impairment to function to his or her maximum capacity in his or her living environment. In this overview, we have just glanced at the world of OT. In the remainder of this text, we will study in greater detail the specific territories that make up this world.

PHOTOGRAPHIC ESSAY

For years, the annual AOTA calendar brought the profession's diversity to the attention of practitioners—but time moves on. Although calendars are no longer produced, pictures from calendars of past years, as well as photography from other sources, illustrate the wonderful diversity of OT. The following photographic essay is a visual answer to the question, "What types of people will I work with as an OT practitioner?"

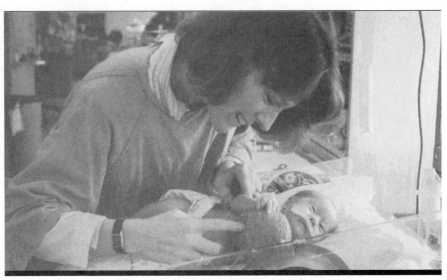

PREMATURE AND AT-RISK INFANTS OFTEN NEED SPECIAL HELP TO PROMOTE NORMAL DEVELOPMENT. THE OT PRACTITIONER STIMULATES HEALTHY MOVEMENT PATTERNS IN THIS NEWBORN. (PHOTOGRAPH BY DEBORAH HENSLEY. COURTESY OF AOTA. SUBMITTED BY THE OCCUPATIONAL THERAPY DEPARTMENT, UNIVERSITY OF VIRGINIA HOSPITAL, CHARLOTTESVILLE, VIRGINIA.)

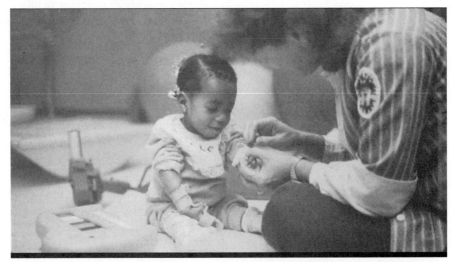

SPLINTS FABRICATED BY AN OT PRACTITIONER PREVENT DEFORMITY AND PROMOTE FUNCTION FOR A CHILD WITH A CONGENITAL DISABILITY. THROUGH OCCUPATIONAL THERAPY, CHILDREN WITH DISABILITIES CAN DEVELOP INDEPENDENCE IN FEEDING, BATHING, AND DRESSING, AND AT HOME, SCHOOL, AND PLAY, OFTEN PARTICIPATING IN REGULAR CLASSROOM ACTIVITIES. (PHOTOGRAPH BY MARIE STRAIGHT. COURTESY OF AOTA. SUBMITTED BY CAROL DECKER, OTR, ORLANDO PEDIATRIC MULTI-THERAPY CLINIC, MAITLAND, FLORIDA.)

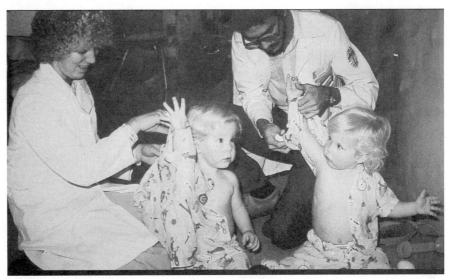

THE OT PRACTITIONER IS ASSESSING THE DEVELOPMENTAL SKILLS OF TWINS.
SCREENING FOR DEVELOPMENTAL PROBLEMS PERMITS TIMELY DELIVERY OF
OCCUPATIONAL THERAPY SERVICES, IF NECESSARY. (PHOTOGRAPH COURTESY OF
AOTA AND ST. JOHN'S IN CLEVELAND, OHIO, JOE ROSENDAUL.)

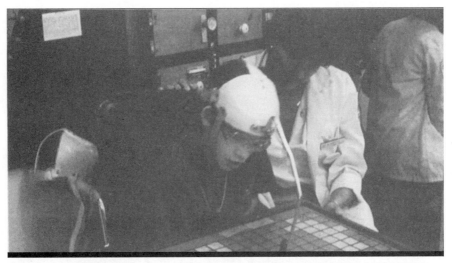

A HELMET AND HEAD STICK ADAPTED BY AN OCCUPATIONAL THERAPIST ALLOW A CHILD
WITH CEREBRAL PALSY TO COMMUNICATE BY USING A COMPUTER. THROUGH OCCU-
PATIONAL THERAPY, INDIVIDUALS WITH CEREBRAL PALSY CAN IMPROVE MOTOR SKILLS;
DEVELOP SOCIAL, COGNITIVE, AND ORGANIZATIONAL ABILITIES FOR SUCCESS AT SCHOOL
AND WORK; INCREASE THE ABILITY TO CARE FOR PERSONAL NEEDS; FUNCTION MORE
INDEPENDENTLY USING ADAPTIVE EQUIPMENT, COMMUNICATION DEVICES, AND OTHER
AIDS. (PHOTOGRAPH BY KAY COOPER, OTR/L. COURTESY OF AOTA. SUBMITTED BY KAY
COOPER, NORTH CAROLINA MEMORIAL HOSPITAL, CHAPEL HILL, NORTH CAROLINA.)

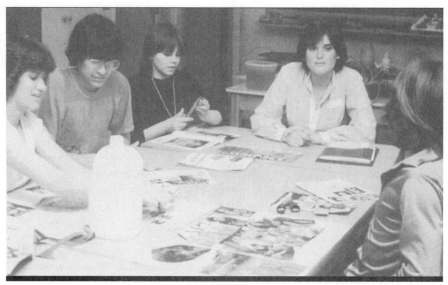

UNDER THE SUPERVISION OF AN OCCUPATIONAL THERAPIST, CLIENTS IN AN ADOLESCENT CHEMICAL DEPENDENCY UNIT CARRY OUT A GROUP ACTIVITY. THIS ACTIVITY TEACHES DAILY LIVING, LEISURE PLANNING, AND PREVOCATIONAL SKILLS TYPICALLY LACKING IN CLIENTS WITH CHEMICAL DEPENDENCY. (PHOTOGRAPH COURTESY OF AOTA.)

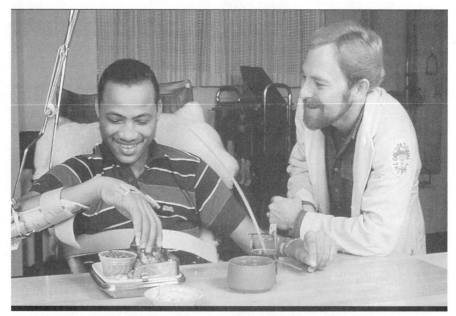

INDEPENDENTLY PERFORMING PERSONAL TASKS PROMOTES A HEALTHY SELF-IMAGE FOR THE INDIVIDUAL WITH A DISABILITY. THIS OT PRACTITIONER HAS PROVIDED A SPECIALIZED DEVICE THAT ALLOWS THIS PATIENT WITH A SPINAL CORD INJURY TO FEED HIMSELF. (PHOTOGRAPH COURTESY OF AOTA.)

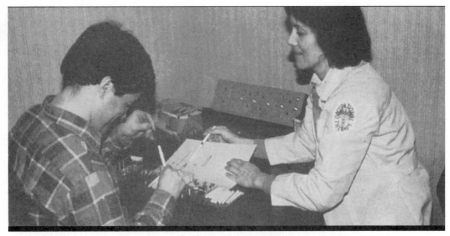

AN ASSEMBLY TASK PROVIDED BY AN OT PRACTITIONER TO A CLIENT WITH A DEVELOPMENTAL DISABILITY CAN IMPROVE PHYSICAL AND MENTAL FUNCTIONING, DEVELOP SELF-CARE SKILLS NEEDED FOR SCHOOL AND WORK TASKS, ADAPT A MORE POSITIVE SELF-IMAGE, AND INTERACT MORE EFFECTIVELY WITH FAMILY, PEERS, AND CO-WORKERS. (PHOTOGRAPH BY BECKY LEVENS, OTR. COURTESY OF AOTA. SUBMITTED BY CHRIS FURY, OTR, REHABILITATION SPECIALISTS CORP., CUSTOM CONTRACTS AND SERVICES, DAC, ST. PAUL, MINNESOTA.)

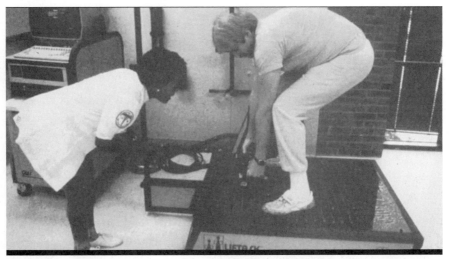

AN OT PRACTITIONER MONITORS A TEST TO ASSESS A CLIENT'S ABILITY TO MEET THE DEMANDS OF HIS JOB. THROUGH OCCUPATIONAL THERAPY, PEOPLE WITH WORK-RELATED INJURIES CAN LEARN PROPER BODY MECHANICS TO PREVENT RE-INJURY, TASK ORGANIZATION AND ENERGY CONSERVATION TO SPEED A RETURN TO WORK, AND SKILLS TO COMPENSATE FOR LOST FUNCTION. PEOPLE WITH WORK-RELATED INJURIES ARE AIDED IN SKILLS ASSESSMENT WHEN A JOB CHANGE IS INDICATED. (PHOTOGRAPH BY DAN SMITH. COURTESY OF AOTA. SUBMITTED BY BARBARA PIEL, OTR, PRODUCTIVE REHABILITATION INSTITUTE OF DALLAS FOR ERGONOMICS, DALLAS, TEXAS.)

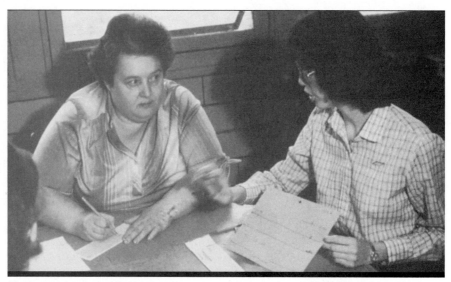

MENTAL HEALTH CLIENTS PRACTICE THE MECHANICS OF MANAGING A CHECKING ACCOUNT AS PART OF A COMMUNITY READINESS PROGRAM. REAL-LIFE SITUATIONS ARE SIMULATED TO PROVIDE CLIENTS WITH THE OPPORTUNITY TO PREPARE FOR INDEPENDENT LIVING. (PHOTOGRAPH BY SAMUEL A. TAYLOR. COURTESY OF AOTA.)

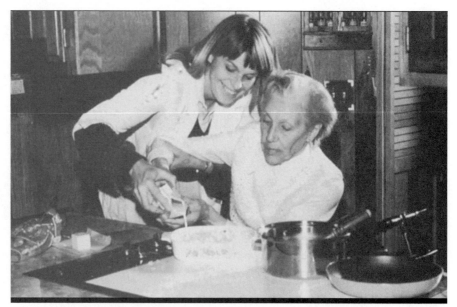

MANY INDIVIDUALS RECOVERING FROM STROKE CAN RETURN TO INDEPENDENT LIVING WITH THE AID OF OCCUPATIONAL THERAPY. VISITING A CLIENT IN THE HOME, AN OT PRACTITIONER PROVIDES GUIDANCE IN SAFE COOKING TECHNIQUES. (PHOTOGRAPH BY BOB PLUNKETT. COURTESY OF AOTA. SUBMITTED BY MYRNA KOOP HARRINGTON, OTR, CENTRAL DISTRICT HOME HEALTH, BOISE, IDAHO.)

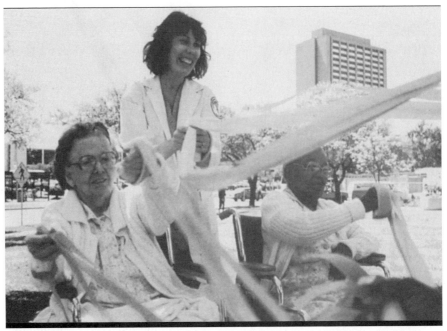

A PLEASURABLE GROUP ACTIVITY STIMULATES SENSORY AWARENESS AND PROMOTES SOCIALIZATION FOR THIS OLDER CLIENT. THROUGH OCCUPATIONAL THERAPY, OLDER INDIVIDUALS WITH HEALTH PROBLEMS ARE MORE SELF-SUFFICIENT AND OFTEN REQUIRE LESS NURSING CARE. THEY MAINTAIN A HIGHER DEGREE OF MENTAL ALERTNESS, ARE ABLE TO PARTICIPATE MORE ACTIVELY IN SOCIAL AND RECREATIONAL ACTIVITIES, AND MAY EXPERIENCE LESS PHYSICAL AND MENTAL DETERIORATION. (PHOTOGRAPH BY ADAM GILLUM. COURTESY OF AOTA. SUBMITTED BY ELISE SULTON, OTR, AND MARY ALICE PETERS, OTC, ST. LUKE'S EPISCOPAL HOSPITAL, HOUSTON, TEXAS.)

REFERENCES

1. American Occupational Therapy Association: Occupational therapy: its definition and function, *Amer J Occup Ther* 26:204, 1972.

2. Hopkins HL: Current basis for theory and philosophy of occupational therapy. In Hopkins HL, Smith HD, editors: *Willard & Spackman's occupational therapy,* ed 8, Philadelphia, 1993, JB Lippincott.

3. Mish F, editor: *Merriam-Webster's collegiate dictionary®,* ed 10, Springfield, Mass, 1994, Merriam-Webster.

*Y*ears ago, I chose to become an occupational therapist after observing other therapists at work. I was impressed by their creativity and people orientation. Back then and today, if you were to ask me what I like most about being an occupational therapist, I would list two reasons. Since my education, I have learned to appreciate our holistic roots that are based on some of the principles of the Moral Treatment Movement. I have also recognized that our meaningful beginning and most of our current literature and research comes from this theme. Intrinsic to our field is the emphasis on function and the promotion of client independence. I have tried to incorporate these central themes in my practice over the years, and I could cite many examples of how I have applied them. Although the field continues to grow and change with the times, I have always recognized our roots, which continue to remain inherent to practice. ◼

Helene Lohman, MA, OTR/L
Assistant Professor
Department of Occupational Therapy
School of Pharmacy and Allied
    Health Professions
Creighton University
Omaha, Nebraska

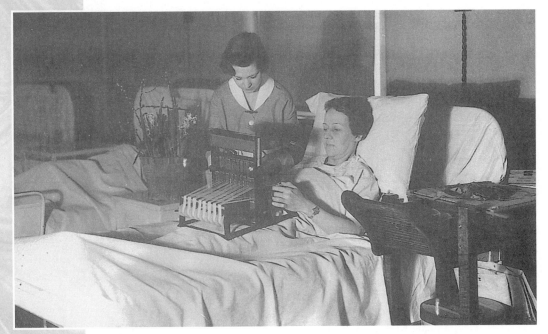

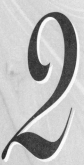

Looking Back: A History of Occupational Therapy

Objectives

After reading this chapter, the reader will be able to:

❖ Identify major social influences that preceded and gave rise to the field of occupational therapy (OT)

❖ Learn the dates of the birth of the profession and the individuals who were involved in its inception

❖ Recognize how influences in the society at large have helped shape the developing field of OT

Key terms

Moral Treatment
Phillippe Pinel
William Tuke
Benjamin Rush
Herbert Hall
George Edward Barton
William Rush Dunton, Jr.
Eleanor Clarke Slagle
Susan Tracy
National Society for the Promotion of Occupational Therapy
Adolf Meyer
Holistic
Reconstruction Aides
Vocational Rehabilitation Act
Medicare
Rehabilitation Act of 1973
Education for all Handicapped Children Act of 1975 (PL 94-142)
Handicapped Infants and Toddlers Act (PL 99-457)
Technology Related Assistance for Individuals with Disabilities Act
Americans with Disabilities Act

To characterize the profession of OT as we know it today, it is necessary to examine the past and understand how the profession originated and developed. Robert Bing, an author who has done extensive research on the history of OT advises, "We exist in the present, yet are future oriented. To make sense of the present or future, we must have knowledge about and an appreciation of the past."[1] Toward this purpose, Chapter 2 presents a general overview of the development of OT. (For more detailed historical accounts, the reader is referred to the references listed at the end of this chapter.)

Chapter 2 photo: Courtesy of the Archives of the American Occupational Therapy Association, Inc.

When the history of OT is traced, there are two threads that are intertwined. The social and cultural thread identifies many currents of human events that have influenced the development of OT through time. The second thread introduces the individuals who set in motion specific events that identified a new approach to health care—an approach called occupational therapy. The individuals who contributed to the development of the profession had backgrounds in a variety of disciplines that included psychiatry, medicine, nursing, arts and crafts, rehabilitation, teaching, and social work. Their backgrounds served to enrich the depth and breadth of the profession of OT.[12]

EIGHTEENTH AND NINETEENTH CENTURIES

The late 1700s and early 1800s can be distinguished by an awakening of a social consciousness, an awareness that social structures lead to vast inequities. A new sense emerged—a measure of life's goodness should be available to all people. This awakening can be seen in many ways, as in the novels of Charles Dickens or in the founding of various welfare organizations. It was also demonstrated by the Civil War, which eliminated the practice of slavery, a previously accepted practice that extended back through all of human history. This social conscience is one thread in the course of human history.

This awakening brought many previously ignored and cruel practices to light, one of which was the treatment of those with mental disorders. Thought to be possessed by the devil, the "insane" were feared by society, locked away like criminals, and often chained, abused, and ignored. With a focus specifically on this group of suffering humanity, the concept of Moral Treatment was initiated.

MORAL TREATMENT

Moral Treatment was grounded in the philosophy that all people, even the most challenged, are entitled to consideration and human compassion. Whereas previously the "insane" were confined and frequently abused, the Moral Treatment Movement sought ways to make the existence of those confined more bearable. One of the ways was involvement in purposeful activity.

Two men from different parts of the world are credited with conceiving the Moral Treatment Movement: **Phillippe Pinel** and **William Tuke.**[1] Phillippe Pinel, a physician in France, introduced "work treatment" for the "insane" in the late 1700s. He used occupation to divert the patients' minds away from their emotional disturbances and toward improving their skills. He used physical exercise, work, music, and literature in his treatment. In addition, an important element was the use of farming as a part of institutional life.[1]

The Society of Friends, also known as Quakers, had a great influence in England. An English Quaker and wealthy merchant, William Tuke, became aware of the terrible conditions in an asylum in York, England, and suggested establishing the York Retreat.[2] Tuke and Thomas Fowler, the appointed visiting physician, believed that Moral Treatment methods were preferable to using restraint and drugs. The environment at the York Retreat was like that of a family where the patients were approached with kindness and consideration.[2]

After the publication of Pinel's work in 1801 and Tuke's work in 1813 on the use of Moral Treatment, many hospitals in both Europe and the United States implemented the reforms.[2] In the United States a Quaker named **Benjamin Rush** was the first physician to institute Moral Treatment practices.

Participants in the Moral Treatment Movement demonstrated that establishing a structure and having the patients engage in simple work tasks promoted better health. Organizing activities for the patients brought order and purpose to unstructured confinement. For these persons whose day-to-day functioning fell outside the bounds of socially acceptable behavior, there was an individualized routine of personal caretaking and productive involvement.

Though the term "Moral Treatment" began to fade by the mid-1800s, many of the concepts initiated by this movement continued. The practice of OT eventually emerged from this humanitarian concern for each human being and from the use of structured activity that simulated a more normal life for asylum inmates.

EARLY TWENTIETH CENTURY

Looking again at the social and cultural thread, changes occurred in science, technology, medicine, and industry toward the end of the nineteenth century and into the beginning of the twentieth century. New modes of communication and transportation accelerated the pace of everyday life. Machines were first used in the production of goods; in 1913 Henry Ford developed the moving assembly line for the production of automobiles. In reaction to the expanding use of tools and machines, a contingency of proponents of the arts and crafts developed. They were opposed to the production of items by machine, believing this alienated people from nature. It was believed that using one's hands to make items connected people to their work, physically and mentally, and thus was healthier.[12]

At the turn of the twentieth century, another issue arose from a slightly different segment of society. There was a concern for those who were taken from the mainstream of life by injury or illness and thereafter expected to sit on the sidelines. Until this time a disabled person either "got better" or was eliminated from competitive involvement in life. The time came to look beyond these two alternatives; there was a need and desire for other options. An awareness that a "handicapped" person is still productive was surfacing in sanitariums and hospitals for convalescent individuals.

These events also had an effect on the profession of OT. In fact, events at this time brought together several individuals who had an interest in the use of occupation and who eventually founded the profession in the United States.

DEVELOPMENT OF THE PROFESSION

HERBERT HALL

At the turn of the century, chronic illness and disability, such as tuberculosis, neurasthenia, and industrial accidents, were on the rise as people became victims of the urban and industrial life. Adapting the arts and crafts movement for medical purposes was a treatment concept developed by **Herbert Hall**, a physician who graduated from Harvard Medical School.[11] He worked with invalid patients, providing medical supervision of crafts for the purpose of improving their health and financial independence.[12]

In 1904 he established a facility at Marblehead, Massachusetts, where patients with neurasthenia worked on arts and crafts as part of treatment. Neurasthenia, a disorder that was commonly seen in women, caused severe weakness during the performance of work activities. The treatment usually prescribed at the time was total rest. Hall's alternative to the "rest cure" was arts and crafts activities, beginning with participation on a limited basis from bed and gradually increasing the level of activity until the patients went to the workshop where she worked on weaving looms, ceramics, and other crafts.[13] He called this approach the "work cure." In 1906 he received a grant of $1000 to study the "treatment of neurasthenia by progressive and graded manual occupation." Hall was also a prolific writer. He later served as President of the National Society for the Promotion of Occupational Therapy from 1920 to 1923.

GEORGE EDWARD BARTON

George Barton was a dynamic and resourceful architect who studied in London under the leader of Britain's arts and crafts movement. Later, he returned to Boston to incorporate the Boston Society of Arts and Crafts. After personally experiencing a number of disabling conditions—tuberculosis, foot amputation, and paralysis of the left side of his body—Barton was determined to improve the plight of convalescent individuals. In 1914 Barton opened Consolation House for convalescent patients in Clifton Springs, New York, where occupation was used as a method of treatment.

Barton studied rehabilitation courses available at the time and made contact with people dedicated to reforming the conditions in asylums, many of whom were influenced by the Moral Treatment Movement. Barton established contact with Dr. William R. Dunton, Jr., a psychiatrist known for his writings on the value of occupation for treatment; Eleanor Clarke Slagle, a social worker who developed a method of treatment called "habit training" (she eventually became a guiding force in the organization of the OT profession); Susan Tracy, a nurse and teacher who published *Studies in Invalid Occupations*[16]; and Susan Cox Johnson, an arts and crafts teacher who wrote a textile textbook and later became the Director of Occupations for the Department of Public Charities of New York.

WILLIAM DUNTON

William Rush Dunton, Jr., considered the father of OT, was a psychiatrist who spent his career treating psychiatric patients. In 1891 he was hired as the assistant staff physician at the Sheppard Asylum (later named the Sheppard and Enoch Pratt Hospital) in Towson, Maryland. Having studied the treatment programs of Pinel and Tukes, he was interested in implementing a similar program at the Sheppard Asylum.

In the early 1910s the hospital introduced a regimen of crafts for its patients. While hospital staff performed necessary medical procedures and provided a structured environment, the patients were expected to actively participate in their rehabilitation by working in the workshop.[12] In 1915 Dunton published, *Occupational Therapy: A Manual for Nurses.* It describes simple activities that the nurse can use or adapt in the treatment of patients.[4] Dunton served as Treasurer and President of the National Society for the Promotion of Occupational Therapy and edited the association's journal for 21 years.

ELEANOR CLARKE SLAGLE

Often referred to as the mother of OT,[12] **Eleanor Clarke Slagle** began her career as a student in social work (Figure 2-1). She attended training courses in curative occupations in 1908 at the Chicago School of Civics and Philanthropy, which was affiliated with Hull House and Jane Addams. After this training, she worked at state hospitals in

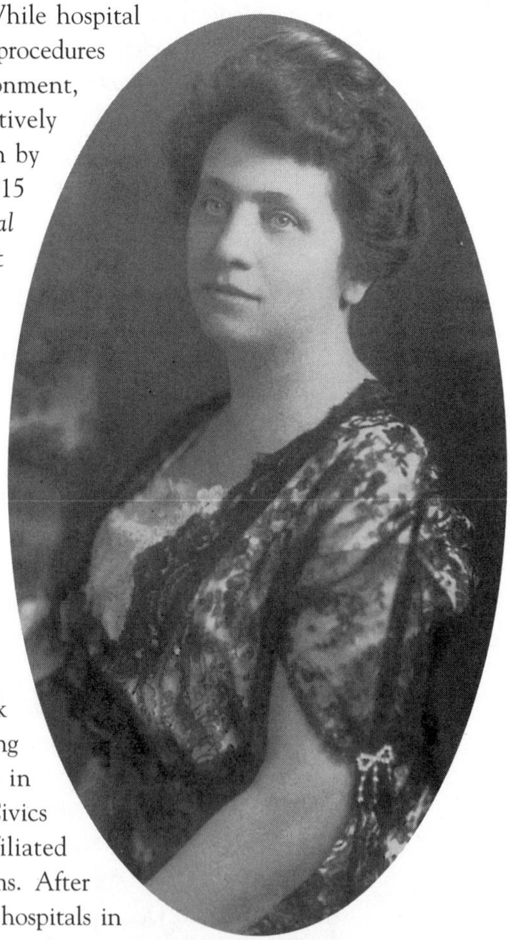

FIGURE 2-1. ELEANOR CLARKE SLAGLE. (PHOTO COURTESY OF THE ARCHIVES OF THE AMERICAN OCCUPATIONAL THERAPY ASSOCIATION, INC., BETHESDA, MD.)

Michigan and New York. In 1912 she was asked by Adolf Meyer to direct a new OT department at the Henry Phipps Psychiatric Clinic of Johns Hopkins Hospital in Baltimore, Maryland. It was at this time that Slagle developed the area of work for which she is most noted, "habit training." Habit training is described as a "re-education program designed to overcome disorganized habits, to modify other habits, and to construct new ones, with the goal of restoring and maintaining health."[1,2] Habit training involved all hospital personnel and took place 24 hours a day. Slagle summarized it as a "…directed activity, and [it] differs from all other forms of treatment in that it is given in increasing doses as the patient improves."[7]

In 1914 Slagle returned to Chicago where she lectured at the Chicago School of Civics and Philanthropy and started a workshop for the chronically unemployed.[12] Soon after, she organized the first professional school for OT practitioners, the Henry B. Flavill School of Occupations.

Slagle's dedication to the profession can be illustrated by the fact that her home was the American Occupational Therapy Association's (AOTA) first unofficial headquarters. During her lifetime she held each office within the Association and served as Executive Secretary for 14 years! In 1953 AOTA established the Eleanor Clarke Slagle Lectureship Award, named in her honor. Today, the AOTA awards this prestigious honor to therapists who have made significant contributions to the profession.

SUSAN TRACY

Susan Tracy was an occupational nurse involved in the arts and crafts movement and in the training of nurses in the use of occupations. She was hired in 1905 to work at the Adams Nervine Asylum, a small mental institution in Jamaica Plain, Massachusetts. While at this institution she supervised the nursing school, developed the occupations program, and conducted postgraduate course for nurses.[12] Tracy's book, *Studies in Invalid Occupations*,[16] is the first-known book written on OT. She describes the selection and practical use of arts and crafts activities for patients. Throughout her career, Tracy was involved in teaching many training courses. She believed only nurses were qualified to practice occupations and tried to make patient occupations a nursing specialty. Tracy was involved with her work and not able to attend the first meeting of the National Society for the Promotion of Occupational Therapy, but she actively served as Chair on the Committee of Teaching Methods.

NATIONAL SOCIETY FOR THE PROMOTION OF OCCUPATIONAL THERAPY

The formal "birth" of the profession of OT can be traced to a specific event. In March, 1917, an assembly of a small group of people from varied backgrounds incorporated the **National Society for the Promotion of Occupational Therapy,** in Clifton Springs, New York. Included in this group were George Barton, William Dunton, Eleanor Clark Slagle, Susan Cox Johnson (Director of Occupations at New York State Department of Public Charities), Thomas Kidner (Vocational Secretary of the Canadian Military Hospital Commission and friend and fellow architect-teacher of George Barton), and Isabel Newton, who attended in the capacity as Barton's secretary (later his wife) and was, in fact, made Secretary of the new organization. Miss Tracy could not attend, but was made a charter member of the Association. These people convened the initial organizational meeting on March 15, 1917 (Figure 2-2).

The meeting produced the Certificate of Incorporation of the National Society for the Promotion of Occupational Therapy. In September, 1917, twenty-six men and women held the first annual meeting of the organization. In 1921 the membership voted to change the name of the organization to the American Occupational Therapy Association. Early in these formative years, a set of principles were developed (Box 2-1). The principles were presented by Dunton in 1918 at the second annual meeting of the National Society for the Promotion of Occupational Therapy.

PHILOSOPHICAL BASE: HOLISTIC PERSPECTIVE

There was another person whose influence helped shape the emerging profession of OT, though he was not present at the first organizational meeting. **Adolf Meyer,** a Swiss physician who immigrated to the United States in 1892 and later became professor of psychiatry at Johns Hopkins University, expressed a point of view that eventually formed the philosophical base of the profession (Figure 2-3).

Box 2-1

DUNTON'S PRINCIPLES OF OCCUPATIONAL THERAPY*

1. ANY ACTIVITY SHOULD HAVE A CURE AS ITS OBJECTIVE.
2. THE ACTIVITY SHOULD BE INTERESTING.
3. THERE SHOULD BE A USEFUL PURPOSE OTHER THAN TO MERELY GAIN THE PATIENT'S ATTENTION AND INTEREST.
4. THE ACTIVITY SHOULD PREFERABLY LEAD TO AN INCREASE IN KNOWLEDGE ON THE PATIENT'S PART.
5. ACTIVITY SHOULD BE CARRIED ON WITH OTHERS, SUCH AS A GROUP.
6. THE OCCUPATIONAL THERAPIST SHOULD MAKE A CAREFUL STUDY OF THE PATIENT AND ATTEMPT TO MEET AS MANY NEEDS AS POSSIBLE THROUGH ACTIVITY.
7. ACTIVITY SHOULD CEASE BEFORE THE ONSET OF FATIGUE.
8. GENUINE ENCOURAGEMENT SHOULD BE GIVEN WHENEVER INDICATED.
9. WORK IS MUCH TO BE PREFERRED OVER IDLENESS, EVEN WHEN THE END PRODUCT OF THE PATIENT'S LABOR IS OF POOR QUALITY OR IS USELESS.[5]

---

*Presented in 1918 at the second annual meeting of the National Society for the Promotion of Occupational Therapy.

OCCUPATIONAL THERAPY HISTORICAL HIGHLIGHTS

LATE 1700s TO EARLY 1800s
USE OF OCCUPATIONS
MORAL TREATMENT
MOVEMENT

EARLY 1900s
CONSOLATION HOUSE
ARTS AND CRAFTS MOVEMENT
INTERVENTION WITH
CONVALESCENT INDIVIDUALS

1914–1918
WORLD WAR I
RECONSTRUCTION AIDES
REHABILITATION
PHYSICAL
DISABILITIES

MARCH 1917
INCORPORATION OF THE
NATIONAL SOCIETY FOR
PROMOTION OF
OCCUPATIONAL
THERAPY

GEORGE BARTON
WILLIAM DUNTON, JR.
ELEANOR CLARKE SLAGLE
SUSAN TRACY (ABS) • SUSAN C. JOHNSON • THOMAS KIDNER • ISABEL G. NEWTON

SEPTEMBER 3, 1917—FIRST ANNUAL MEETING
1918—SECOND ANNUAL MEETING
Principles of Occupational Therapy presented
1921—FIFTH ANNUAL MEETING
Adolf Meyer delivers keynote address, "The Philosophy of Occupational Therapy"

AOTA DEVELOPMENTS	SOCIETAL CHANGES
1922 Occupational therapy publications begin	
1923 Association name becomes AOTA	
1932 First National Registry is established	Depression slows development
1935 Essentials are adopted	
WWII OT services recognized by Armed Services	
1945 Registration examination is required	Rehabilitation movements begin
1947 Examination becomes objective test	Antibiotics gain widespread use
1950s Eleanor Clarke Slagle Lectureship is awarded	Neuroleptic drugs are developed
AOTA reorganizes	Plastics technology impacts therapeutic equipment
	Retardation programs are instituted
	Deinstitutional Plan releases many people
1960s New COTA category is established	Medicare and Medicaid are enacted
State regulatory laws are introduced	Community mental health programs begin
	Diagnostic-related groups change health care delivery
1970s Standards and Ethics are written	Education for All Handicapped Children Act is enacted
AOTA lobbies for public policy	
1980s AOTA moves into new headquarters	Technology-Related Assistance for Individuals with
Occupational therapy publications increase	Disabilities Act
Certification and membership separate	
1990s AOTA publications and membership continue to increase; AOTA moves headquarters to new building in Bethesda, Md	Americans with Disabilities Act

FIGURE 2-2. HISTORIC HIGHLIGHTS OF OCCUPATIONAL THERAPY.

Meyer was committed to a **holistic** perspective and developed the psychobiological approach to mental illness. He advocated that each individual should be seen as a complete and unified whole, not merely a series of parts or problems to be managed. He maintained that involvement in meaningful activity was a distinct human characteristic. Further, he believed that providing an individual with the opportunity to participate in purposeful activity promoted health.

In 1921 at the fifth annual meeting of the National Society for the Promotion of Occupational Therapy in Baltimore, Meyer delivered the keynote address. "The Philosophy of Occupational Therapy"[11] was later published in the organization's first journal in 1922. In his keynote address he stated that:

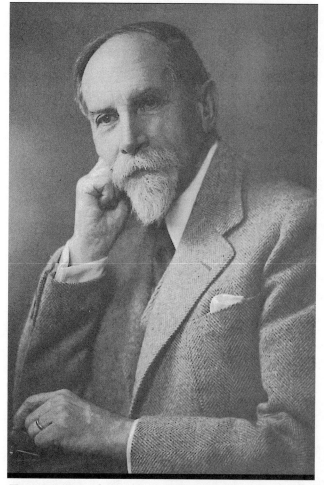

"There are many... rhythms which we must be attuned to: the *larger rhythms* of night and day, of sleep and waking hours...and finally the big four—work and play and rest and sleep, which our organism must be able to balance even under difficulty. The only way to attain balance in all this is *actual doing, actual practice*, a program of wholesome living as the *basis* of wholesome feeling and thinking and fancy and interests".[11]

Thus Adolf Meyer provided the initial fundamental philosophical statement of the field and the foundation on which the profession of OT was built.

GROWTH THROUGH PUBLICATION

An emphasis upon publication greatly shaped the new profession of OT and continued to mold its emerging character. Within 5 years of the organization's founding, it began to publish a journal devoted to the profession. Credit for the emphasis on publication is given to Dr. Dunton. His articles on the use of occupation for treatment purposes first caught the attention of George Barton, before the plans of an organization had been laid, and he later played a leadership role in journal developments. Dr.

FIGURE 2-3. ADOLF MEYER. (PHOTO COURTESY OF THE ARCHIVES OF THE AMERICAN OCCUPATIONAL THERAPY ASSOCIATION, INC., BETHESDA, MD.)

Dunton directed publicity and its publications for the newly formed organization. His interest in writing had an early influence upon the nature of the organization.

As reported in Reed and Sanderson's *Concepts of Occupational Therapy*,[14] "In 1921, he [Dunton] proposed that a journal be developed for OT because the *Maryland Psychiatric Quarterly* and *Modern Hospital* could not devote enough space to the growing profession. The *Archives of Occupational Therapy* began publication in 1922 with Dr. Dunton as editor, a position he held until 1947 when he retired. The name of the journal changed to *Occupational Therapy and Rehabilitation* in 1925 with volume 4." At the time of Dunton's retirement, Reed and Sanderson continued, "...the Association had elected to start a journal that would be owned by the Association. This new journal was named the *American Journal of Occupational Therapy*" and began its publication in 1947.[14] Over the years the journal has become known informally as *AJOT* (pronounced ā-jot).

It should be noted that since 1925, membership in the national organization has automatically included the journal subscription as a membership benefit. Regular distribution of the latest information in the field has been a binding force for OT's diverse membership.

Now that the individuals who influenced the founding and formation of the professional organization have been discussed, attention returns to the events that shaped both the world at large and the new profession of OT.

WAR YEARS

Beyond the use of occupations for the "insane" and the early sheltered workshops for convalescent individuals, such as Barton's Consolation House, World War I and **Reconstruction Aides** made up another thread that was woven into the tapestry of the profession's formation.

After the onset of World War I, a reconstruction program was initiated by the U.S. military. The purpose of the program was to rehabilitate soldiers who had been injured in the war so that they could either return to active military duty or be employed in a civilian job. The program was placed under the direction of orthopedic professionals and included OT practitioners, at that time called curative or bedside therapists, as well as physiotherapists and vocational evaluators.

In early 1918 on a trial basis, the program began at Walter Reed Hospital in Washington, D.C. with a group of physiotherapists and OT practitioners who were civilian women with no military ranking.[6] Several training programs were implemented, and hundreds of women were trained to be practitioners. The program was implemented overseas when the first group of reconstruction aides were sent to France to assist in the rehabilitation of soldiers. Under appalling working conditions—no rank, no uniforms, no materials or equipment, no prepared working areas—the reconstruction aides demonstrated to the Army that involvement in activities had a beneficial effect on hospitalized soldiers suffering from "shell shock."[1] The approach proved to be beneficial to the Army, and the demand for the aides' services increased throughout the war.

As the need for reconstruction aides increased, so did the need for training. Not only did existing schools and hospitals add quick training courses, new schools were started to meet the need. Typically, the programs consisted of instruction in arts and crafts, medical lectures, and hospital etiquette, as well as practical experience in a hospital or clinic. Although only a high school diploma was required, many of the women accepted into these programs had previous training in social work, in teaching, or in the arts.[12] (It was later, in 1923, that AOTA established education standards. See Chapter 7.)

At the end of World War I, many of the women who trained to become reconstruction aides left the field. Only some of the aides were OT practitioners. Others eventually became OT practitioners, and some went back to their prior roles (e.g., artist, teacher).[10] Many of the training programs closed.

There is some controversy about the era of the reconstruction aide, because training programs were hastily developed in response to the war. The historical significance of the reconstruction aides, however, is that they were the means by which OT became linked with physical disabilities.

The Great Depression impacted all aspects of life, which further slowed the development of OT, bringing additional program closures and cuts in OT staff. Attention to such rehabilitative care, which began with World War I, did not re-emerge until World War II brought new and similar needs.

World War II created a new demand for more OT practitioners. Because they had not achieved military status during World War I, few OT practitioners were employed in the Army or in Army hospitals when World War II broke out.[13] Once again, war emergency training courses were implemented to quickly train needed OT personnel. As a result, the number of employed practitioners increased significantly.[13] During World War II the U.S. Armed Forces officially recognized the field of OT as a vital rehabilitative service, and OT practitioners attained military status.

POST WORLD WAR II

After the 1940s the pace of change accelerated, and the changes that were brought to the profession were vast and rapid.

NEW DRUGS AND TECHNOLOGY

The discovery of the neuroleptic drugs (tranquilizers and antipsychotics) in the mid-1950s completely changed the course of psychiatric treatment. As psychotic behavior yielded to chemical control, it became possible to discharge many people, eventually leading to a national plan to release clients—the national

"Deinstitutionalization Plan." In anticipation of local care needs, community mental health programs were developed.

Other pharmacologic advances also affected the delivery of OT services. As antibiotics gained widespread use and new vaccines were developed, diseases such as tuberculosis and poliomyelitis were nearly eliminated. These advancements changed the focus of long-term rehabilitative services.

On the technical side, new fabrication materials—increasingly easier to use—were being developed in rapid succession, having an impact on splint making. New therapeutic equipment was being developed, requiring special training in their use.

EFFECTS OF LEGISLATION

Legislation and regulations passed by lawmakers during the postwar period also have had an effect on health care and the delivery of OT services. In this section, legislation and its impact on the practice of OT are examined.

The **Vocational Rehabilitation Act** and its amendments of 1943 provide for the payment of medical services to persons injured by accident or illness while employed. Occupational therapy is covered as a part of these services.

Medicare (PL 89-97) was enacted in 1965. It covers OT services in the inpatient setting and limited coverage for outpatient services. Initially, this legislation did not provide for services given by OT practitioners in independent private practice. However, government involvement in health care eventually led to new reimbursement procedures for Medicare recipients. In this system of fixed payment for diagnostic-related groups (DRGs), massive changes in hospital organization and care delivery have occurred. (In 1988, legislation granted Registered Occupational Therapists [OTRs] the right to Medicare provider numbers, permitting direct reimbursement for OT services.)

The **Rehabilitation Act of 1973** establishes several important principles. The first of these is the concept of reasonable accommodation. The Act mandates that employers and institutions of higher education receiving federal funds must accommodate the needs of employees and students with disabilities. The Act also prohibits discrimination in employment or in admissions criteria to academic programs solely on the basis of handicapping condition.

The **Education for All Handicapped Children Act of 1975** (PL 94-142) establishes the right of all children to a free and appropriate education, regardless of handicapping condition. This law includes OT as a related service. Before the passage of PL 94-142, many children with disabilities were not in school programs, let alone receiving therapy services. Under the requirements of this law, an individual education plan (IEP) must be written for each student. The IEP describes the student's specialized program and identifies measurable goals. The **Handicapped Infants and Toddlers Act** (PL 99-457) was passed in 1986 as an amendment to the Education for All Handicapped Children Act. The amendment extends the provision of PL 94-142 to include children from 3 to 5 years of age and initiates new early intervention programs for children from birth to 3 years of age. A primary service included in the amendment is OT. The result of these two laws has been an increase in OT services provided to children and an increase in the number of OT personnel employed within the school environment.

The **Technology Related Assistance for Individuals with Disabilities Act of 1988** (PL 100-407) addresses the availability of assistive technology devices and services to individuals with disabilities. Many OT practitioners are involved in providing these services.

The **Americans with Disabilities Act** (ADA) (PL 101-336) passed in 1990 provides civil rights to all individuals with disabilities. It guarantees equal access to and opportunity in employment, transportation, public accommodations, state and local government, and telecommunications for individuals with disabilities. Occupational therapy personnel provides consultation to private and public agencies to assist them in meeting these guidelines.

Government legislation and regulation has affected who receives OT services and how these services are delivered. There will continue to be governmental influence on the delivery of OT services in the future.

CHANGES IN THE PROFESSION

With the ebb and flow of society's changes, the profession has continued to adapt and meet the demands of the external environment. The outer or external changes of society have often meant changes in the profession. One of the greatest strengths of the field of OT is its well-run national organization. Throughout its history, AOTA has continued to expand and mature. To complete this brief history of the field, see Figure 2-2 for a few postwar highlights of AOTA's internal events.

Beginning in 1945, successful completion of an examination became a requirement for registering as an OT practitioner. The examination was initially an essay format; in 1947 it adopted the format of an objective test.

After World War II a number of OT practitioners were practicing in medical and rehabilitation facilities; this caused a shortage in psychiatric settings. Aides and technicians working under OT practitioners in psychiatric settings became knowledgeable in the techniques used and were often some of the most stable employees. As Shirley Holland Carr reports, "Supportive personnel knew how to do things, but lacked goal-oriented intervention methods necessary to work without immediate supervision".[3] This factor motivated a drive toward organizing courses for OT assistants. In the late 1950s a new category of practitioner was initiated— the Certified Occupational Therapy Assistant (COTA). The introduction of this new level of practitioner required many years of experimentation and study by AOTA to determine the appropriate interface and regulation. This was an important issue throughout the 1960s.

The 1950s and 1960s also brought organizational changes to accommodate and improve both the overall function of and membership representation in the ever-growing and expanding organization. AOTA data banks indicate that in 1945 there were 2177 members. The membership census in 1997 exceeded 59,000.

A controversial issue of the 1970s was state regulatory laws. Individual states began to introduce laws requiring OT practitioners to become licensed in order to practice. AOTA initially opposed this action, then took a neutral position, and finally affirmed licensing to ensure quality OT care. Since these laws are individually determined by each state, licensure of OT services has taken place gradually. (Regulation and licensure are discussed in greater detail in Chapter 7.)

Also during the 1960s and 1970s, AOTA expended great efforts to ensure that OT would be appropriately included in the onslaught of new federal governmental legislation directed at the delivery of health care. Lobbying for the interests of OT became a function of AOTA.

In the 1980s, AOTA moved into its own building, thus signifying a new era that began to yield results of AOTA's long-standing emphasis on research. This decade witnessed a wealth of new books and publications, including a new research journal, *The Occupational Therapy Journal of Research*. The latter part of the decade also brought a significant change in professional membership in AOTA. AOTA separated certification from its membership in 1986. On completion of all requirements, an OT practitioner is certified through the National Board of Certification of Occupational Therapy (NBCOT), subject to certification regulations, whereas AOTA membership is separate and voluntary.

UNIQUE IDENTITY

Occupational therapy has sought its own separate identity as a health care service, and change has been continual. There are, however, consistent elements throughout its history that confirm the unique identity of OT. From its beginning, OT has been based on a holistic point of view. The profession believes that the individual needs to engage in occupations, and that treatment must be based on the use of purposeful activities and on a commitment to support and encourage the independence of the client. The total function of the person is the focus of treatment, and the interpersonal relationship between the client and OT practitioner is vital to the process.

In the fiftieth anniversary commemorative issue of the *American Journal of Occupational Therapy*, Margaret Rerek states, "Most striking in a historical review of occupational therapy is the dramatic consistency of its basic assumption that man has a need to self-actualize through his work and/or leisure. While techniques have altered considerably over the years, there is an equal consistency in the goals of correcting or ameliorating whatever dysfunction prevents self-actualization...occupational therapy has been focused since its birth on health and function."[15]

SUMMARY

The new profession of OT officially came into being as the result of a meeting of incorporation in March 1917. It grew out of the rising social consciousness of the early twentieth century wherein consideration was given to Moral Treatment in psychiatric facilities, rehabilitation in sanitariums, and restoration for soldiers injured in battle, and attention was given to the use of activities as a course of treatment. The profession was forged by adapting to changing needs in a changing world. As a field of practice, OT has evolved through merging theory and research while focusing on health and function.

Activities

1. Research and write a short paper on the Moral Treatment Movement of the 1800s.
2. Compile short biographies on the founders of OT by reading three or four sources.
3. Search back volumes of *American Journal of Occupational Therapy* (and the older *Archives of Occupational Therapy* and *Occupational Therapy & Rehabilitation*, if available). Use lists of article titles to show the changes in emphasis from decade to decade.
4. Research and write a short paper on any single social influence, legislation, or technical development. Elaborate on how the event affected the practice and profession of OT.
5. Research and make a wall chart with a time line that depicts significant events and changes in AOTA since its inception.

REFERENCES

1. Bing R: Living forward, understanding backward. In Ryan S, editor: *The certified occupational therapy assistant: principles, concepts, and techniques*, ed 2, Thorofare, NJ, 1993, Slack.

2. Bing R: Occupational therapy revisited: a paraphrasatic journey, *Amer J Occup Ther* 35:(8)499, 1981.

3. Carr SH: The COTA heritage: proud, practical, stable, dynamic. In Ryan S, editor: *The certified occupational therapy assistant: principles, concepts, and techniques*, ed 2, Thorofare, NJ, 1993, Slack.

4. Dunton WR: *Occupational therapy: a manual for nurses*, Philadelphia, 1915, WB Saunders.

5. Dunton WR: The principles of occupational therapy. In *Proceedings of the National Society for the Promotion of Occupational Therapy: second annual meeting*, Catonsville, Md, 1918, Spring Grove State Hospital Press.

6. Gutman SA: Looking back—influence of the US military and occupational therapy reconstruction aides in World War I on the development of occupational therapy, *Amer J Occup Ther* 49:256, 1995.

7. Kidner TJ: Occupational therapy: its development, scope, and possibilities, *Occup Ther Rehabil* 10:3, 1931.

8. Levine RE: The influence of the arts-and-crafts movement on the professional status of occupational therapy, *Amer J Occup Ther* 41:248, 1987.

9. Licht S: The founding and founders of the American Occupational Therapy Association, *Amer J Occup Ther* 21:269, 1967.

10. Low JF: The reconstruction aides, *Amer J Occup Ther* 46:38, 1992.

11. Meyer A: The philosophy of occupation therapy, *Arch Occup Ther* 1:1, 1922. (Reprinted *Amer J Occup Ther* 31: 10, 1977.)

12. Quiroga V: *Occupational therapy: the first 30 years 1900 to 1930*, Bethesda, Md, 1995, American Occupational Therapy Association.

13. Reed KL: The beginnings of occupational therapy. In Hopkins HL, Smith HD, editors: *Willard & Spackman's occupational therapy*, ed 8, Philadelphia, 1993, JB Lippincott.

14. Reed KL, Sanderson SR: *Concepts of occupational therapy*, ed 3, Philadelphia, 1992, Williams & Wilkins.

15. Rerek MD: The depression years 1929-1941: occupational therapy—a historical perspective, *Amer J Occup Ther* 25(5):15, 1971.

16. Tracy SE: *Studies in invalid occupation*, Boston, 1910, Whitcomb & Barrows.

I am celebrating 3 years in the field of occupational therapy as a Certified Occupational Therapy Assistant. It has been a fulfilling 3 years, and this career has awarded me the opportunity to meet a number of very courageous and inspiring individuals.

There is nothing more rewarding than witnessing a patient's progress toward independent living. Occupational therapy enables people to achieve their potential by maximizing their assets and minimizing their dysfunction. This is what I find so unique about this field and what initially attracted me to it. ■

The human ability to dream, plan, experience, and master one's environment embodies the philosophy of occupational therapy. The practitioner's ability to recognize, explore, and facilitate a person's intrinsic motivators is the essence of the occupational therapy process. ■

Diane Bertolotti, AAS, COTA
The Rusk Institute of Rehabilitation
    Medicine
New York, New York

Mary Sands, MSEd, OTA, FAOTA
Chairperson
Occupational Therapy Assistant
    Department
Orange County Community College
Middletown, New York

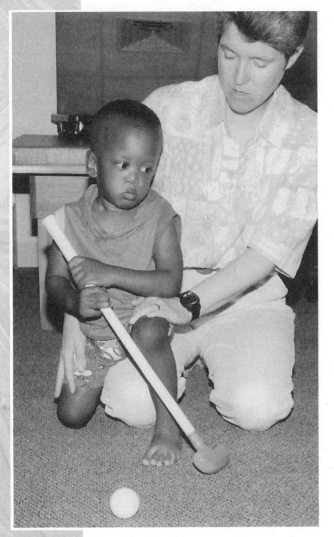

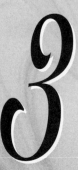

*Philosophy of
Occupational Therapy*

Objectives

After reading this chapter, the reader will be able to:

✤ Understand the importance of a profession's philosophical base
✤ Describe the components of a philosophy, in general; more specifically, describe the philosophy of occupational therapy (OT)
✤ Explain the meaning of *occupation* in the context of the profession
✤ Identify the two premises underlying the model of human occupation
✤ Describe purposeful activity
✤ Describe adaptation as used in OT
✤ Recognize the underlying general goal of all OT treatment

Key terms

Philosophical base	Mechanistic	Equality
Metaphysical component	Occupation	Freedom
Epistemology component	Model of human occupation	Justice
Axiology component	Purposeful activity	Dignity
Holistic approach	Adaptation	Truthfulness
Active being	Humanism	Prudence
Organismic	Altruism	

When defining OT, it is necessary to examine the philosophical base from which it is derived. Workable philosophies are not imposed from the outside; rather, they unfold from a historic base. As Chapter 2 is read, some central themes within the early practice of OT emerge. This important history is the foundation of OT as it is today. In recent years, individuals in the field have focused on the task of weaving the implications from past theory and practice into a sound, identifiable philosophical base. This has not been the task of one person alone. Some of those involved in this undertaking have included Mary Reilly, Gail Fidler, Wilma West, Elizabeth Yerxa, Gary Kielhofner, Anne Mosey, and Lela Llorens. Each have added to the work from their different areas of interest.

In this chapter the components of philosophy, in general, are examined first; then the philosophy of OT is introduced, and the central themes of the profession are discussed.

UNDERSTANDING PHILOSOPHY

Familiarity with and understanding of the **philosophical base** of one's profession is important for several reasons. A profession's philosophy serves as a set of values, beliefs, truths, and principles that guide the practitioner's actions.[13] It helps define

---

Chapter 3 photo: Ratliffe KT: *Clinical pediatric physical therapy: a guide for the physical therapy team,* St Louis, 1998, Mosby.

the nature of the existence of the profession, guides the actions of the practitioners of the profession, and helps practitioners substantiate the reason for existence.

It is helpful to understand what contributes to philosophy before applying it to a specific profession. In studying philosophy in general and the philosophical basis of a profession in particular, it is necessary to address questions related to three components.[13] The first is the **metaphysical component,** and it concerns questions such as, "What is the nature of man?" The second is the **epistemology component,** and it is related to the development of a professional philosophy. The epistemology component "investigates critically the nature, methods, limits, and validity of human knowledge."[8] Questions such as, "How do we know things?" and "How do we know that we know?" are addressed in the epistemology component. **Axiology** is the third component of philosophy, and it is concerned with the study of values. There are two types of questions represented in this component—questions of aesthetics (e.g., "What is beautiful or desirable?") and questions of ethics (e.g., "What are the standards and rules of right conduct?")[13] Using these four types of questions as guidelines, the philosophical base of the OT profession can be examined.

PHILOSOPHICAL BASE

In 1979 the Representative Assembly adopted a philosophical base of OT (Box 3-1). The four questions related to the components described above explain the philosophical base of OT and identify the evolution of its concepts in the profession's history. There are several key concepts that are explored in-depth.

Box 3-1

PHILOSOPHICAL BASE OF OCCUPATIONAL THERAPY

MAN IS AN ACTIVE BEING WHOSE DEVELOPMENT IS INFLUENCED BY THE USE OF PURPOSEFUL ACTIVITY. USING THEIR CAPACITY FOR INTRINSIC MOTIVATION, HUMAN BEINGS ARE ABLE TO INFLUENCE THEIR PHYSICAL AND MENTAL HEALTH AND THEIR SOCIAL AND PHYSICAL ENVIRONMENT THROUGH PURPOSEFUL ACTIVITY. HUMAN LIFE INCLUDES A PROCESS OF CONTINUOUS ADAPTATION. ADAPTATION IS A CHANGE IN FUNCTION THAT PROMOTES SURVIVAL AND SELF-ACTUALIZATION. BIOLOGICAL, PSYCHOLOGICAL, AND ENVIRONMENTAL FACTORS MAY INTERRUPT THE ADAPTATION PROCESS AT ANY TIME THROUGH THE LIFE CYCLE. DYSFUNCTION MAY OCCUR WHEN ADAPTATION IS IMPAIRED. PURPOSEFUL ACTIVITY FACILITATES THE ADAPTIVE PROCESS.

OCCUPATIONAL THERAPY IS BASED ON THE BELIEF THAT PURPOSEFUL ACTIVITY (OCCUPATION), INCLUDING ITS INTERPERSONAL AND ENVIRONMENTAL COMPONENTS, MAY BE USED TO PREVENT AND MEDIATE DYSFUNCTION AND TO ELICIT MAXIMUM ADAPTATION. ACTIVITY AS USED BY THE THERAPIST INCLUDES BOTH INTRINSIC AND THERAPEUTIC PURPOSE.[4]

WHAT IS MAN?

Much of the health care system in the Western world has been developed from a reductionistic approach, wherein humankind is reduced to separately functioning body parts. Specialties have been designed to separately treat these body functions for greater expediency and efficiency; their purpose is to isolate, define, and treat body functions and to focus on a specific problem. This reductionistic approach has proved valuable in producing many cures and amazing technological developments. In more recent years, however, the trend in medicine has been to move away from the specialist and return to the family practitioner who addresses all the bodily functions of the client.

In contrast, since its beginning, OT has viewed humans holistically and has adhered to a **holistic approach.** The holistic perspective can be traced to Adolf Meyer. In *The Philosophy of Occupation Therapy*, he states, "Our body is not merely so many pounds of flesh and bone figuring as a machine, with an abstract mind or soul added to it. [Rather, it is a live organism acting] in harmony with its own nature and the nature about it."[9] The holistic approach emphasizes the organic and functional relationship between the parts and the whole being. This approach maintains that a person is a whole, an interaction of physical, psychological, sociocultural, and environmental elements. If any element (or subsystem) is negatively affected, a disruption or disturbance will be reflected throughout the whole.

OT also views a human as an **active being.** Again looking to Meyer, "Our conception of man is that of an organism that maintains and balances itself in the world of reality and actuality by being in active life and active use."[9] Humans are actively involved in controlling and determining their own behavior and are capable of changing behavior as desired.[10] This view is referred to **organismic.** A **mechanistic** view, on the other hand, sees the human as passive in nature and controlled by the environment in which he or she lives.[10]

Related to the belief that the human is an active being, at the core of OT is the belief that **occupation** is critical to the existence of human beings. Occupation is the central word to the profession's identification, and it is a word often misunderstood by those outside the profession. As stated earlier the dictionary defines the word *occupation* as "An activity in which one engages." It refers to all the *doing* that fills one's time. In contemporary communication the word occupation has been commonly and frequently used to refer to one's job, as in the question, "What is your occupation?" People often overlook its more fundamental meaning. In the profession of OT there is a return to the more basic meaning. From the perspective of OT, occupation refers to "the ordinary and familiar things that people do everyday."[1]

Throughout the history of the profession, human occupation has been typically categorized by OT practitioners into the areas of self-care (self-maintenance), work, play, and leisure.[1] At a given time an individual may be occupied with caring for oneself by washing, dressing, or eating. A person may be occupied with productive tasks, such as paid employment or tasks that are necessary for the care of one's family. At other times, occupational involvement may be with activities that one simply finds pleasurable, such as playing cards, watching a movie, or exercising.

A model other than the medical model is needed to understand the field of occupational therapy. Kielhofner, Burke, and others, building on the ideas of Mary Reilly, point to a model that incorporates the philosophy upon which occupational therapy is built. This is the **human occupation model,** which holds that it is through activity—active engagement with the environment—that the human being becomes what he or she is.[7] There are two major premises underlying the human occupation model:

(1) Individuals are open systems, both influenced by and influencing the environment in which they exist

(2) Mind and body are interrelated and cannot be regarded as "separate parts."

With these two assumptions, the human occupation model provides a structure for understanding a person's interaction with his or her environment through activity or occupational behavior.

On the surface it may seem as if the concept of occupation is a simple one; in fact, the nature of occupation contains many dimensions and is rather complex.[1] The dimensions that comprise occupation include (1) the performance of the act, (2) the context in which the act is performed, (3) the psychological dimensions that include the individual's intrinsic need for mastery, competence, and self-identity, (4) the sociocultural and symbolic dimensions of the act, (5) the spiritual dimensions (nonphysical and nonmaterial aspects) related to the meaning of the occupation to the individual, and (6) the temporal dimension of the occupation, which relates to the fact that many occur over a period of time.[1] In Chapter 9, these dimensions are discussed in greater detail.

HOW DOES MAN KNOW WHAT HE KNOWS?

OT believes that a human learns through experience and by "doing." This concept is found in many of the early writings of the founding members of the profession.[9, 12, 14] For OT practitioners, this "doing" is referred to as **purposeful activity.** Purposeful activity involves the client on many levels. Coordination between the person's sensorimotor, cognitive, and psychosocial systems is necessary and elicited when an individual engages in purposeful activities.[3]

Purposeful activity is often used synonymously with the term *occupation.* However, recent position papers published by the American Occupational Therapy Association (AOTA) have been developed with the intent of making a distinction between the two terms. In AOTA's 1993 *Position Paper: Purposeful Activity,* purposeful activity is defined as the "goal-directed behaviors or tasks that comprise occupations."[3] Goal-directed behavior implies that the person is focused on the goal of the activity rather than the processes involved in achieving the goal.[3] The goal of the activity should be seen as meaningful by the client, and as a result, the client's participation would be active and voluntary.

Through this "knowing by doing," a human also learns to adapt. As seen in the philosophical base of OT, **adaptation** is defined as "a change in function that promotes survival and self-actualization."[4] In OT, purposeful activity is used to promote adaptation. Through purposeful activity the individual achieves mastery over the environment, which contributes to the individual's feeling of competency.[5] Gail Fidler and Jay Fidler describe purposeful activity and the development of competence. They write, "The ability to adapt, to cope with the problems of everyday living, and to fulfill life roles requires a rich reservoir of experiences gathered from direct engagement with both human and non-human objects in one's environment." They continue, "It is through such action with feedback from both human and non-human objects that an individual comes to know the potential and limitations of self and the environment and achieves a sense of competence and intrinsic worth."[6]

The philosophical base mentions the use of purposeful activity to improve or maintain health. Mary Reilly summarizes this concept in her Eleanor Clarke Slagle lectureship when she states, "Man through the use of his hands as they are energized by mind and will can influence the state of his own health."[11] OT practitioners use purposeful activity as a means to help a client learn a new skill, restore a deficient ability, compensate in the presence of a functional disability, maintain health, or prevent dysfunction.[3] The therapeutic use of purposeful activity requires that the OT practitioner analyze activity from a number of different perspectives. Activity analysis is a skill specific to OT and is discussed in detail in Chapter 16.

WHAT IS DESIRABLE?

As mentioned earlier, OT works in, around, and with the medical field but belongs to a different model. The purpose of medicine is to treat, medicate, and apply life-saving techniques and technology; its purpose is to fill the needs that a person cannot. OT believes that the quality of life is important. Therefore the purpose of OT is independent functioning. Whatever can be achieved, the goals are to teach and foster independence and to seek ways for the client to regain or find the capacity to function independently, depending less on the care provided by others and more on the self.

OT seeks to improve the quality of life for any person whose functional ability is impaired or limited. This goal is achieved by helping the client develop greater independence in the performance of any area of occupational behavior. For example, a goal of treatment may be to enable a client to independently brush his or her teeth, or to manage a checkbook, or to become more alert to the body mechanics that help avoid injury on the job. Likewise, the goal of treatment may ensure that the client increases the strength in the body part needed to perform a necessary task, or achieve better coordination for all activities, or be better able to enjoy life by developing a hobby, or more fully participate in life by developing social skills. Together, the OT practitioner and client focus on maximizing occupational performance.

WHAT ARE THE "RULES OF RIGHT CONDUCT?"

As discussed in Chapter 2, the profession of OT emerged from the era of Moral Treatment, which valued the humanitarian treatment of individuals who were mentally ill. OT is still based on **humanism,** a belief that the client should be treated as a person, not an object. The humanistic perspective is one of the pillars of the profession. From this humanistic perspective, values and attitudes central to the profession have evolved. The paper, *Core Values and Attitudes of Occupational Therapy Practice*,[2] identifies the concepts of altruism, equality, freedom, justice, dignity, truth, and prudence as the core values and attitudes of OT.

Altruism is the unselfish concern for the welfare of others. It is demonstrated through the commitment of the OT practitioner to the profession and to one's client with caring, dedication, responsiveness, and understanding. **Equality** is treating all individuals equally with an attitude of fairness and impartiality and respecting each individual's beliefs, values, and lifestyles in the day-to-day interactions of the OT practitioner.[2]

The OT practitioner also values **freedom,** an individual's right to exercise choice and to "demonstrate independence, initiative, and self-direction."[2] Freedom is demonstrated through nurturing, which is very different from controlling or directing. OT practitioners nurture their clients by providing support and encouragement, enabling the client to develop his or her inherent potential. Nurturing encourages the development of independence in the client, rather than retaining all direction and control in the hands of the practitioner.

Justice is the need for all OT practitioners to abide by the laws that govern the practice and legal rights of the client. Through the value of **dignity,** the uniqueness of each individual is emphasized. OT practitioners demonstrate this value through empathy and respect for each person. **Truthfulness** is a value demonstrated through behavior that is accountable, honest, and accurate, and that maintains one's professional competence. **Prudence** is the ability to demonstrate sound judgment, care, and discretion.[2]

SUMMARY

The philosophical base of a profession represents its core beliefs, values, and principles. The history of OT provides the foundation for the philosophy that represents the current practice of OT. This history helps address questions such as: "What is humankind?" "What is truth?" "What is ethical or right conduct?" "What is desirable?"

When exploring the diversity of the field of OT, it is important to maintain an awareness of the concepts of holistic approach, occupation, purposeful activity, adaptation, independent function, and improving the quality of life, for these concepts embody the philosophical roots of the field (Figure 3-1).

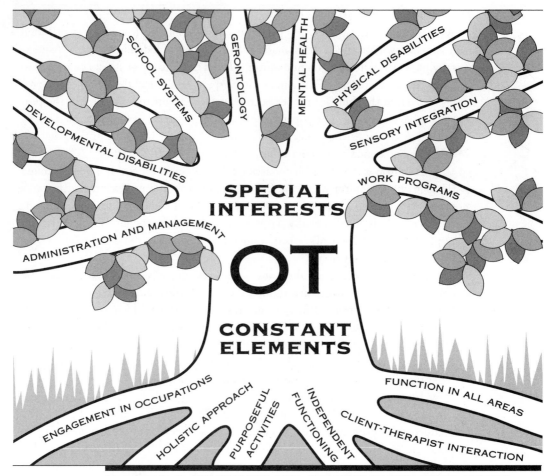

FIGURE 3-1. PHILOSOPHICAL BASE: THE ROOTS OF OCCUPATIONAL THERAPY.

OT views humans as active beings and from a holistic perspective. *Occupation* is seen as an essential part of human existence and refers to all the daily activities that people do. *Purposeful activity* is any goal-directed behavior that engages the person on a sensorimotor, cognitive, or psychosocial level. There are three categories of occupational performance: self-care, work and productivity, and play and leisure. The underlying goal of all OT is to increase the individual's independence in any area of occupational performance, thus the OT practitioner must recognize inhibitors of activity and be able to design a plan for correction.

Humans learn by doing and, through the process of adaptation, develop a mastery of self and competence. Improving a client's quality of life (particularly increasing a person's independence) is the focus of the services provided by OT practitioners. OT provides the client with opportunities to adapt and improve one's quality of life.

Activities

1. Identify your values and beliefs. Do they relate to the values and beliefs of the occupational therapy profession?
2. Review Chapter 2 and research other historical occupational therapy resources to trace consistencies between the early and current philosophies of the profession.
3. From case study articles (i.e., *OT Week*), gather examples of quality-of-life changes that result from occupational therapy intervention.
4. In your own words, write a description of occupational therapy.

REFERENCES

1. American Occupational Therapy Association: Position paper: occupation, *Amer J Occup Ther* 49:1015, 1995.
2. American Occupational Therapy Association: Core values and attitudes of occupational therapy practice, *Amer J Occup Ther* 47:1085, 1993.
3. American Occupational Therapy Association: Position paper: purposeful activity, *Amer J Occup Ther* 47:1080, 1993.
4. American Occupational Therapy Association: The philosophical base of occupational therapy, *Amer J Occup Ther* 33:785, 1979.
5. Fidler GS: From crafts to competence, *Amer J Occup Ther* 35:567, 1981.
6. Fidler GS, Fidler JW: Doing and becoming: purposeful action and self actualization, *Amer J Occup Ther* 32:305, 1978.
7. Kielhofner G: *A model of human occupation: theory and application*, ed 2, Baltimore, 1995, Williams & Wilkins.
8. Landau SI: *The Doubleday dictionary®*, New York, 1975, Doubleday.
9. Meyer A: The philosophy of occupation therapy, *Arch Occup Ther* 1:1, 1922. (Reprinted *Amer J Occup Ther* 31:10, 1977.)
10. Reed KL: The beginnings of occupational therapy. In Hopkins HL, Smith HD, editors: *Willard & Spackman's occupational therapy*, ed 8, Philadelphia, 1993, JB Lippincott.
11. Reilly M: Occupational therapy can be one of the great ideas of 20th century medicine, *Amer J Occup Ther* 16:2, 1962.
12. Robeson HA: How can occupational therapists help the social service worker? *Occup Ther Rehabil* 5:279, 1926.
13. Shannon PD: Philosophical considerations for the practice of occupational therapy. In Ryan SE, editor: *The certified occupational therapy assistant: principles, concepts, and techniques*, ed 2, Thorofare, NJ, 1993, Slack.
14. Slagle EC: Training aides for mental patients, *Arch Occup Ther* 1:13, 1922.

The most memorable aspects of my career in occupational therapy education are the wonderful students I am privileged to know and the opportunity to share with them my beliefs and philosophy about the health-giving value of occupation. My students teach me so much about life, teaching, and learning. It is richly rewarding to facilitate and witness the evolution of the college student to the professional. ▪

Lorraine Williams Pedretti, MS, OTR
Professor Emeritus
Department of Occupational Therapy
San José State University
San José , California

As an occupational therapy educator, I find it rewarding to facilitate learning and observe the transition from student to clinician. The profession of occupational therapy has provided me opportunities to interact with many individuals including clients and their families, other members of the health care team, and occupational therapy practitioners. Occupational therapy has provided me with many opportunities for professional growth and learning, while collaborating with other occupational therapy practitioners. Occupational therapy is a way of life—not just a profession!" ▪

Sue Byers-Connon, BA, COTA/L, ROH
Instructor
Occupational Therapy Assistant
    Program
Mount Hood Community College
Gresham, Oregon

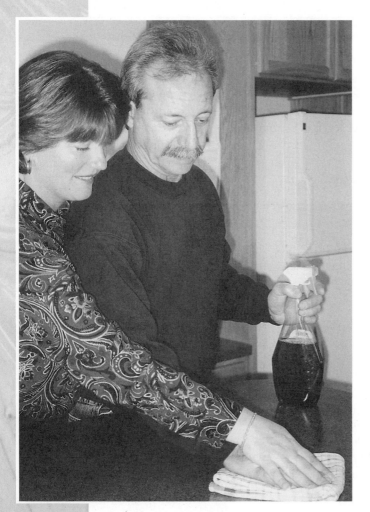

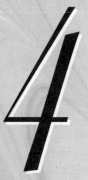

4 Occupational Therapy
Personnel and Educational
Requirements

Objectives

After completing this chapter, the reader will be able to:

✤ Identify the categories of occupational therapy (OT) personnel
✤ Delineate the educational requirements for each personnel category
✤ Identify the common roles performed by OT practitioners
✤ Describe the three levels of performance for OT practitioners
✤ Understand the types of supervision required for the different levels of performance
✤ Describe service competency

Key terms

National Board for Certification of Occupational Therapy
Accreditation Council for Occupational Therapy Education
Fieldwork
Registered Occupational Therapist
Certified Occupational Therapy Assistant
Entry level
Intermediate level
Advanced level
Close supervision
Routine supervision
General supervision
Minimum supervision
Service competency
Occupational Therapy Aide

There are two levels of educational preparation and two corresponding levels of OT practitioners in the field of OT. At the professional level—the most highly trained—is the Registered Occupational Therapist (OTR). At the technical level is the Certified Occupational Therapy Assistant (COTA). A third category of worker, who does not receive specialized training before working in the field, is the Occupational Therapy Aide. To be consistent with the terminology used by the American Occupational Therapy Association (AOTA), the term *occupational therapy personnel* is used when referring to *all* personnel (including Aides) who work in OT, and the term *occupational therapy practitioner* refers to any individual who is certified by the **National Board for Certification of Occupational Therapy** (NBCOT) as either an OTR or a COTA. When it is necessary to distinguish the two levels of practitioner, the respective titles are used.

Chapter 4 photo: Early MB: *Physical dysfunction practice skills for the occupational therapy assistant*, St Louis, 1998, Mosby.

ENTRY-LEVEL EDUCATIONAL PREPARATION

The entry level education for both OTR and COTA programs is regulated in all parts of the United States by the **Accreditation Council for Occupational Therapy Education** (ACOTE) of the AOTA. (See Chapter 7 for further information.) ACOTE sets the guidelines for accredited programs. These guidelines are published in *The Essentials and Guidelines for an Accredited Program for the Occupational Therapist*[9] and in *The Essentials and Guidelines for an Accredited Program for the Occupational Therapy Assistant*.[10] ACOTE evaluates each programs' compliance with "the essentials," and schools that meet these guidelines become accredited.

As of 1997 there are 105 accredited OTR programs and 128 accredited COTA programs in the United States and Puerto Rico.[1] In selecting a school the prospective student is advised to seek information about the school's accreditation status, mission statement, and philosophy, as well as the emphasis of its educational program. This information enables a student to make an informed choice, ensuring the best selection.

Many similarities exist when comparing the accreditation criteria for the OTR and COTA. The curricula for both consist of a similar combination of classroom and clinical learning experiences. At both levels, students complete anatomy, physiology, medical conditions, kinesiology, and general education courses that lead to a degree awarded by the respective college or university. Courses in the professional areas of the curricula are also similar in content. Students at both levels learn OT principles, practices, and processes. The difference in the education for the OTR is the depth of theory provided in both the core and professional curricula.

Each level of training requires practical experience, or what is referred to as **fieldwork.** The purpose of fieldwork is to "provide occupational therapy students with the opportunity to integrate academic knowledge with the application of skills at progressively higher levels of performance and responsibility."[3] For this reason, two levels of fieldwork are provided. The initial level is referred to as Level I fieldwork and is completed concurrently with the academic courses. The purpose of Level I fieldwork is to introduce the OT student to the profession and to the various applications of treatment intervention. The amount of time required at this level varies from program to program.

Level II fieldwork requires that the OTR student complete full-time fieldwork at a facility for a minimum of 24 weeks, and it requires that the COTA student complete 12 weeks of full-time fieldwork. At Level II, both OTR and COTA students are immersed in the OT practice, and by the end of his or her fieldwork, each is expected to be minimumly functioning at the entry level.

After completing this educational requirement, candidates at each professional level are eligible to sit for the national certification examination, which is administered by the NBCOT. For those candidates who pass the certification examination, NBCOT issues an identification number that indicates the professional status in the field of OT;

the graduate is then entitled to use the appropriate professional designation after her or his name—*Registered* Occupational Therapist or *Certified* Occupational Therapy Assistant. Candidates residing in states that have licensure are then eligible to apply for a state license to practice. (See Chapter 7 for further information.)

If the examination is not passed, a candidate can pay the fee and take the examination again. The number of times a candidate can take the test is limited to three administrations. If the person is working under a temporary license and fails the examination, he or she may not continue working in the capacity of an OT practitioner. He or she may work as an Aide until the test is passed. The national examination for each level of practitioner is offered two times per year on the same day throughout the country.

EDUCATIONAL PREPARATION FOR THE OTR

To be an OTR an individual must complete at least 4 years of college and, at a minimum, hold a Bachelor of Sciences or Arts degree. However, there have been some exceptions to this rule. For a brief time, experienced COTAs were permitted to challenge the OTR certification examination and, if successful, to become an OTR without fulfilling formal educational requirements. This option, however, is no longer an available.

One path to becoming an OTR is to earn a 4-year Bachelor of Sciences or Arts degree in OT. A second path to becoming an OTR is earning a degree in another related field (i.e., psychology, child development) and then completing a certificate program—an intensive year of OT academics plus an internship. The person who completes this program earns an *Occupational Therapy Certificate* and is eligible to take the certification examination. A third way to become an OTR is to complete a degree in a related field and then enter a basic Master's degree OT program.

EDUCATIONAL PREPARATION FOR THE COTA

The first COTA training programs were structured differently than they are today. As discussed in Chapter 2, training for the COTA originated in psychiatric settings. The first program to implement training in general practice occurred in Maryland in 1960. Early training programs were operated by various organizations rather than the higher educational system.[12] In 1965, AOTA implemented several changes in COTA programs, one of which being the establishment of programs in junior or community colleges.

To become a COTA, with the exception of those under the earlier training programs previously noted, an individual must complete at least 2 years of postsecondary education in an accredited program. This program could be either in a community or junior college or in a technical training school. Whether an Associate of

Sciences or Arts degree is awarded depends on the institution's ability to grant degrees. The COTA must also complete Level I and Level II fieldwork. The educational requirements for the OTR and the COTA are summarized in Box 4-1.

ROLES OF OT PRACTITIONERS

OT practitioners may operate in many different roles, as identified in Table 4-1. The major functions of each role and the scope of the role, performance areas, qualifications, and supervision are described in detail in a 1993 AOTA document entitled, "Occupational Therapy Roles." (See Appendix A.)

Direct patient care is the primary role carried out by the OT practitioner. Other roles include educator, fieldwork educator, supervisor, administrator, consultant, fieldwork coordinator, faculty, program director, researcher, and entrepreneur. Frequently, OT practitioners function in more than one role—at times within the same job. For example, an OTR may provide client treatment and perform the functions of an administrator; a COTA may hold positions as both a faculty member and clinician. As the career of an OT practitioner progresses, he or she may wish to advance within the role or transition into a different role.

Box 4-1

EDUCATIONAL REQUIREMENTS FOR OTRs AND COTAs

OTR

COMPLETED ONE OF THE FOLLOWING PROGRAMS FROM AN ACCREDITED COLLEGE:

- 4-YEAR BACHELOR OF SCIENCES OR ARTS DEGREE IN OCCUPATIONAL THERAPY

- 4-YEAR BACHELOR OF SCIENCES OR ARTS DEGREE IN A RELATED FIELD WITH A POSTGRADUATE CERTIFICATE IN OCCUPATIONAL THERAPY

- 4-YEAR BACHELOR OF SCIENCES OR ARTS DEGREE IN A RELATED FIELD WITH A BASIC MASTER'S DEGREE IN OCCUPATIONAL THERAPY

COMPLETED AT LEAST 6 MONTHS OF LEVEL II FIELDWORK

PASSED NATIONAL OTR CERTIFICATION EXAMINATION

COTA

GRADUATED WITH A 2-YEAR ASSOCIATE SCIENCES OR ARTS DEGREE FROM AN ACCREDITED COMMUNITY OR JUNIOR COLLEGE OR TECHNICAL TRAINING SCHOOL

COMPLETED AT LEAST 12 WEEKS OF LEVEL II FIELDWORK

PASSED NATIONAL COTA CERTIFICATION EXAMINATION

OTR, Registered Occupational Therapist; COTA, Certified Occupational Therapy Assistant.

TABLE 4-1	OCCUPATIONAL THERAPY ROLES*

ROLE	MAJOR FUNCTION
Practitioner—OTR	Provides quality occupational therapy services, including assessment, intervention, program planning and implementation, discharge–planning-related documentation, and communication. Service provision may include direct, monitored, and consultative approaches.
Practitioner—COTA	Provides quality occupational therapy services to assigned individuals under the supervision of an OTR.
Educator (consumer, peer)	Develops and provides educational offering or training related to occupational therapy to consumer, peer, and community individuals or groups.
Fieldwork Educator (practice setting)	Manage Level I or II fieldwork in a practice setting. Provides occupational therapy assistant students with opportunities to practice and carry out practitioner competencies.
Supervisor	Manages the overall daily operation of occupational therapy services in defined practice area(s).
Administrator (practice setting)	Manages department, program, services, or agency providing occupational therapy services.
Consultant	Provides occupational therapy consultation to individuals, groups, or organizations.
Fieldwork Coordinator (academic setting)	Manages student fieldwork program within the academic setting.
Faculty	Provides formal academic education for occupational therapy or occupational therapy assistant students.
Program Director (academic setting)	Manages the occupational therapy educational program.
Researcher/Scholar	Performs scholarly work of the profession, including examining, developing, refining, and evaluating the profession's body of knowledge, theoretical base, and philosophical foundations.
Entrepreneur	Entrepreneurs are partially or fully self-employed individuals who provide occupational therapy services.

*NOTE: Many jobs involve more than one role, and job titles vary by setting.

From American Occupational Therapy Association: Career exploration and development: a companion guide to the occupational therapy roles document. In COTA *information packet: a guide for supervision*, Bethesda, Md, 1993, AOTA.

LEVELS OF PERFORMANCE

The profession recognizes that not every practitioner performs at the same level. In the 1970s in an attempt to delineate these differences, AOTA identified six practitioner classifications: OTR specialized, OTR experienced, OTR entry level, COTA experienced, COTA entry level, and Occupational Therapy Aide. In the 1980s these classifications were expanded to include the categories of OTR intermediate and COTA intermediate, but the Occupational Therapy Aide was excluded because it was not considered a professional category. These classifications were based on the amount of time a practitioner performed in the field. Recognizing that time in the field is not a valid indicator of a person's level of performance, this criterion becomes problematic. Consequently, these categories and descriptions have been further revised.

Currently, the three levels of performance for all OT practitioners are identified as entry, intermediate, and advanced. The practitioner's level of expertise is based on attaining a higher skill level through work experience, education, and professional socialization.[8]

Table 4-2 shows the level of expertise and describes the professional development required at each level. The person at the **entry level** is expected to be responsible for and accountable in professional activities related to the role. At the **intermediate level,** the practitioner has increased responsibility and typically pursues specialization in a particular area of practice. The person functioning at the **advanced level** is considered an expert, or a resource, in the respective role. For each role delineated in *Occupational Therapy Roles*[8] (Appendix A), job expectations for all three performance areas are listed.

Each individual progresses along this continuum at a different pace. Some individuals never progress past the entry level in a particular role, or a person may transition to a new role, wherein his or her level of performance is classified at entry level. For example, an individual who has worked as an OTR at the advanced level may transfer into an administrative role at the entry level. A COTA at the intermediate level may transition to the role of an entry-level faculty member. Even at the entry level, individuals in both situations may need to acquire additional knowledge and skill to satisfactorily perform the new job functions. It is also possible for an individual to function in two roles at different levels. For example, a COTA intermediate level practitioner may assume new responsibilities as a fieldwork educator. In the new role, this COTA would initially perform the job function at the entry level.

SUPERVISION

With the increased use of COTAs and Occupational Therapy Aides, questions regarding the amount and type of supervision frequently arise. In the document *Guide for Supervision of Occupational Therapy Personnel,*[6] recommendations for supervision are provided. However, individual states, accreditation bodies, and third party payers may have regulations that may supersede these guidelines.

TABLE 4-2	LEVELS OF ROLE PERFORMANCE	
ROLE	**MAJOR FOCUSES**	**SUPERVISION**
Entry	• Development of skills • Socialization in the expectations related to the organization, peer, and profession. *Acceptance of responsibilities and accountability for role-relevant professional activities is expected.*	Close
Intermediate	• Increased independence • Mastery of basic role functions • Ability to respond to situations based on previous experience • Participation in the education of personnel *Specialization is frequently initiated, along with increased responsibility for collaboration with other disciplines and related organizations. Participation in role-relevant professional activities is increased.*	Routine or general
Advanced	• Refinement of specialized skills • Understanding of complex issues affecting role functions *Contribution to the knowledge base and growth of the profession results in being considered an expert, resource person, or consultant within a role. This expertise is recognized by others inside and outside of the profession through leadership, mentoring, research, education, and volunteerism.*	Minimal

From American Occupational Therapy Association: Occupational Therapy Roles, *Amer J Occup Ther* 47:1087, 1993.

TABLE 4-3	TYPES OF FORMAL SUPERVISION
TYPE	**DESCRIPTION**
Close	Daily, direct contact at the site of work
Routine	Direct contact at least every 2 weeks at the site of work, with interim supervision through other methods such as telephone or written communication
General	Monthly direct contact with supervision available as needed by other methods
Minimal	Contact only on an as-needed basis; may be less than monthly

From American Occupational Therapy Association: Occupational Therapy Roles, *Amer J Occup Ther* 47:1087, 1993.

Formal supervision is described along a continuum as shown in Table 4-3.[8] At one end of the continuum is **close supervision,** which is the greatest amount of supervision and requires direct, daily contact. **Routine supervision** follows, in which there is direct contact at least every 2 weeks. **General supervision** is next, which is described as at least monthly contact. Finally, **minimal supervision** is at the other end of the continuum, providing supervision on an as-needed basis.[8]

Supervision is closely tied to role function and level of performance. Looking again at Table 4-2, the degree of supervision changes for each level of performance. Although not required, it is recommended that close supervision be provided to an entry level OTR by an experienced OTR. If an entry level OTR is working in an independent practice, he or she should seek out an experienced OTR to provide some consultation at a minimum. Routine or general supervision is recommended for an intermediate level OTR.[6]

The COTA at each level requires at least general supervision by an OTR. Although the entry level COTA typically requires close supervision, the intermediate level practitioner requires routine supervision, and the advanced level practitioner requires general supervision.[6] The OTR is ultimately responsible for the services provided by either the COTA or Occupational Therapy Aide.

SERVICE COMPETENCY

Because the OTR is responsible for the performance level of the COTA, he or she must have confidence that the COTA will obtain the same results when performing service provision. **Service competency** is a useful mechanism to ensure that services are provided with the same high level of confidence. AOTA provides the following definition:

> "Service competency is the determination, made by various methods, that two people performing the same or equivalent procedures will obtain the same or equivalent results. In test development this is known as interrater reliability. The same concept can be applied to professionals working together in the service provision process. It stems from the assumption that the OTR employs currently acceptable practices."[11]

The methods and standards to establish service competency vary depending on the task or procedure involved. Methods such as independent scoring of standardized tests, observation, videotaping, and co-treatment can be used. For frequently used procedures, service competency is more easily established; procedures that are used less frequently may require closer supervision. Before service competency is established for a particular procedure, it is recommended that the acceptable standard of performance be met on three successive occasions between an OTR and COTA or between an experienced OTR and an entry level OTR who lacks experience in particular procedures.[11]

INTERRELATED ROLES

In establishing levels of supervision and service competency, it is important that the OTR and COTA work together in a collaborative relationship that promotes quality service and professional development.[8] Beyond the practical need to determine appropriate duties and supervision, each OT practitioner needs to be aware that the roles of the OTR and COTA are intended to be interrelated. Any suggestion of power struggle, job competition, or jealousy between the two is indicative of internal problems or poor department management. Ideally, collaboration between the OTR and COTA is an example of today's interdisciplinary health care teams. The team approach is one in which various disciplines meet and plan the overall care of the client, maintaining an awareness of his or her needs, responses, and goals. Team members become mutual sources of information and support in treatment.

OCCUPATIONAL THERAPY AIDE

The use of Aides in health care is becoming more commonplace because of the implementation of cost-cutting measures. It is an area that has resulted in many questions and concerns. A recent position paper developed by AOTA defines the **Occupational Therapy Aide** as "an individual assigned by an OT practitioner to perform delegated, selected skilled tasks in specific situations under the intense close supervision of an OT practitioner."[5]

As mentioned earlier, the person working as an Aide is not expected to have special training. The Aide performs delegated tasks, receiving on-the-job training. Because the level of training is limited, it is important that supervision remain close. The Occupational Therapy Aide may be supervised by either an OTR or a COTA; however, the OTR remains the individual ultimately responsible for the actions of the Aide.

DEMOGRAPHICS OF OT PRACTITIONERS

The latest membership data from AOTA show that within the OTR classification, 94% are women and 6% are men; within the COTA classification, 92% are women and 8% are men.[7] For the highest level of OTR in any field, 70% had earned a Baccalaureate degree, 26% a Master's degree, 2% an undergraduate degree with an OT certificate, and 1% a Doctorate degree. For the COTA, 81% had earned an Associate degree, 11% a Baccalaureate degree, 6% an undergraduate degree with an OT certificate, and 2% a Master's degree.[2] The highest percentage of OT practitioners are employed in California and New York.[4] In Chapter 5 the types and demographics of employment settings in which OT personnel work are discussed.

SUMMARY

The OTR and COTA are the two official levels of professionals in the field of OT. Untrained personnel working in OT departments are called Occupational Therapy Aides. OT personnel are hired and salaried according to education and experience, in accordance with AOTA guidelines, which recognize an increased level of expertise with increased knowledge and skill. The formal education of the OTR and COTA are similar in content, but a greater investment of time and a greater depth of knowledge are required of the OTR.

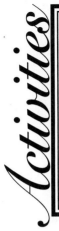

Activities

1. Interview an occupational therapy administrator in a large department; chart the staffing patterns of the occupational therapy personnel.
2. Prepare a report on the national certification examination (when, where, cost).
3. Write a short paper on the history of occupational therapy education.
4. Interview an occupational therapy practitioner. Determine his or her motivation for entering the field. How did he or she learn about occupational therapy? Why did he or she decide to pursue the field? What is his or her educational background? Ask him or her to describe their fieldwork experiences.

REFERENCES

1. American Occupational Therapy Association: Accreditation council completes full agenda, *OT Week*, September 25,1997.

2. American Occupational Therapy Association: Percent of registered occupational therapists and certified occupational therapy assistants by highest-level education degree, 1980 and 1996. *AOTA 1990 member data survey*, 1990, Bethesda, Md, AOTA; and AOTA *1995-96 member data survey*, 1996, Bethesda, Md, AOTA.

3. American Occupational Therapy Association: Statement: purpose and value of occupational therapy fieldwork education, *Amer J Occup Ther* 50:845, 1996.

4. American Occupational Therapy Association: *Estimated numbers of occupational therapy personnel*, Bethesda, Md 1995, AOTA.

5. American Occupational Therapy Association: Position paper: use of occupational therapy aides in occupational therapy practice, *Amer J Occup Ther* 49:1023, 1995.

6. American Occupational Therapy Association: Guide for supervision of occupational therapy personnel, *Amer J Occup Ther* 48:1045, 1994.

7. American Occupational Therapy Association: Demographic information occupational therapy practitioners, *1994 AOTA membership files*, Bethesda, Md, 1994, AOTA.

8. American Occupational Therapy Association: Occupational therapy roles, *Amer J Occup Ther* 47:1087, 1993.

9. American Occupational Therapy Association: Essentials and guidelines of an accredited educational program for the occupational therapist, *Amer J Occup Ther* 45:1077, 1991.

10. American Occupational Therapy Association: Essentials and guidelines of an accredited educational program for the occupational therapist, *Amer J Occup Ther* 45:1085, 1991.

11. American Occupational Therapy Association: Entry-level role delineation for registered occupational therapists (OTRs) and certified occupational therapists (COTAs), *Amer J Occup Ther* 44:1091, 1990.

12. Hirama H: *Occupational therapy assistant: a primer*, Baltimore, 1996, Chess Publications.

I chose the field of occupational therapy because the profession seemed limited only by the individual professional. As an occupational therapist, I have had numerous choices of work settings and ages of clients with whom I have interacted. I have worked in acute care hospitals, comprehensive outpatient and adult day care settings, public school settings, regular day care settings, preschool settings for children with special needs, as well as home environments. I have had the pleasure of working with clients of all ages from diverse cultural backgrounds. I am currently teaching in a community college. Our typical COTA student is nontraditional in age and historical background.

While working in the direct service arena, I was rewarded on a regular basis as my clients progressed, gaining more active interaction and control of themselves and their environment. I believe I have been able to significantly impact the quality of life of my clients. In essence, it is not how long we live (quantity) but rather how we live (quality). Occupational therapists are in a unique position to assist in improving the quality of life of the persons for whom we serve. ◼

Jean W. Solomon, MHS, OTR/L, BCP
Clinical Coordinator and Instructor
Occupational Therapy Assistant
    Program
Department of Rehabilitative Services
Trident Technical College
Charleston, South Carolina

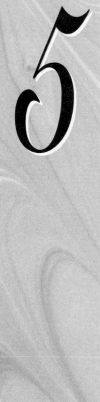

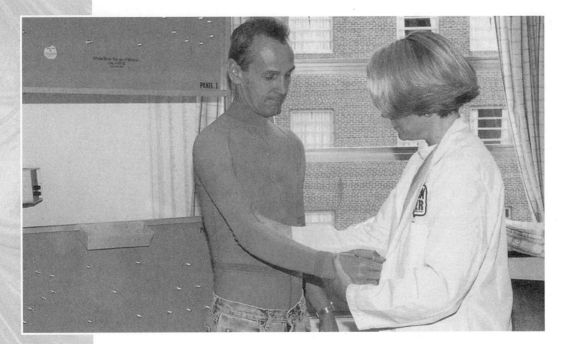

Employment Settings

Objectives

After reading this chapter, the reader will be able to:

✤ Describe how the holistic approach influences the ways in which occupational therapy (OT) practitioners practice

✤ Characterize settings in which OT practitioners are employed by types of administration, levels of care, and spheres of practice

✤ Understand the meaning of spheres of practice and identify each

✤ Identify the primary health problems and treatment aims addressed in each sphere of practice

✤ Identify various OT employment settings

Key terms

Public agencies
Private not-for-profit agencies
Private for-profit agencies
Continuum of care
Acute care
Diagnostic-related groups
Subacute care
Long-term care
Biological (medical) sphere
Psychological sphere
Sociological (social) sphere

As discussed in Chapter 3, OT subscribes to a holistic approach, which contends that correction of a problem promotes health. In OT the holistic approach extends to the improvement of function for all types of disability; as a result, the application of services is not confined to a particular kind of setting. Employment settings vary greatly. Settings wherein therapy usually occurs can be identified, but there are other settings not mentioned that also employ OT practitioners. Further, there are settings not yet discovered where OT services will be offered.

CHARACTERISTIC OF SETTINGS

The different types of settings in which OT practitioners are employed can be characterized in three ways. These characterizations categorize and identify the many employment settings available to the practitioner. For the purposes of this text, employment settings are characterized according to: (1) administration of the setting, (2) levels of care, and (3) spheres of practice.

Chapter 5 photo: Pedretti LW: *Occupational therapy: practice skills for physical dysfunction*, ed 4, St Louis, 1996, Mosby.

ADMINISTRATION OF SETTING

A health care agency can be categorized as a public agency, a private not-for-profit agency, or a private for-profit agency (also called proprietary). The type of agency affects the mission and purpose of the agency, its reimbursement mechanisms, and its organizational structure.

Public agencies include those that are operated by federal, state, or county governments. Agencies at the federal level include the Veteran's Administration Hospitals and Clinics, Public Health Services Hospitals and Clinics, and Indian Health Service. Agencies at the state level include correctional facilities, state hospitals for persons who are mentally ill or have developmental disabilities, and state medical school hospitals and clinics. The county may operate county hospitals, clinics, and rehabilitation facilities. These hospitals and clinics deliver services to clients in the same way as federal and state facilities. However, the administration comes under different regulations, which may affect employment or how services are reimbursed.

Private not-for-profit agencies receive special tax exemptions available to not-for-profit organizations. These agencies typically charge a fee for services and maintain a balanced budget so they can continue to provide services. These agencies include hospitals and clinics with religious affiliations, private teaching hospitals, and organizations such as the Easter Seal Society and United Cerebral Palsy.

Private for-profit agencies are owned and operated by individuals or a group of investors. These agencies are in business to make a profit. In the last several years, many agencies have been purchased by large for-profit corporations to form multi-hospital–facility systems. This has significantly changed health care. Multi-hospital–facility systems allow the corporation to buy supplies and equipment in bulk at a lower volume rate. Because these systems provide a wider range of services, they have an advantage when it comes to developing contracts with third-party payers to provide health care services.

LEVELS OF CARE

Another way of characterizing health care settings is the level of care that is required by the individual client. Health care is provided to the consumer along a continuum, as the client's needs dictate. Often, this is referred to as a **continuum of care.** The point where the client falls along this continuum dictates the type of setting and the services provided.

Acute care is the first level on the continuum. A client at this level has a sudden and short-term need for services and is typically seen in a hospital. Services provided in the hospital are expensive because of the high cost of technology and the number of services provided. For years, hospitals billed and were paid for the services they provided. The *Prospective Payment System*, introduced under Public Law 98-21 and passed in 1983, changed the way in which hospitalization for the beneficiaries of Medicare was paid. Under this system, a nationwide schedule was implemented, defining how much hospitals would be paid for treatment of the Medicare client. Depending on the client's diagnosis, hospitals are paid a predetermined, fixed fee, based on **diagnostic-related groups** (DRGs), regardless of the services provided. The system provides an incentive for hospitals and physicians to reduce costs and discharge a client from the hospital as soon as possible. As a result, the average length of a hospital stay has decreased since 1983.[5] Further, short hospital stays and measures to contain costs have affected the utilization of OT practitioners, decreasing the number of practitioners practicing in hospital-based settings[7,8] (Figures 5-1 and 5-2).

Shorter hospital stays created a need for an interim level of care, referred to as **subacute care.** Initiated in response to the DRGs, subacute care provides a lower level of care. At this level, the client still needs care but does not require an intensive level or specialized service; thus the costs can be reduced. The National Subacute Care Association defines persons that need subacute care as "medically complex cases requiring a longer period of rehabilitation and recovery, usually from 1 to 4 weeks."[4] Hospitals with excess acute care beds have converted many to less expensive subacute care beds, whereas skilled nursing facilities have upgraded some beds to the subacute level.[4] In addition, freestanding subacute care facilities have been established.[1] The client typically served by a subacute care facility is a person who has sustained a stroke or hip fracture, has undergone hip replacement, or has cancer. Rehabilitation services, including OT, are a major component in subacute care.

The next interim level is referred to as **long-term care.** At this level the client has stabilized medically but has a condition that is chronic in nature. This client needs services over a long period of time, potentially throughout his or her life. Persons requiring this level of care include those who have developmental disabilities, a long history of mental illness, or sustained an injury resulting in a severe disability. Elderly persons, who are living longer and need more care, may also require long-term care. Services provided at this level may take place in an institution, a skilled nursing or extended care facility, a residential care facility, the client's home, an outpatient clinic, or a community-based program.

SPHERES OF PRACTICE

Finally, employment settings in OT can be characterized according to a concept called "spheres of practice." In their book, *Concepts of Occupational Therapy,* Reed and Sanderson employ spheres of practice to group categories of problems addressed in OT. This grouping is valuable; it enables the OT practitioner to begin to interpret the nature of the problem being addressed.[6]

As this text elaborates on the concept of spheres of practice, it is important for the student to understand that the categories mix and overlap. Only in the "ivory tower" of theoretical speculation are these ideas studied separately—the positions held by OT practitioners and the people they meet usually embody a mixture.

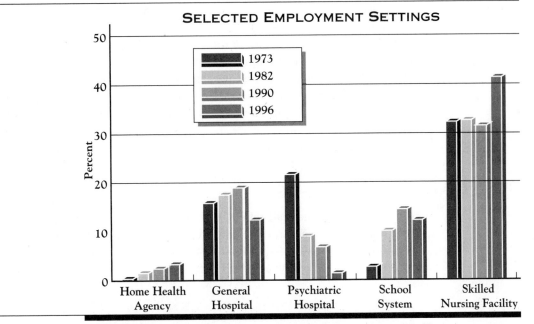

FIGURE 5-1. COTA EMPLOYMENT SETTINGS. (FROM STEIB PB: TOP EMPLOYMENT SETTINGS FOR COTAS, <u>OT WEEK</u>, NOVEMBER 21, 1996, AOTA.)

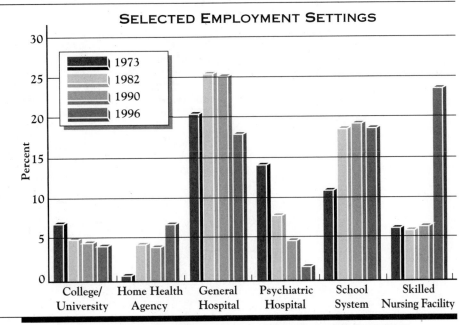

FIGURE 5-2. OTR EMPLOYMENT SETTINGS. (FROM STEIB PA: GROWTH IN GERIATRIC CARE REFLECTED IN OTR SURVEY, <u>OT WEEK</u>, NOVEMBER 14, 1996, AOTA.)

The spheres of practice, as identified by Reed and Sanderson, are (1) biological (medical), (2) psychological, and (3) sociological (social). As the concept is illustrated (Figure 5-3), the center of these three overlapping spheres is a region identified as "occupational performance," the profession's central concern. As health problems occur from any of the possible spheres, they affect the person's ability to engage in occupations (or activities) required in his or her life. Help in making the adjustment and finding new ways to function is often needed. OT practitioners operate in all three spheres; their role is that of problem solvers. Practitioners plan and guide improvement of function.

WITHIN THE SPHERES OF PRACTICE

Within the **biological (medical) sphere,** medical problems usually caused by disease, disorder, or trauma are encountered. Primary limitations addressed by the OT prac-

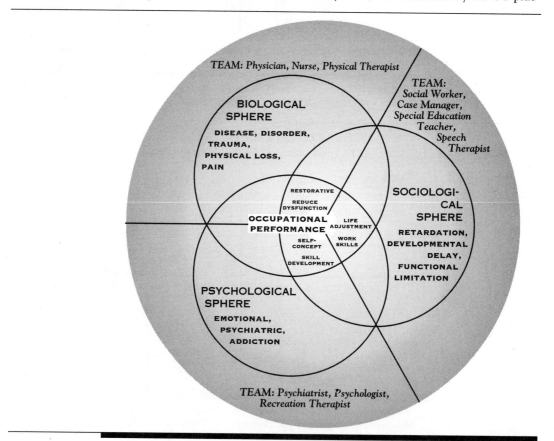

FIGURE 5-3. SPHERES OF PRACTICE DIAGRAM. (DATA FROM REED K, SANDERSON SR: CONCEPTS IN OCCUPATIONAL THERAPY, ED 3, BALTIMORE, 1992, WILLIAMS & WILKINS.)

titioner include loss of capacity, loss of sense, limitation in development or growth, limitation in movement, pain, damage to body systems, or neuromuscular disorders.

Within the **psychological sphere,** problems identified as emotional disorders, cognitive disorders, or psychiatric problems are encountered. These problems may be caused by an inability to cope with stress, a biochemical imbalance, a disease process, or a combination of developmental and environmental factors. OT practitioners address problems that affect thinking, memory, attention, emotional control, judgment, or self-concept.

Within the **sociological (social) sphere,** problems meeting the expectations of society are encountered. These problems may result from a severe physical or cognitive disability that limits functioning, developmental delays, mental retardation, long-term emotional problems, or any combination of the above. OT practitioners address the absence of the ability to take care of one's own needs, a lack or loss of life skills, poor interpersonal skills, a failure to properly adapt to environmental changes, a lack of capacity for independent functioning, and improper or detrimental behavior patterns. In general, these problems require long-term life adjustment.

To illustrate the difference between these three spheres, consider the client who is in therapy to improve work skills with a long-term goal of employment. It makes a difference whether his or her lack of work skills is due to biological (paralysis), psychological (severe depression), or sociological problems (mental retardation). The treatment plan in each case calls for a very different set of goals and objectives.

It is important to be aware that these practice spheres are *not* mutually exclusive. If the OT practitioner is employed in a medical setting, he or she should not ignore the psychological and sociological spheres when treating a client with a biological limitation. To provide therapy to the whole person means including all spheres in treatment planning. For example, a person who has undergone an amputation (biological sphere) may exhibit a psychological problem associated with denial and anger, which must be addressed before a prosthesis (artificial limb) is accepted and a restoration program is successful. Another example is the OT practitioner who works in a setting that is primarily sociological (social) in focus—a group home with a program to teach life skills to adults who have mental retardation. Because of the limitations in their communication skills, specific problems of mentally retarded adults often go undetected. While working with the client in hygiene and simple job skills, the OT practitioner may discover specific upper extremity weakness. Even though the program goals are life-skills training, the discovery of a weakness in the upper extremity requires further evaluation of and work on a goal that is considered biological—strengthening. It is important not to get locked into one sphere because of the work setting and forget to include the total range of needs of the person being served.

The sphere of practice concept can be used as a guide to categorize and identify the settings that typically employ OT practitioners. Many employment settings may be grouped according to the prevalent kind of treatment emphasis, either biological, sociological, or psychological (Table 5-1). In reality, the kinds of setting frequently involve an overlap of treatment concerns, but distinctions of emphasis can be made, and this arrangement of relational groups will be useful.

There are other employment opportunities that do not lend themselves to the spheres division, and some of those will also be identified. Because the intent of this chapter is to focus on employment settings, many different therapy skills are mentioned for illustration purposes but are not elaborated on. These skills are discussed in other sections of this book.

BIOLOGICAL EMPHASIS

The first OT employment setting that generally comes to mind is a medical facility where rapid client turnover is expected. Therefore the discussion begins here, considering short-term medical care in the treatment of acute illness or trauma.

HOSPITALS

Many large and some smaller general hospitals have OT departments. The clients are inpatients who are receiving care for acute illnesses. The usual focus of OT treatment in hospitals is evaluation and general medical and functional concerns. For example, the OT practitioner in this setting may provide evaluations, such as assessing independence in self-care, determining range of motion, and providing muscle and perceptual tests. The practitioner may program activities to increase strength, coordination, or independent self-care. With shortened hospital stays, the

TABLE 5-1	EMPLOYMENT SETTINGS (GROUPED BY THE SPHERES OF PRACTICE CONCEPT)	
BIOLOGICAL (medical)	**SOCIOLOGICAL (social)**	**PSYCHOLOGICAL**
HOSPITALS	**SCHOOLS**	**INSTITUTIONS**
General	Public	Psychiatric
State and federal	Special	Mental retardation
Specialty	● Visual impairment	
	● Hearing impairment	
	● Cerebral palsy	
CLINICS	**DAY TREATMENT**	**COMMUNITY MENTAL HEALTH**
HOME HEALTH	**WORKSHOPS**	**SUPERVISED LIVING**
ALL INCLUSIVE	Long-term care	
PRIVATE PRACTICE	Self-defined	
OTHER	Correctional, industry, hospice, national societies	

NOTE: The categories do not indicate specialization. There are overlapping services in all spheres; the classification highlights the setting's primary concern.

OT practitioner immediately addresses concerns regarding the client's ability to return home (e.g., home equipment needs, family training). The skilled practitioner who is alert to a holistic perspective will also address health-promoting concerns.

In addition to inpatient acute care, some hospitals provide rehabilitation services, which are performed over a longer period of time. OT is used in these specialty units within the general hospital. A typical rehabilitation unit provides services to adult clients who have sustained some type of disabling condition, such as a stroke, head trauma, or spinal cord injury. Another area where these types of services are provided is the neonatal unit for infants at risk as a result of premature birth. The OT practitioner in a neonatal unit provides infant stimulation and testing of reflexes and motor functioning. Feeding is evaluated, and corrective training is given when needed. Range of motion is monitored and positioning is recommended to prevent deformities. Some infants are hospitalized for months receiving specialized treatment.

OT practitioners are also employed at specialty hospitals designed to provide services to a particular group of clients, such as those with spinal cord injuries, head traumas, or burns. Children's hospitals are also included in this category of specialty hospitals. Through reading, workshops, and on-the-job training, the OT practitioner acquires the special skills needed to practice in such settings.

CLINICS

A clinic is another employment setting with a medical focus. A clinic gives treatment strictly on an outpatient basis. Clients are often (but not necessarily) those who have been recently released from a hospital but need, after discharge, more therapy for the same disabling condition. Outpatient clinics may be affiliated with a hospital, or they may be a separate entity. In a clinic, long-term functioning is an important consideration. The OT practitioner may be expected to teach adaptive behavior and develop mechanical adaptations in addition to the usual tasks performed for inpatient clients.

Physical disability rehabilitation clinics have existed for a long time. Notable examples are the Easter Seal Society Clinics found in many cities. Specialty clinics, such as hand clinics, orthopedic clinics, or children's developmental clinics, have emerged more recently.

HOME HEALTH AGENCIES

Spurred on by changes in our national health care delivery system, home health agencies are becoming increasingly prevalent. The client temporarily resides and is treated in a hospital; in a clinic, the client comes to the therapy department; in a home health agency (as the name implies), the treatment is administered in the client's home. Many home health agencies employ OT practitioners of various disciplines, as well as nurses and nurses aides.

An advantage of working in home health is that the OT practitioner is providing therapy in the client's natural setting. This is especially important for the practitioner because he or she is frequently working with the client on problems related to performance in self-care, work and school, or play and leisure. The disadvantage of working in a home health setting is that it is more difficult or at least more time-consuming to communicate with other members of the team. The OT practitioner may not have the day-to-day contact with other team members and may need to make a point of communicating with them regarding treatment plans and progress. Another disadvantage is the time it takes to drive from the employment setting to the client's home; the practitioner needs to plan ahead for the treatments to be certain that he or she has all the necessary equipment and supplies for the day.

There are different ways to work for home health agencies, depending on how the particular agency is run. An OT practitioner may be employed full time at regular hours and go wherever assigned, or the practitioner may be an independent contractor with an agency and take specific referrals as desired.

SOCIAL EMPHASIS

Beyond individuals with medical concerns are those whose functional limitations infringe on their ability to satisfactorily interact with others. These clients have needs that are long-term, since they are usually permanently disabled in some way. Therapy is concerned with life adjustments that will increase the individual's daily functioning despite limitations. Thus the main concern is a social focus rather than a medical one, and therapy is directed toward a way of "being in the world."

SCHOOLS AND SPECIAL EDUCATION

In 1975 a new law passed, the Education for All Handicapped Children Act, known as Public Law PL 94-142. This law makes public school education available to all children, regardless of handicap or disability. Since public schools are required to educate children with special needs, it is necessary to provide for those needs by employing OT practitioners in the areas of physical therapy, OT, and speech therapy. Not every school employs practitioners. How a school system provides these services is determined by state and local policies, but every county in every state must have some therapy services available for children with disabilities in order to receive federal funding.

Many special education schools founded before the passage of PL 94-142 continue to exist to meet specific needs. There are special schools for children with visual impairment (blind or low vision), hearing impairment (deaf), and cerebral palsy (CP). Frequently, OT practitioners are employed at these schools.

DAY TREATMENT

Day treatment facilities are provided for groups of people who need daytime supervision, people who are able to live in the community (rather than in an institution or full-care facility) but require some assistance. Some individuals may live at home with families whose members work, whereas others live in boarding homes but cannot plan their own activities. Day treatment facilities provide structured programs of activities. These facilities are in place for children with behavioral disorders, for persons who have mental illness, for persons with Alzheimer's disease, and for the elderly.

WORKSHOPS

Some progressive communities provide special workshops for people who are not able to seek employment in the competitive job market. These may be sheltered workshops, training centers, or retirement workshops. Many clients in sheltered workshops have some type of developmental disability. Here, OT practitioners may be employed for work-skill development, work hardening, adapting to the environment, task modification, or a variety of other functions.

PSYCHOLOGICAL SETTINGS

The next cluster of settings has its main focus in the psychological sphere. In these settings, social problems are also addressed, but the settings are regarded primarily as psychiatric, or mental health, settings.

INSTITUTIONS

Although there was a national deinstitutionalization plan implemented in the 1970s, there are still some state hospitals that provide services for those with severe developmental or emotional disabilities. These institutions (or state hospitals) are a source of employment for OT practitioners and frequently offer traditional psychiatric OT programs wherein the practitioner plans activities (e.g., crafts, recreation, outings) for the purposes of skill development, self-awareness, and social interaction.

COMMUNITY MENTAL HEALTH CENTERS

Community mental health centers emerged with the closing of institutions and are organized differently from region to region and from town to town. Some centers have only medication clinics and counseling, some have crisis units, and many have day treatment programs. In settings that use OT, a practitioner individually works with a client or with a group to develop life skills, plan an outing, or run arts and crafts workshops.

SUPERVISED LIVING

Supervised living refers to partially or fully supervised housing for people whose problems do not warrant institutional care but who are not ready or able to manage on their own. Programming may vary from limited guidance to fully structured programs. Supervised living includes substance-abuse programs (often with a specific time limit) for alcoholics or drug addicts; half-way houses, which are usually a temporary living arrangement for someone leaving an institution but before going on to independent living; or group homes, which are expected to be more or less permanent for the client. In these settings the OT practitioner may work with the client on general planning, such as organizing household chores, outings, and recreational activities, engaging the residents in life-skills training.

ALL-INCLUSIVE SETTINGS

A provider of OT services that combines and addresses needs from all three spheres—biological, psychological, and sociological—is a long-term care facility. A long-term care facility provides a residence for people for a prolonged period of time or even permanently. Included are extended, residential, and specialty long-term care, as well as skilled nursing facilities. The special skills needed by the OT practitioner in these settings depend on the nature of the facility and probably include any of the previously mentioned kinds of focus.

PRIVATE PRACTICE

Another kind of employment for consideration is self-employment or private practice, which can be designed to fit any or all the previously mentioned spheres. Although private practice is not new, it is a growing area within the profession. The 1980s produced a sizable increase in OT practitioners in private practice, indicating that this concept will be especially important for the future.

Private practice opened for practitioners in 1988 when the federal government, through the Health Care Financing Administration, implemented Medicare Part B coverage. This enabled OT practitioners to fully participate in Medicare programs by permitting qualified practitioners to apply for Medicare provider numbers. A provider number allows a practitioner to become an independent provider and bill directly for services.

As the field of OT becomes more self-directing, OT practitioners are finding new ways to market their expertise through private practice. An individual may make his or her skills independently available on a one-on-one basis, or practitioners may group together and market therapy services. There are many legal ramifications that must be explored when choosing private practice, and a person needs good administrative skills to pursue such a venture.

One of the advantages of private practice is that the OT practitioner can design a practice according to personal interests or desires. Some Registered Occupational Therapists (OTRs) take individual referrals and administer treatment in private homes, whereas others ask clients to come to their facilities. Some OTRs sell services in blocks of time. For example, an OT practitioner may contract to spend a specific number of hours at a school or a number of days at a nursing home,. Yet, another practitioner, with a similar or differing discipline, may incorporate and market therapy services as a business enterprise, employing practitioners from both professional and assistant levels.

OTHER SETTINGS

Other employment possibilities exist—correctional facilities, industrial settings, hospices, health maintenance organizations, and community transition, case management, and academic and research programs. As expressed in Jaffe and Epstein's

Occupational Therapy Consultation: Theory, Principles, and Practice, "Today's health care delivery system has changed the role of the OT practitioner. It has expanded from practice in traditional clinical arenas to broader health care settings. As we move into new or nontraditional arenas, there is a growing need for increased communication skills, information, and expertise in the field of consultation."[3]

Consulting is mentioned only to make the reader aware of the expanding possibilities within the field of OT. Consultation requires highly developed professional expertise and management skills; the consultant and agency negotiate the parameters of service and set their own limits.

There are also potential employers of OT services that use job titles other than "occupational therapist." For example, a nursing home or day-treatment program may employ an OT practitioner as an Activity Director or Activity Coordinator. Although these facilities choose to use another title (and are not regulated by the state laws that govern the practice of OT), they regard OT education (especially that of a Certified Occupational Therapy Assistant [COTA]) as desirable preparation for positions of leadership in activity programs.

OTHER PROFESSIONALS IN THE HEALTH CARE SETTING

A chapter on employment settings would not be complete without a discussion of the other professionals that are partners with OT practitioners in the delivery of health care services. These members include, but are not limited to, professionals in the fields of physical therapy, speech therapy, nursing, rehabilitation engineering, special education, vocational rehabilitation counseling, medicine, social work, and psychology. Each individual team member contributes knowledge and skills from his or her area of expertise to the delivery of quality patient care.

For the best results, it is important that all professionals involved with a client's care work together as a team to meet the treatment goals of the client. Ongoing communication among team members regarding treatment plans and their progress is essential. For quality and cost-effective delivery of services, team members should enhance each other's treatment and avoid a duplication of services.

OCCUPATIONAL THERAPY EMPLOYMENT TRENDS

Employment trends for both the OTR and COTA demonstrate a shift away from employment in psychiatric and general hospital settings toward skilled nursing settings. In 1996 over 40 percent of all COTAs worked in a skilled nursing facility, almost double the number of COTAs employed in this setting in 1990 (see Figure 5-2). Although approximately 19 percent of COTAs worked in the school systems in 1990, this number decreased to 9 percent in 1996; the number of COTAs working in psychiatric and general hospitals declined as well.[7]

Since 1990, employment trends for the OTR (see Figure 5-3) also show a significant increase in employment in skilled nursing facilities, as well as an increase in employment in home health agencies. However, employment for the OTR has experienced a decline in psychiatric and general hospitals, as well as a slight decline in school systems. Schools, general hospitals, and skilled nursing facilities each employed approximately 18 percent of the OTR population in 1996.[8]

SUMMARY

The holistic approach affirms a mind-body link and in doing so seeks to improve any limitation in functioning. As a result of the diversity that this entails, different employment settings dictate different primary treatment aims. One way to organize this diverse range-of-work possibilities is by using the spheres of practice concept. The three traditional spheres of practice are biological (medical), sociological (social), and psychological. A medical setting is geared for a short-term stay; as a result, OT treatment focuses on the immediate acute needs to enhance the client's functioning during illness and recovery. A social setting focuses on the individual with a long-term handicap or disability; as a result, treatment is aimed at ameliorating functional limitations and at training for long-term life adjustment. A psychological setting is one in which mental illness, emotional disorders, and substance abuse are treated; as a result, treatment is aimed at skill development, self-awareness, and learning appropriate interaction skills. In addition to the traditional spheres, a multitude of possibilities exist in nontraditional arenas for the OT practitioner.

An employment setting can also be distinguished by its administration and the level of care it provides. The administration of the setting can be either a public agency; a private, not-for-profit agency; or a private for-profit agency. The level of care provided to the client also distinguishes the type of setting. Care can be characterized as acute, subacute, or long-term.

There are certain trends that can be identified when the demographics of OT practitioners in various employment settings are studied. With the increasing number of elderly individuals, one trend is an increase in the number of practitioners employed in skilled nursing or long -term care settings. This trend has been accompanied by a decline in the number of OT practitioners employed in psychiatric and general hospitals.

Activities

1. Research the kinds of OT employers in your area; determine which kind employs the greatest number of OT practitioners.
2. Make a list of all specific facilities within a designated area that use OT services.
3. Trace the history and current status of a specific kind of employer; interview an OT practitioner working in that area.
4. Make salary comparisons for entry level practitioners (OTR and COTA) in different kinds of employment settings. (Note: These data may not be available in some states.)
5. Review a series of case studies (many can be found in *Willard & Spackman's Occupational Therapy*[2] and *American Journal of Occupational Therapy*). Photocopy the narrative history (minus any treatment plan); identify and group the occupational problems according to the sphere from which they arise.

REFERENCES

1. Hirama H: *Occupational therapy assistant: a primer,* Baltimore, 1996, Chess Publications.
2. Hopkins HL, Smith HD, editors: *Willard & Spackman's occupational therapy,* ed 8, Philadelphia, 1993, JB Lippincott.
3. Jaffe EG, Epstein CF: *Occupational therapy consultation: theory, principles and practice,* St Louis, 1992, Mosby.
4. Joe B: Subacute care fills growing niche, *OT Week,* Feb 27, 1997, American Occupational Therapy Association.
5. Levy LL: Occupational therapy's place in the health care system. In Hopkins HL, Smith HD, editors: *Willard & Spackman's occupational therapy,* Philadelphia, 1993, JB Lippincott.
6. Reed K, Sanderson SR: *Concepts in occupational therapy,* ed 3, Baltimore, 1992, Williams & Wilkins.
7. Steib PA: Top employment settings for COTAs, *OT Week,* Nov 21, 1996, American Occupational Therapy Association.
8. Steib PA: Growth in geriatric care reflected in OTR survey, *OT Week,* Nov 14, 1996, American Occupational Therapy Association.

My training as a COTA has benefited me in every venture that I have undertaken. I treat it as a birth certificate. No matter what title I take in my place of employment, I will forever consider myself an occupational therapy practitioner. My skills and experience speak for themselves. I do not need a title to define who I am or what I can do. I am proud to be a COTA, and I am confident in my abilities to provide quality services to the individuals with whom I work. One of the most exciting things about working in the field of occupational therapy is that I am not limited to one environment. I can be a clinician, an educator, an administrator, or an entrepreneur. The only boundaries are those I set for myself or allow others to set for me. ■

Robin A. Jones, BS, COTA/L, ROH
Director
Great Lakes Disability and Business
    Technical Assistance Center
University of Illinois at Chicago
Chicago, Illinois

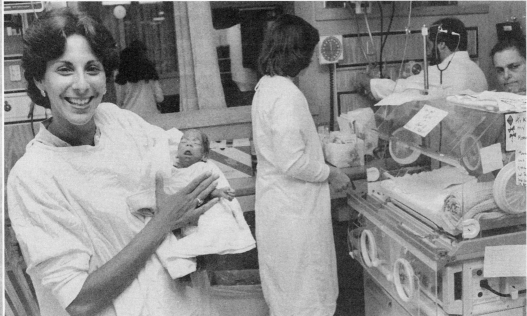

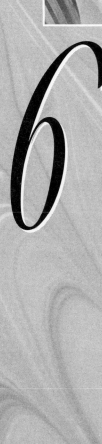

6 Ethics of the Profession

Objectives

After reading this chapter, the reader will be able to:

✤ Understand the purpose of a Code of Ethics
✤ Differentiate between ethics and laws
✤ Describe the function of the Commission on Standards and Ethics
✤ Identify the American Occupational Therapy Association's (AOTA) principles of ethics
✤ Demonstrate an ability to pose solutions to ethical dilemmas

Key terms

Professional judgment
Morals
Ethics
Code of Ethics
Commission on Standards and Ethics
Beneficence
Nonmaleficence
Autonomy
Confidentiality
Veracity
Fidelity
Ethical dilemma

On a daily basis, occupational therapy (OT) practitioners are confronted with situations that require a decision. The practitioner uses clinical reasoning skills to make therapeutic decisions. However, these clinical decisions, as well as decisions unrelated to therapeutic intervention, both require what is called **professional judgement.** Although a part of clinical decision-making, professional judgement extends beyond direct caregiving. Similar to clinical judgment, professional judgement is characterized by the wisdom of the choices made.

Morals and ethics guide professional judgment. **Morals** are related to "character and behavior from the point of view of right and wrong."[3] Morals develop as a result of background, values, religious beliefs, and the society in which a person lives. **Ethics** is the study and philosophy of human conduct. As defined by Purtilo, ethics is "a systematic reflection on and an analysis of morals."[4]

The **Code of Ethics** of a profession is the primary influence on professional judgment. Ethical codes "do not tell you what to do when conflicts or problems arise, rather they outline the moral dimensions of health care practice in your

Chapter 6 photo: Wallace HM, Biehl RF, MacQueen JC, Blackman JA: *Mosby's resource guide to children with disabilities and chronic illness,* St Louis, 1997, Mosby.

field."[4] A Code of Ethics provides guidelines for making choices and decisions that are regarded as correct or proper. These guidelines are usually stated in the form of principles. A person or group may be guided by unwritten ethical principles, or a group may develop a formal or written Code of Ethics. When a Code of Ethics is formalized as a written document, it is directed to the specific group of individuals that occupy an identifiable role.

Ethics differs from laws and rules in that ethical standards are more general, and their intent is to give positive guidance rather than impose binding and nega-tive limits to specific situations. However, because ethics today has been blended with law to form professional standards, ethical misconduct may also constitute a violation of the law.[5] In this chapter ethics is discussed. The standards and regula-tions that govern the practice of OT are discussed in Chapter 7.

AOTA ETHICAL CODE

For many years the OT practitioner functioned under unwritten, informal ethical principles, but in the 1970s, AOTA took steps to develop a formal code. *Occupational Therapy Code of Ethics*[1] was initially adopted by the Representative Assembly in April 1977 and revised in 1979, 1988, and 1994. With its adoption, this code became the formal and official voice of the profession on the subject of the proper rendering of OT services to the public, of conduct between and among professionals, of documentation, and of other activities, such as education and pro-fessionalism in general. (See Appendix B.)

The latest revision of this AOTA document is in the form of six principles, each addressing a different aspect of professional behavior. The **Commission on Standards and Ethics** was established to ensure compliance with the Code. "Acceptance of membership in the American Occupational Therapy Association commits members to adherence to the [profession's] Code of Ethics and its enforce-ment procedures."[1] (In Chapter 7, enforcement of the code is discussed in greater detail.)

For introductory purposes, a listing of the six principles follows, with a brief description of each and an example that relates to an aspect of professional behavior addressed by the principle.

PRINCIPLE 1: BENEFICENCE AND NONMALEFICENCE

In general terms, the principle of **beneficence** means that the OT practitioner shall contribute to the good health and welfare of the client, whereas the principle of **nonmaleficence** means that the practitioner shall not inflict harm to the client. Principle 1 of the Code of Ethics has four parts, each of which are related to the well-being of the recipient of services. This principle highlights the need for OT practitioners to (1) treat each client equitably; (2) not exploit a client sexually, physically, financially or socially; (3) avoid bringing harm to the client; and (4) charge fees that are reasonable and commensurate with the services provided.[1]

Example A: Mr. Parker was receiving OT services, but his ability to pay for services has run out. Therapist A had begun a daily self-feeding program for Mr. Parker. She visits his room at mealtime and introduces herself to the hospital aide assigned to him during lunch. Therapist A explains the proper use of the adaptive equipment that has been given to Mr. Parker. She speaks with Mr. Parker and the aide about how to work on independence and discusses what assistance may still be needed, as as well as the tasks he can accomplish alone. Therapist A does not bill for this instructive visit, knowing that both the client and the hospital aide will give better support to the program when personally addressed about the issue.

Example B: When serving as a consultant to a residence facility for individuals who have severe mental retardation, Therapist B becomes aware that another therapist is submitting charges to the home for one-half-hour individual treatments. In reality, the therapist is only passing through the unit and briefly talking with the clients; no treatments are given. After observing the pattern for several weeks, Therapist B speaks with the therapist who then brushes off the inquiry, "Look, we all have plans on file, but these kids aren't going to progress no matter what we do." Therapist B brings the matter to the attention of the administrator.

Example A illustrates the OT practitioner's concern for the client by ensuring the hospital aide had been properly trained in feeding so that harm would be avoided and the client would benefit from the therapy. Example B illustrates that an OT practitioner is expected to address a situation in which the residents of a facility are being financially exploited or receiving services not commensurate with what is being billed.

PRINCIPLE 2: AUTONOMY AND PRIVACY AND CONFIDENTIALITY

The need for the OT practitioner to respect the rights of the recipients of services is the topic of Principle 2, which protects the right of autonomy and the rights of privacy and confidentiality. **Autonomy** is the freedom to decide and the freedom to act.[2] **Confidentiality** refers to the expectation that information shared by the client with the OT practitioner, either directly or through written or electronic forms, will be kept confidential and private. Confidentiality also stipulates that the client will determine how and to whom confidential information may be shared.

There are five parts to Principle 2 that address the rights of autonomy and privacy and confidentiality. The OT practitioner must collaborate with the recipients of services (including other caregivers and family members) to (1) determine the goals; (2) inform them of the nature, possible risks, and outcomes of services; (3) receive informed consent when the recipient is involved in a research study; (4) respect a recipient's decision to refuse treatment; and (5) maintain confidentiality with regards to information known about the recipient of services.[1]

Example: Mrs. Jones, who is indigent and lives in a nursing home, will not participate in any activities and resists going to therapy. When out of her room, she constantly asks to be returned. Therapist B speaks with Mrs. Jones and learns that she does not want to leave her room for fear someone will "steal her things." Therapist B does not laugh or dismiss the concern but deals with the issue by making a treatment plan to address her fear. Therapist B first determines the "things" about which Mrs. Jones is worried and learns that this woman, who has almost nothing to claim as her own, fears she will lose her hair-brush, an old mirrored compact, a brocade change purse, a bottle of toilet water, and a pair of underpants. Mrs. Jones does not want to tell anyone, but with her consent Therapist B makes plans for a wheelchair carrier and identifies a goal. Part of Mrs. Jones' reality orientation program is the use of a checklist to "pack" her carrier with these few treasured belongings each morning and to "unpack" it at the end of each day when she retires to her room for the night. The staff is informed that using a daily checklist is part of her OT program. Now Mrs. Jones and her carrier go to activities and therapy without protest.

This example illustrates a respect for the rights of both autonomy and confidentiality. Therapist B respects Mrs. Jones' right to decide if and how she will participate in therapy and allows her to contribute to the treatment planning process. The practitioner respects Mrs. Jones' right to confidentiality by not discussing with others the reasons she refuses to go to therapy.

PRINCIPLE 3: COMPETENCE

Principle 3 stipulates that all OT practitioners maintain a high standard of competence. This principle provides that a practitioner must have the appropriate credentials to practice, participate in continuing education and professional activities, use procedures that meet AOTA's Standards of Practice, use procedures that are accurate and current, ensure that OT practitioners receive appropriate levels of supervision, ensure that practitioners perform duties that are appropriate to their qualifications and experience, and know when to consult or refer to other service providers.[1]

Example: Therapist C has accepted a new job in a school system that occasionally uses Sensory Integration (SI) as a technique of treatment. Therapist C's only exposure to SI had been in school several years earlier. He informs his supervisor of his plans to take an SI workshop and, until then, requests guidance in any SI treatment programs for the students to whom he is assigned.

In this example, Therapist C is in compliance with Principle 3 by asking a qualified OT practitioner to closely supervise every SI treatment program, an area in which he does not have the level of competence required. Therapist C is aware that he needs further education and experience before he is competent to practice in this area.

PRINCIPLE 4: COMPLIANCE WITH LAWS AND POLICIES

Principle 4 focuses on the obligation of OT practitioners to comply with the laws and regulations that guide the profession. This principle stipulates that the practitioner must be aware of federal, state, and local laws, as well as institutional policies, and abide by them. The practitioner is also directed to inform employers, employees, and colleagues about these laws and policies. In addition, this principle addresses the requirement that those under supervision adhere to the Code of Ethics. Another component of this principle is the importance of accurately reporting and documenting information related to professional activities.

Example: Therapist D has moved to a new state. Before moving she requests a copy of the licensure law and notes the limits that the new state places on the use of treatment modalities. After employment, she reads the employer's policies and procedures guide regarding facility records and acquaints herself with the department's style of recordkeeping. The facility uses a specific style for documenting treatment. Although not familiar with the style of charting, Therapist D refreshes her understanding with the format and implements it in her documentation.

This example demonstrates Therapist D's compliance with the state laws related to treatment procedures and with the documentation policies delineated by the facility where she works.

PRINCIPLE 5: ACCURACY IN INFORMATION ABOUT SERVICES

Principle 5 is related to the issue of **veracity,** or the duty of the health care professional to tell the truth. Therefore it focuses on the need for OT practitioners to accurately represent their qualifications, education, training, and competence. Practitioners are directed not to use any form of false advertising or exaggerated claims. This principle also addresses the need to disclose instances that may pose actual or potential conflicts of interest.

Example: Therapist E, who is opening a private practice, makes certain that the advertising circulars promoting the center do not the make any exaggerated claims about the center's ability to "cure" or make promises of a "new life that therapy will bring." The principle of veracity is illustrated in this example through the OT practitioner's concern that her private practice uses truthful advertising to promote its services.

PRINCIPLE 6: PROFESSIONAL RELATIONS

The theme of Principle 6 is **fidelity,** or faithfulness, in professional relationships. Principle 6 deals with the relationships between an OT practitioner and his or her colleagues and other professionals. This principle deals with the importance of maintaining confidentiality in matters related to colleagues and staff, accurately representing qualifications, views, and findings of colleagues, and reporting any misconduct to the appropriate entity.

Example: An OT student has just completed her thesis for her Master's degree. Her faculty advisor wants to present the results at the national conference. The faculty advisor asks the student for permission to submit a conference proposal that discusses the results of the student's thesis with the understanding that the student will be listed as the principal author. The student is also encouraged to present the paper with the faculty advisor, if accepted.

In this example the professor demonstrates the principle of fidelity to her student colleague. By ensuring that both the faculty advisor's name and the student's name are on the paper, she is accurately reporting who has been involved in both gathering the data and reporting the findings.

ETHICAL DILEMMAS

Unfortunately, many of the ethical issues that OT practitioners confront are not as clear cut as the examples presented. When speaking of ethical issues or ethical behavior, the issue of *appropriate* conduct is discussed, which always requires interpretation. In a given situation, two or more ethical principles may collide with one another, making it difficult to determine the best or highest moral action. The result is an **ethical dilemma**.[2]

Carol Davis suggests in *Patient Practitioner Interaction* that five steps be taken to resolve an ethical dilemma:

1. Gather all the facts that can be known about the situation.
2. Determine which ethical principles are involved (e.g., beneficence, nonmaleficence, justice, veracity, autonomy, confidentiality).
3. Clarify your professional duties in this situation (e.g., do no harm, tell the truth, keep promises, be faithful to colleagues). Duties such as these are often outlined in one's Code of Ethics.
4. Describe the general nature of the outcome desires or the consequences. Which seems most important in this case—an outcome which is most beneficial for the patient, for society, for a particular group, or for oneself?
5. Describe practical features that are pertinent to this situation—one or more of the following: the disputed facts, the law, the wishes of others, the resources available, the effectiveness and efficiency of action, the risks, the resources available, the Code of Ethics and Standards of Practice, the degree of certainty of the facts on which a decision is based, the predominant values of the others involved (which may or may not coincide with the values predominant in health care in the United States).[2]

The ability to decide which action is the highest ethical alternative can be developed by considering situations in which there are conflicting elements and questions to which there are no set *correct* answers. By considering ethical dilemmas, one value is weighed over another, justifying the decision on the basis of the ethical reasoning process. Following are two ethical dilemmas. Using the suggested principles and process, how would each be resolved?

DILEMMA 1

A young client has just completed a series of treatments, and his goals have been reached. He was injured in an automobile accident wherein the driver had excellent insurance coverage, so the insurance has not run out. You know that his home situation is not good; there is concern for his welfare because the parents are both alcoholics. The client gets great pleasure from the attention he receives in therapy and works hard on his program. In the time you have been working with him, his whole attitude has improved. He wants to keep coming, but your goals have been reached. Do you discharge him or continue treatment?

DILEMMA 2

You have a private practice. Another Registered Occupational Therapist (OTR), who works as a consultant to a new, attractive, well-equipped nursing home, requests that you come for a splinting consultation. (She is not confident of her skill in this area.) You return with the splint on a day when the OTR who requested your consultation services is not there; the director calls you into his office. He offers *you* the consultant job on a regular basis, explaining that he will terminate the other OTR because he likes your splinting skills and believes such skills will benefit his clients. What do you do?

SUMMARY

The purpose of a professional Code of Ethics is to provide standards of conduct to the practitioners of a profession. These standards are not laws, but they are guidelines that require professional judgment. The AOTA Code of Ethics identifies a set of six principles that apply to all occupational therapy personnel in all types of roles. The Commission on Standards and Ethics enforces the Code. The Code covers issues of beneficence toward the recipients of service, recipients' autonomy and privacy and confidentiality, professional duties, professional justice, veracity to the public, and fidelity and veracity to colleagues. By nature, ethical issues are usually not black-and-white issues. Typically, ethical dilemmas arise when the best action is unclear. Following simple guidelines will help the practitioner make a decision and justify the ethics of the decision.

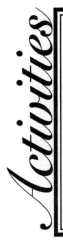

1. Gather and write out a series of ethical dilemma situations. If needed, ask faculty members and practicing therapists to supply the situations along with suggested solutions. Divide the class into small groups and hand out the printed scenarios without any suggested resolutions. After a time period in which each group identifies the ethical principle in question and discusses the issue, have each group report their solutions to the class. After each group reports, share the suggested solutions and lead a class discussion. (Remember, the solution given is not necessarily the correct or best one.)

2. Secure a copy of the Code of Ethics of two other allied health professions. Compare them to the AOTA Code of Ethics (see Appendix B).

REFERENCES

1. American Occupational Therapy Association: Occupational therapy code of ethics, *Amer J Occup Ther* 48:1037, 1994.

2. Davis CM: *Patient practitioner interaction: an experiential manual for developing the art of health care*, ed 2, Thorofare, NJ, 1994, Slack.

3. Landau SI, editor: *The Doubleday dictionary®*, New York, 1975, Doubleday.

4. Purtilo R: *Ethical dimensions in the health professions*, ed 2, Philadelphia, 1993, WB Saunders.

5. Scott RW: *Promoting legal awareness in physical and occupational therapy*, St Louis, 1997, Mosby.

Occupational therapy is by far the most unique of allied health care professions. The delicate balance of art, science, and human interaction on which the profession is based contributes not only to this uniqueness but to the obvious effectiveness of occupational therapy intervention throughout the life span. ■

Glen Gillen, MPA, OTR/L, BCN
Supervisor, Inpatient Rehabilitation
Occupational Therapy, Department of
Rehabilitation Medicine
Columbia–Presbyterian Medical Center
Clinical Instructor, Program in
    Occupational Therapy
College of Physicians and Surgeons
Columbia University
New York, New York

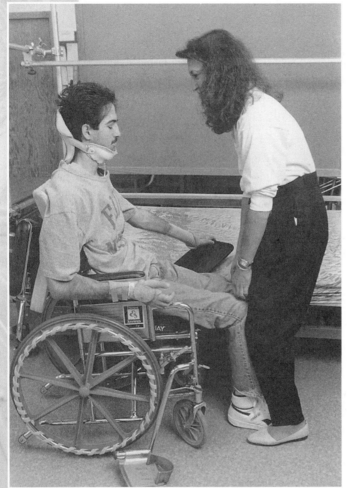

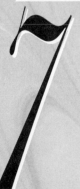

7

Standards and Regulations of Occupational Therapy Practice

Objectives

After reading this chapter, you will be able to:

❖ Understand the importance of standards in occupational therapy (OT)

❖ Distinguish between accreditation, certification, and state regulation

❖ Describe the disciplinary processes developed by state regulatory boards, the professional association, and the certification board

Key terms

Accreditation

Joint Commission on the Accreditation of Hospital Organizations

Rehabilitation Accreditation Commission

The Essentials

Accreditation Council for Occupational Therapy Education

Certification

Registration

National Board for Certification in Occupational Therapy

Specialty certification

Licensure laws

Statutory certification

Trademark laws

Standards of practice

Disciplinary Action Information Exchange Network

Standards that define the criteria, or expectations, for the delivery of services are important in the health care field. Standards of practice and their enforcement help ensure that the consumer receives quality services delivered by competent practitioners. There are several mechanisms in place that develop and regulate standards for organizations and individuals in the practice of OT. These mechanisms are accreditation, certification, licensure, and standards of practice. It is important that the OT practitioner is aware of these mechanisms and their effect on the practitioner's delivery of services, including third-party reimbursement for such services. They serve as a "seal of approval," ensuring that the individual or organization meets standard qualifications.

ACCREDITATION

Accreditation is a form of regulation that determines whether an organization or program meets a prescribed standard. Although accreditation is voluntary, there is external pressure for organizations to be accredited, such as obtaining reimburse-

Chapter 7 photo: Early MB: *Physical dysfunction practice skills for the occupational therapy assistant*, St Louis, 1998, Mosby.

ment from third-party payers. The first step of the accreditation process entails the development of the standards. Experts knowledgeable in the field and representatives of the public are brought together to develop these standards. Standards are continually reviewed and updated to reflect current practice.[8]

Organizations seeking accreditation first submit an application for a review or survey.[5] A self-study completed by the organization is then required by most accrediting bodies. Through this self-study, the organization reviews the standards and addresses how it meets them. Once the self-study is complete, a team representing the accrediting body visits the facility. Though often arduous for the organization, the accreditation process should be viewed as a learning experience with the goal to improve the quality of services that the organization provides, based on the standards established.

ACCREDITATION OF HEALTH CARE AGENCIES

Many of the organizations in which OT practitioners work will likely be influenced by some type of accreditation. In health care, the two most widely known accreditation bodies are the **Joint Commission on the Accreditation of Hospital Organizations** (JCAHO) and the **Rehabilitation Accreditation Commission** (CARF).

JCAHO develops standards and accredits health care organizations in the United States. These organizations include hospitals, health care networks, and organizations that provide long-term care, behavioral care, and laboratory and ambulatory services.[7]

CARF sets standards and accredits organizations that deliver rehabilitation services. CARF's standards and guidelines are separated into three areas: behavioral health, employment and community services, and medical rehabilitation. The CARF accreditation process is aimed at improving the quality of services provided to individuals with disabilities.[10] CARF is also involved in research related to outcomes measurement and management. CARF's standards specifically address the utilization of OT in rehabilitation.

ACCREDITATION OF EDUCATIONAL PROGRAMS

Accreditation of an OT educational program means that the standards of the profession have been met in the school's curriculum and the school has received the formal approval of the American Occupation Therapy Association (AOTA). This approval ensures that graduates of an accredited program will have met the prescribed minimal entry level standards and are qualified to take the national certification examination. To qualify to sit for the national certification examination, a candidate must graduate from an accredited educational program (see Chapter 4).

Since 1935 AOTA has set standards for educational programs. Over the years these standards have been modified several times (including the adoption of standards for Certified Occupational Therapy Assistant [COTA] programs in 1958) with the latest revision published in 1991. These standards exist today as the *Essentials and Guidelines for an Accredited Program for the Occupational Therapy Assistant* and the *Essentials and Guidelines for an Accredited Program for the Occupational Therapist*. Many people refer to these standards as **The Essentials**. The Essentials are periodically reviewed and revised as the educational requirements for the profession change.

The **Accreditation Council for Occupational Therapy Education** (ACOTE) of AOTA accredits both Registered Occupational Therapist (OTR) and COTA educational programs. There is a standard procedure that every school must follow to become accredited and to maintain accreditation. First, the school must inform AOTA of its intention to begin a new program. Next, the school must build its curriculum around The Essentials. Each school has some freedom to arrange the necessary content areas as it chooses, but all programs must cover the areas included in The Essentials.

Initial accreditation occurs in two stages: (1) review of the program design, and (2) on-site inspection after at least 1 year of operation. After passing these two stages, the program becomes fully accredited, subject to review on a regular basis. The review board has the power to grant or withhold approval. If it is demonstrated that program changes are needed for compliance with The Essentials, the review team will make recommendations; the school has a limited time to comply. Failure to comply will result in withdrawal of accreditation. An educational program currently undergoes an on-site evaluation for accreditation at 5 years after its initial accreditation and at 7 years thereafter.

ENTRY-LEVEL CERTIFICATION

Certification refers to the acknowledgement that an individual has the qualifications to be an entry-level practitioner. The two levels of certification in OT are OTR and COTA. As stated previously, a person must first fulfill the educational requirements and clinical training requirements before becoming eligible to sit for the appropriate national examination. The individual who passes the certification examination receives initial certification, which demonstrates eligibility for entry-level practice.

Certification and registration has a long history in AOTA. In 1931, AOTA initiated the registration of OT practitioners. **Registration** is the listing of qualified individuals by a professional association or government agency. Individuals who had approved professional training and 1 year of subsequent work experience were placed on the Main Register. With the publication of the first National Register in 1932, there were 318 OTRs who qualified. A Secondary Register was also used to register those individuals who had practical experience but not the formal education. In 1937 this Secondary Registry was eliminated, and only graduates of accredited programs were admitted to the Register. In 1939 the standards for registration were expanded to include the passage of a written essay examination. In 1947 the essay examination was converted to an objective multiple-choice examination. This format is still in use today.[6]

After the development of COTA programs in the late 1950s, certification for COTAs was implemented for those individuals who graduated from an approved educational program. A plan to "grandfather" those who did not graduate from an approved program but had worked a minimum of 2 years in one disability area and had recommendations from three qualified individuals was implemented by AOTA in 1957.[6] This plan was eliminated in 1963. The first COTA certification examination was administered in 1977.

During the 1970s, continued certification based solely on AOTA membership came under criticism. Arguments against such recertification maintained that in a changing field like OT, it is important to determine if the practitioner's abilities are keeping pace with professional advances. It was argued that each member's certification should come under periodic review rather than be automatically issued with an AOTA membership. No acceptable means for recertification was developed, in spite of many studies to this end. However, as a result of these discussions, a category called "certified only" was created in the 1980s for members who wanted to be certified without being a member of AOTA.[1] Additionally, during this time, state regulatory laws were focusing on the issue of competency in recertification.

In the early 1980s the issue of recertification was at a standstill; yet because of antitrust concerns, AOTA wanted to proceed with reorganizing the process. The certification process underwent a major administrative change in 1986 when an autonomous certification board was created, separating AOTA membership and certification. This board was initially named the American Occupational Therapy Certification Board (AOTCB). In 1988 the AOTCB was incorporated as a separate entity from AOTA.[1]

In 1996, AOTCB changed its name to the **National Board for Certification in Occupational Therapy** (NBCOT). It has a fifteen-member board of directors composed of eight OT practitioners and seven public members. It functions independently in all aspects of certification.

It was also at this time that NBCOT implemented a certification renewal program, establishing procedures for renewal of certification every 5 years. The first phase of the program is intended to screen illegal and incompetent behavior. To renew certification the OT practitioner is required to complete a screening questionnaire relating to illegal or incompetent behavior and pay a fee. NBCOT reviews each questionnaire and, when appropriate, renews certification to the practitioner for 5 years. In Phase II of the program, recertification will involve some form of self-appraisal, although this program has yet to be delineated. Frequently, the recertification procedures have met some resistance from OT practitioners, and as of this writing the final result is not clear. One question remains. How will NBCOT's procedures mesh with those of state regulatory boards, which are responsible for issuing state licenses to practice?

SPECIALTY CERTIFICATION

Many OT practitioners gain advanced knowledge, skill, and experience in a special area of practice. Through **specialty certification** these individuals can voluntarily seek to be recognized for their particular expertise. At this time, most of these specialty certifications are available only to the OTR. A mechanism to recognize COTAs with advanced knowledge and skill is under development by AOTA.

Several organizations offer voluntary certification based on the passage of an examination, evidence of experience, or both. AOTA offers specialty certification in neurorehabilitation and pediatrics. Sensory Integration International offers a specialty certification in sensory integration (SI). The American Society of Hand Therapists certifies individuals in hand therapy and those who pass the examination are allowed to use the designation, Certified Hand Therapist (CHT) after their name. The Rehabilitation Engineering and Assistive Technology Society of North America (RESNA) offers a specialty certification in assistive technology. These are just a few examples of the many specialty certifications currently available.

Since many OT practitioners specialize in a particular area of practice, specialty certification provides a credential to the individual that designates a certain level of expertise and the qualifications to practice in that specialty area. This is important information for consumers and third-party payers.

STATE REGULATION

The final area to consider is that of regulation by the state in which the practitioner is employed. This is a relatively new aspect of regulation in the field. Whereas certification has been part of the profession since 1932, state regulation has been in place only since the 1970s.

As of June 1996, all 50 states had some form of regulation for OT practitioners. These state regulations are not a function of AOTA but rather are under the auspices of each individual state or province. This regulation takes the form of licensure (39 states, District of Columbia, and Puerto Rico), statutory certification laws (5 states), registration (3 states), or trademark laws (3 states and Guam). Of these states, three do not regulate COTAs (Rhode Island, Colorado, and Virginia).[3]

In addition to listing the qualifications needed for a person to practice, **licensure laws** also define the scope of practice of a profession and, therefore, are often referred to as practice acts. In the states with licensure laws, it is illegal to offer OT services without a license. Under **statutory certification** or registration, a person may not use the title of or proclaim to be *certified* or *registered* unless he or she has met specific entry-level requirements. State **trademark laws** are similar to statutory certification in that they also prevent non-OT practitioners from representing and charging for OT services. Neither statutory certification nor trademark laws define the practice of the profession.

A license to practice is a state's way to ensure the public that the person delivering services has obtained the minimum degree of competency required by the profession and has the government's permission to engage in that service. In most cases there is no formal test or examination required other than presenting to the state substantiated proof that the applicant possesses the expertise so claimed. After being certified by NBCOT, the OT practitioner must write to the state in which he or she wishes to practice for an application that will explain what is needed. The state OT association can provide information on where to apply. The OT practitioner fills out the forms, supplies the required data, and pays the fee. Upon satisfying all legal requirements, the practitioner is issued a license to practice. Each state requires its own licensing, and it is permissible to be licensed in as many states as one wishes.

States with licensure laws (and some with statutory certification) have a board that executes the regulations. Licensure boards may vary from state to state and range from an advisory board to an autonomous body. Most states have an autonomous licensure board that is responsible for writing the regulations that govern the license, collecting fees and issuing licenses, investigating complaints, and delineating requirements for continuing competency.[5]

To renew one's license, many state regulations require that the practitioner complete a number of continuing education hours, the number of which varies from state to state. Regardless of whether the state requires continuing education units, it is extremely important that the OT practitioner continue learning throughout his or her career. It is the responsibility of the practitioner to keep his or her knowledge base up-to-date with current practice. Continuing education programs are offered throughout the country by AOTA, state associations, and many other public and private agencies. Programs are offered as self-study courses, in person, or through the Internet.

STANDARDS OF PRACTICE

The AOTA has established **standards of practice** that are to be used by OT practitioners as guidelines for the delivery of OT services. The *Standards of Practice for Occupational Therapy* were last revised in 1994 and can be found in Appendix C. The standards are delineated in ten areas: (1) professional standing, (2) referral, (3) screening, (4) assessment, (5) intervention plan, (6) intervention, (7) transition services, (8) discontinuation, (9) continuous quality improvement, and (10) management.

DISCIPLINARY PROCESSES

There is no point in having ethical codes and standards for the profession unless they are enforced. AOTA, NBCOT, and state regulatory boards have jurisdiction over the profession. Each has developed policies and procedures for the enforcement of the standards.

AMERICAN OCCUPATIONAL THERAPY ASSOCIATION

The professional association, AOTA, has jurisdiction over complaints against members who are suspected of unethical conduct. The Standards and Ethics Commission (SEC) of AOTA is responsible for the Code of Ethics, the Standards of Practice, and The Essentials for accreditation of educational programs. The responsibilities of the SEC include upholding the practice and educational standards of the profession, educating members on current ethical issues, monitoring members' behavior, and examining allegations of unethical conduct.[4]

The SEC only reviews claims that are made against a member of AOTA; it has no jurisdiction over nonmembers. Complaints filed with the SEC are given a preliminary investigation by a committee. If evidence warrants a formal complaint, the President of AOTA is notified and appoints a judicial counsel to hear the case. If the member is found to have committed an ethical violation, one of the following disciplinary sanctions are imposed: reprimand, censure, membership suspension, or permanent revocation of membership in AOTA.[2]

NATIONAL BOARD FOR CERTIFICATION OF OCCUPATIONAL THERAPY

NBCOT has jurisdiction over all certified practitioners in addition to those eligible for certification. A complaint can be filed with NBCOT against any practitioner who has failed to engage in the "safe, proficient, and/or competent practice of occupational therapy." As spelled out in NBCOT's *Procedures for Disciplinary Action*,[9] grounds for discipline fall under the categories of incompetence, unethical behavior, or impairment. A complaint received by NBCOT goes through a review process to determine whether the allegations are justified. If so, one of six sanctions is imposed by NBCOT, depending upon the seriousness of the misconduct (Box 7-1).

STATE REGULATORY BOARDS

As discussed earlier, state regulation of OT practitioners is under the jurisdiction of an appointed state regulatory board. Its responsibility is to protect the public from potential harm that may be caused by unqualified or incompetent practitioners. Therefore it typically limits its review of complaints to those involving a threat of harm to the public. If the regulatory board determines that a practitioner has violated the law, one of several disciplinary sanctions are employed. Sanctions taken by regulatory agencies include public censure, suspension and revocation of licensure or practice privileges. Each state has jurisdiction only over practitioners licensed in the state.

Box 7-1

POSSIBLE SANCTIONS IMPOSED BY NBCOT

REPRIMAND

FORMAL EXPRESSION OF DISAPPROVAL OF CONDUCT, PRIVATELY COMMUNI-
CATED, RETAINED IN THE INDIVIDUAL'S CERTIFICATION FILE, AND NOT PUB-
LICLY ANNOUNCED.

CENSURE

FORMAL EXPRESSION OF DISAPPROVAL, PUBLICLY ANNOUNCED.

INELIGIBILITY

INELIGIBILITY FOR CERTIFICATION FOR AN INDEFINITE OR SPECIFIED PERIOD
OF TIME.

PROBATION

REQUIREMENT THAT THE INDIVIDUAL FULFILL CERTAIN CONDITIONS
(EDUCATION, SUPERVISION, COUNSELING) TO REMAIN CERTIFIED.

SUSPENSION

LOSS OF CERTIFICATION FOR A SPECIFIED PERIOD OF TIME, AFTER WHICH
THE INDIVIDUAL MAY BE REQUIRED TO APPLY FOR REINSTATEMENT.

REVOCATION

PERMANENT LOSS OF CERTIFICATION.

Modified from National Board for Certification in Occupational Therapy: *Procedures for Disciplinary Action*, Gaithersburg, Md, 1995, NBCOT.

It is at the discretion of the professional association and its board whether it communicates formally with state regulatory boards.[11] However, it is the policy of AOTA and NBCOT to communicate with state regulatory boards when disciplinary actions have been taken against OT practitioners. The formal mechanism used for this is the **Disciplinary Action Information Exchange Network (DAIEN).** This is a list of individuals, published quarterly in NBCOT's newsletter, who have been subject to disciplinary action and have been reported by NBCOT, AOTA, or a state regulatory board.[4]

SUMMARY

Standards of practice are important in the field of OT because they help ensure that practitioners are competent and are delivering quality services to the consumer. There are several mechanisms in place for the development and regulation of the standards related to OT practice. These mechanisms are:

Accreditation: Health care institutions receive accreditation by JCAHO or CARF; OT educational institutions are accredited by AOTA.

Certification: NBCOT grants individuals the right to entry-level practice at one of two levels, OTR or COTA, depending on formal education.

State regulation: All states provide regulation, whether it be licensure law, trademark law, or statutory certification. State licensure law defines not only the minimum qualifications for a person to practice but also the scope of the OT practice (practice acts). In states with licensure law, it is illegal to offer services without a state license. State trademark laws prevent nonpractitioners from providing and charging for OT services. Similarly, under statutory certification, an OT practitioner cannot claim to be certified or registered without meeting specific entry-level requirements.

Disciplinary procedures have been established by AOTA, NBCOT, and state regulatory boards to review and investigate claims of misconduct. Depending on the nature of the misconduct, disciplinary sanctions may include reprimand, censure, or suspension or revocation of one's membership, certification, or license.

Activities

1. Obtain a copy of The Essentials from the director at your educational program; make a chart to show in which courses The Essentials are addressed.
2. Research and report to the class the history of the different mechanisms of regulation in the field of occupational therapy at both the professional and technical levels.
3. Determine the procedure for obtaining a state license under the following circumstances: (1) upon graduation from a program; (2) upon moving from one state to another where you do not have a license; and (3) when professional standing has been obtained in a country other than the United States.

REFERENCES

1. American Occupational Therapy Association: Chronology of certification issues dated through January 29, *OT Week*, Feb 13, 1997, AOTA.

2. American Occupational Therapy Association: *Enforcement procedure for occupational therapy code of ethics*, Bethesda, Md, 1996, AOTA.

3. American Occupational Therapy Association: *Summary of state regulation of occupational therapy practitioners*, Bethesda, Md, 1996, AOTA.

4. American Occupational Therapy Association: Ethical jurisdiction of occupational therapy: the role of AOTA, AOTCB, and state regulatory boards, *OT Week*, Apr 15, 1993, AOTA.

5. Fine SB, Bair J, Hoover SP, Acquaviva JD: Regulation and standard setting. In Bair J, Gray M, editors: *The occupational therapy manager*, Rockville, Md, 1985, AOTA.

6. Gray M: The credentialing process in occupational therapy. In Ryan SE, editor: *Practice issues in occupational therapy: intraprofessional team building*, Thorofare, NJ, 1993, Slack.

7. Joint Commission on Accreditation of Healthcare Organizations: *What advantages does our JCAHO accreditation offer you?* Internet, 1996, Medical Data Institute and Millstar Electronic Publishing Group.

8. Kauffmann SH: Occupational therapy consultation for adult rehabilitation program standards and regulations. In Jaffe EG, Epstein CF, editors: *Occupational therapy consultation: theory, principles, and practice*, St Louis, 1992, Mosby.

9. National Board for Certification in Occupational Therapy: *Procedures for disciplinary action*, Gaithersburg, Md, 1995, NBCOT.

10. Rehabilitation Accreditation Commission: *What is CARF?* 1996, Internet.

11. Scott RW: *Promoting legal awareness in physical and occupational therapy*, St Louis, 1997, Mosby.

Choosing a career in occupational therapy is one of the best decisions I have ever made. Joining the American Occupational Therapy Association (AOTA) is another. Becoming an occupational therapist and a member of its professional association are two sides of the same coin—I cannot imagine one without the other.

My 31 years as an occupational therapist have been wonderfully fulfilling, varied, and ever changing. The challenges have been fresh and constant—from how to implement innovative treatment techniques, to ways to measure the impact of interventions, to adapting to new payment and organizational methods. I have tried to keep up with and even help shape these changes through my clinical practice as a fiscal intermediary and through my service to AOTA, where I currently serve as President. As a health care provider and leader of our association, I have advocated confronting managed care head-on, not as an adversary but as a system with the potential to help us hone our skills and deliver more effective and targeted care to patients at the lowest possible cost to them and to society.

Joining our professional association offers so many benefits. On a personal level, it provides members with fellowship, mentoring, and networking opportunities. Collectively, it offers us a voice in the halls of Congress, in federal agencies, and with the public-at-large. The association also provides opportunities for disseminating research and new practice skills through our annual conference, a variety of publications, and continuing education courses, including offerings on our association's web site. Our membership has been growing as occupational therapy practitioners and students realize that in unity there is strength. I feel privileged to have served as President during these challenging times and hope that I have been able to provide some useful guidance to our members. ■

Mary Foto, BS, OT, FAOTA, CCM
Department of Occupational Therapy
University of Southern California
Los Angeles, California
President, American Occupational
    Therapy Association (through April
    1998)

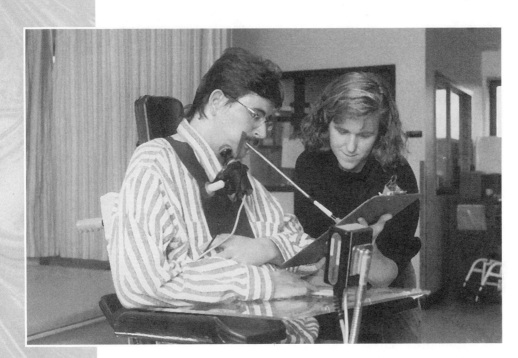

8
American Occupational Therapy Association

Objectives

After reading this chapter, the reader will be able to:

✤ Describe the mission and major activities of the American Occupational Therapy Association (AOTA)
✤ Identify the membership categories and benefits of membership in AOTA
✤ Describe the structure of AOTA
✤ Delineate AOTA activities that are focused on assuring the delivery of quality occupational therapy (OT) services
✤ Identify the ways in which AOTA contributes to the professional development of its members
✤ Describe how AOTA is involved in improving consumer access to health care services

Key terms

American Occupational Therapy Association
Volunteer sector
Executive Board
Representative Assembly
American Student Committee of the Occupational Therapy Association
American Occupational Therapy Foundation
American Journal of Occupational Therapy

It is customary for each profession to establish a professional organization. The stronger and better supported the association is, the greater the benefits for the individual members. A professional association is organized and operated by its members for its members. It exists to protect and promote the profession it represents by (1) providing a communication network and channel for information; (2) regulating itself through the development and enforcement of standards of conduct and performance; and (3) guarding the interests of those within the profession.

The professional organization for OT practitioners in the United States is the **American Occupational Therapy Association** (AOTA). Originally incorporated in 1917 as the National Society for the Promotion of Occupational Therapy, the association's name was changed to its present version in 1923. Each state also has a professional organization for OT practitioners living in the state. Although there is frequent collaboration between AOTA and the individual state associations, the state associations are funded and operated totally independent from the national association. It is a plus for any OT practitioner entering the field to have a good understanding of the national organization, as well as his or her state association. This awareness enables members to learn how to make use of these organizations and the various services they provide. Since it would be impossible to discuss each state association in this text, this chapter focuses on the national association.

MISSION OF AOTA

As a result of a combination of good fortune and wise planning, American OT practitioners have developed a strong and well-run national organization. It was the profession's first and it remains its most influential association. The mission of AOTA is:

> "To support a professional community for members and to develop and preserve the viability and relevance of the profession. The organization serves the interests of its members, represents the profession to the public, and promotes access to occupational therapy services."[1]

In keeping with this mission statement, AOTA has identified three primary areas in which its efforts are directed. These areas are (1) assuring the quality of OT services; (2) improving consumer access to health care services; and (3) promoting the professional development of its members.[1]

MEMBERSHIP IN AOTA

There are three professional membership categories in AOTA: the Registered Occupational Therapist (OTR), the Certified Occupational Therapy Assistant (COTA), and the Occupational Therapy Student (OTS). There are also two non-OT categories for those interested in the profession: the Organizational member and the Associate member. These membership categories differ in several ways, such as who can attend special meetings, hold office and vote, and the level of fees paid for membership and conferences. Organizational and Associate members do not have voting privileges. Membership cost is higher for OTRs, as is appropriate for their ability to command higher salaries. The cost for the OTS is kept low to encourage them to become involved in the organization and to familiarize themselves with membership benefits. In 1997, membership in AOTA reached more than 59,000 members.[2]

Members at all levels are encouraged to become actively involved in AOTA by serving on committees, running for offices, attending the annual conference—or in any way an individual's schedule may allow—to become a knowledgeable and informed professional.

ORGANIZATIONAL STRUCTURE OF AOTA

AOTA is made up of a volunteer sector and paid national office staff. The paid office staff is employed at the headquarters and performs the day-to-day operations under the management of the Executive Director. The national office staff is organized around four divisions: Finance and Operations, Professional Issues and Special Programs, Professional Development, and Professional Affairs. The headquarters for AOTA is in Bethesda, Maryland.*

The **volunteer sector** consists of all the members of the association and is represented by the Executive Board and the Representative Assembly. The **Executive Board** is charged with the administration and management of the association and includes elected officers. There are several standing committees of the Executive Board. The **Representative Assembly** (RA) is the legislative and policy-making body of the AOTA. It is composed of elected representatives from each recognized state, elected officers of the assembly and the association, a representative from the student committee, a COTA representative, the First Delegate of the World Federation of Occupational Therapy, and the Chairpersons of the Commissions. The standing commissions of the RA include the Commission on Education, the Commission on Practice, and the Commission on Standards and Ethics.

Many OT educational programs have a club or organization for OTSs and the student groups in turn may participate in the **American Student Committee of the Occupational Therapy Association** (ASCOTA), a standing committee of the Executive Board of AOTA.

ASSURING QUALITY OF OCCUPATIONAL THERAPY SERVICES

Assuring the delivery of quality OT services is identified by AOTA as one of the major activities of the association. Defining standards is one activity performed by AOTA that promotes the delivery of quality OT services. It is the association's responsibility to develop standards, produce official documents that identify the standards, and review the standards on a regular basis. The formulation and existence of documents and standards are viewed as member benefits because they are potentially valuable to all practitioners. Standards ensure that educational programs will properly prepare the student, that guidelines are set to enable OT practitioners to deal with employers on job descriptions and duty assignments, and that a code of conduct is provided to help clarify ethical issues. AOTA has developed standards of education (The Essentials), standards of practice, and ethical standards. Each are discussed in previous chapters.

Accreditation of entry-level OTR and COTA educational programs is another activity performed by AOTA that is designed to assure the delivery of quality OT services. As discussed in Chapter 7, the Accreditation Council for Occupational

---

*AOTA's address: 4720 Montgomery Lane, Bethesda, Maryland, 20814-3425. Telephone number: (310) 652-2682.

Therapy Education (ACOTE) is the arm of AOTA that is responsible for accrediting educational programs.

In cooperation with the **American Occupational Therapy Foundation (AOTF)**, AOTA conducts research activities that investigate the outcomes of OT services, which contribute to the delivery of quality practice. AOTF was incorporated as a separate not-for-profit organization in 1965. It is a vehicle for providing resources to programs and individuals for the purpose of carrying out OT education and research. AOTF also operates a library that contains most books and journals written on any aspect of OT.

Finally, AOTA lends its support to states for the regulation of practice through licensure and other state laws. As discussed in Chapter 7, state regulatory laws help ensure that practitioners meet certain competencies; they may also define the scope of practice. AOTA collaborates with state agencies to develop and enforce these laws.

PROFESSIONAL DEVELOPMENT OF MEMBERS

Another primary focus of AOTA is promoting the professional development of its members. This responsibility is met through a number of activities, including publications, continuing education, and practice information.

PUBLICATIONS

The association, either by itself or through AOTF, makes available to its members a vast array of information on OT. These publications make an important and nationwide contribution to the professional development of OT practitioners.

The national organization's official publication, **American Journal of Occupational Therapy** (AJOT), is the main artery of information for the field and deserves special attention. Almost since its founding, AOTA has published a professional journal. Although the directorship, title, format, and content have all experienced changes, the intent to produce an informative professional publication has remained constant.

AJOT is distributed monthly (except for bimonthly publications in July/August and November/December) to all AOTA members, and it is also available through subscription to interested nonmembers and libraries. All aspects of the journal, from article content and features to advertisements, pertain to OT. Subjects may include approaches to practice, new programs and techniques, reports of research, educational and professional trends, and areas of controversy in the field. Articles are written by professionals in OT or related fields and must meet the rigid standards set by its editors.

Becoming familiar with AJOT is as much a part of becoming an OT practitioner as learning the steps of the OT process and other fundamental concepts. AJOT follows a standard design and format: the year of publication is identified as a volume and each month is indicated by a number (i.e., 1995 = Volume 49 and March = Number 3; therefore the March 1995 issue is Vol 49, No 3.) The page numbering begins at 1 in the January issue and continues sequentially throughout the year; therefore each year stands as one complete volume. This numbering system allows for easy reference. The last issue of the year, the November/December publication, includes an index of all the year's articles, listed by author and by subject.

It is the aim of the profession to accumulate a body of specific OT research, thereby increasing the strength of the profession's theoretical base. Most of this research has been published through and is chronicled in *AJOT*. In April 1981 the number of research papers reached such a level that AOTA added a new publication, *Occupational Therapy Journal of Research*, to address the need for more research publication opportunities. This journal is published quarterly and has a fee for subscription.

As a part of AOTA membership, each member is eligible to join one Special Interest Section. Each Special Interest Section publishes a quarterly newsletter. Members receive the newsletter for the section they have joined and are eligible to participate in activities such as meetings held by their respective Special Interest Section. The Special Interest Sections include Administration and Management, School System, Developmental Disabilities, Education, Gerontology, Home and Community Health, Mental Health, Physical Disabilities, Sensory Integration, Technology, and Work Programs.

Two fairly recent additions to the list of AOTA publications are *OT Week* and *OT Practice*. These publications are designed to keep members informed about the profession in general and the association in particular. They carry timely and useful clinical information to the members while freeing *AJOT* to focus on more scholarly material of long-term interest. Both are automatically furnished to members. *OT Week*, as the name implies, is published and mailed to members on a weekly basis. Aside from the news articles, its primary purpose is to serve as an employment bulletin. Each issue advertises OT employment opportunities across the nation. *OT Practice* is published on a monthly schedule and is designed to provide practical information of a clinical and professional nature.

Other single title publications are available from AOTA. An extensive catalog of books, videotapes, audiotapes, brochures, official documents, and other materials are available for sale on a broad range of topics related to OT. Depending on the information, materials are available for purchase, rent, loan, or are distributed free of charge.

CONTINUING EDUCATION

AOTA sponsors an annual conference, continuing education workshops across the country, self-study programs, and courses available on the Internet. The most significant among these is the annual meeting that is held in a different city each year, hosted by the area's local or state association. All members are welcome, and there are special sections and presentations that appeal to all participants. The conference is both serious and fun. At every hour of the day, there are events taking place in simultaneous sessions. Papers are presented, research is described, speeches are given by people of national reputation, banquets and workshops are held, outstanding contributions to the field are recognized, business meetings are conducted, the latest materials and equipment are displayed, and old friendships are renewed and new networks are established. The difficult part is narrowing selections to only one per session. This is a major event and a marvelous way for members to remain current on the happenings in the field—if it is important to OT, the participants will hear about it at the conference.

PRACTICE INFORMATION

In addition to all the publications mentioned, AOTA has developed resources for information on all the practice areas. These resources include written practice packets, as well as staff experts and volunteers who provide consultation.

IMPROVING CONSUMER ACCESS TO HEALTH CARE SERVICES

An important activity of any professional association is ensuring that the services of the profession are accessible to the consumer. This is accomplished through an ongoing process of communication with state and federal lawmakers, regulatory bodies, third-party payers, other health care professionals, the media, and the public. For example, the AOTA keeps abreast of proposed legislation and special committees within the government, ensuring that new laws affecting the practice are not passed without hearing the voice of the profession. When the federal government developed legislation outlining what services schools must provide for the Handicapped Children Act, AOTA provided information on OT services and successfully lobbied for the inclusion of OT. This professional vigilance applies not only to the government but also to the private sector. When major insurance companies write or rewrite policies regarding the health services they will cover, AOTA works to ensure OT is included. AOTA has also initiated a toll-free hotline, which consumers can access for information regarding OT.

SUMMARY

A professional organization exists to serve the needs of its members. The AOTA is the national organization representing OT practitioners. Its major activities include assuring the delivery of quality OT services, improving consumer access to health care, and promoting the professional development of its members. Awareness of the services and benefits provided by national and state professional associations is important for the OT practitioner.

Avenues used by AOTA to assure the delivery of quality services include the development and enforcement of standards, accreditation of educational programs, research, and support for regulation. To encourage the professional development of its members, AOTA conducts continuing education programs, publishes materials, and provides practice information. *AJOT* is the main publication of the national organization, through which OT practitioners are kept informed of developments within the field of OT. Consumer access to health care services is improved through AOTA's distribution of information to the federal and state lawmakers, the insurance providers, the media, the public, and other health care providers.

Activities

1. Request information on an aspect of AOTA's operation that is of special interest to you; write a brief paper on your findings.
2. Gather information on the next AOTA conference (e.g., when, where, cost, theme), and prepare a bulletin board display or poster.
3. Hold a class brainstorming session to compile a list of topics appropriate for a 15-minute conference short paper.
4. Gather information on your state occupational therapy association; prepare an informational handout for your class.
5. The following is a recommended series of exploratory *American Journal of Occupational Therapy* investigations. Each stage is a bit more demanding and thus builds an increasing familiarity with both the publication and research techniques. These can become a series of projects over a period of time. Each class member is to:
   a. Locate the place and manner in which *American Journal of Occupational Therapy* is housed (current and back volumes). Briefly report on some aspect of the publication (i.e., any standard feature column, kinds of advertisement, article specifications, indexing style).
   b. Read any article or column of interest from *American Journal of Occupational Therapy*; give a 5-minute oral report on the topic, the source information, and the point of interest.
   c. Research an article on an assigned topic; give a 5-minute oral report. (Further research may be required to gain information on the topic before the article search.)
   d. Read an article from any occupational therapy source; write a half-page original abstract on the topic.
   e. Make a notebook for class use of *American Journal of Occupational Therapy* abstracts, classified by subject headings.

REFERENCES

1. American Occupational Therapy Association: *Personal communication*, Bethesda, Md, Apr 1997, AOTA.

2. Joe B: 80 years of growth and progress, *OT Week*, Bethesda, Md, 1997, AOTA.

In Section II, the student learns the process underlying the practice of occupational therapy. Before an occupational therapist practitioner begins to deliver occupational therapy services to the consumer, it is necessary to learn more than a set of skills. The practitioner must learn to function from internalized concepts, which guide perceptions and thought. These are the elements of practice.

In Chapter 9, occupational therapy theory and its domain of concern is discussed. This serves as a backdrop for the actual process of delivering occupational therapy services. Chapter 10 provides a brief overview of the stages involved in the occupational therapy process. Chapter 11 discusses in depth the assessment stage of the occupational therapy process, whereas Chapter 12 looks further into the areas of treatment planning and intervention. Chapter 13, the final chapter of this section, is devoted to service management functions that are performed by the occupational therapy practitioner but not related to direct client care.

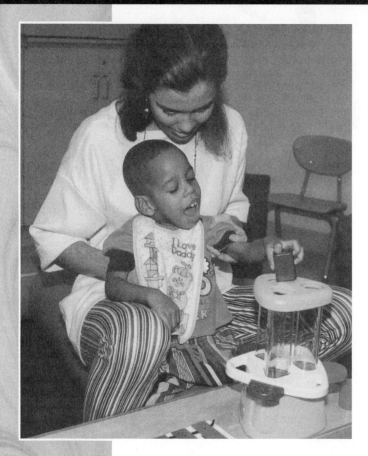

Two

The Practice of Occupational Therapy

Early in my career as an occupational therapist, I treated a woman whose primary goal was to feed her dog—independently. She did not believe that learning to dress or bathe or prepare her own meals was nearly as important as feeding her dog. "You see," she said, "a dog belongs to the person who feeds it." She quickly learned to feed "Mugsy" on her own. Later, I helped her progress from maximal assistance to modified independence in dressing, bathing, and meal preparation. In spite of meeting these goals, she always introduced me to others as "the therapist who figured out how I could feed Mugsy again."

We are individuals who treasure our independence in areas that are unique to our circumstances and our view of the world. As occupational therapists, one of our greatest charges is to respect the wishes, goals, and dreams of our clients. Therapeutic outcomes are only as important as they are to our individual patients. ▪

Maureen Michele Matthews, BS, OTR
Clinical Supervisor, Occupational
    Therapy
Santa Clara Valley Medical Center
San Jose, California

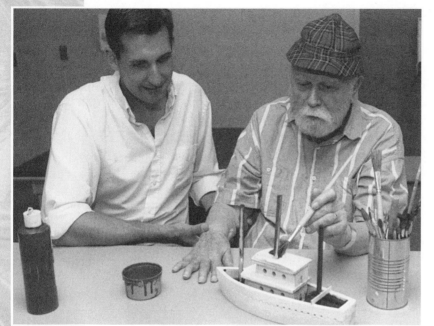

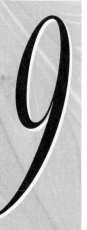

Occupational Performance: Domain of Concern in Occupational Therapy

Objectives

After reading this chapter, the reader will be able to:
- ✤ Differentiate between theory and frame of reference
- ✤ Understand the use of theory and its importance in occupational therapy
- ✤ Identify the domain of concern of occupational therapy
- ✤ Describe occupational performance
- ✤ Delineate the three performance areas
- ✤ Characterize the three performance components
- ✤ Describe the performance contexts

Key terms

Theory
Concepts
Principles
Frames of reference
Domain of concern
Occupational performance
Occupational roles
Performance areas
Activities of daily living
Work and productive activities
Play and leisure activities
Performance components
Sensorimotor components
Cognitive and cognitive integration components
Psychosocial skills and psychological components
Performance contexts
Temporal aspects
Environmental aspects
Model of human occupation

Thus far the attention of this text focuses on elements that provide a backdrop for the profession of occupational therapy (OT). Now, the underlying concepts are examined, and the foundation for understanding the OT process is laid. Before delving into the sequence of steps that make up OT service delivery, it is important to understand the nature of theory, the use of frames of references, and the domain of concern that forms the foundation for the profession.

Section II photo: Case-Smith J, Allen AS, Pratt PN: *Occupational therapy for children,* ed 3, St Louis, 1996, Mosby.

Chapter 9 photo: Lohman H, Padilla R, Byers-Connon S: *Occupational therapy with elders: strategies for the COTA,* St Louis, 1998, Mosby.

This chapter begins by providing the basic terminology and explains the importance of the theory and frames of references in OT practice. Later in the chapter, the domain of concern in OT is described.

UNDERSTANDING THEORY

As defined in *Merriam-Webster's Collegiate Dictionary®*, 10th edition,[16] **theory** is "the analysis of a set of facts in their relation to one another." There are two major structural components to theory: concepts and principles.[14,23] **Concepts** are ideas that represent something in the mind of the individual. These ideas range from simple, concrete ideas to complex, abstract ideas. Concepts are expressed through the use of symbols and language. Children develop categories for different concepts. For example, a child learns that clothing is a category that can be divided into shoes, pants, dresses, and shirts, among others. **Principles** explain the relationship between two or more concepts.[14] For instance, once the concept of color is learned, such as blue and yellow, a child learns the principle that mixing these two colors produces green.

Theory incorporates ideas similar to what has been described and is defined as "a set of interrelated assumptions, concepts, and definitions that presents a systematic view of phenomena by specifying relationships among variables, with the purpose of explaining and predicting the phenomena."[21] It is important to realize that in practice, theories range in scope and complexity along a continuum. At one end are theories that are very broad in scope and attempt to cover many aspects of a discipline, usually making them more complex. At the other end of the continuum are theories that have a very narrow focus and concern only a small portion of the field.[14]

Students frequently resist theory. There is a desire to "get in there and do something" and not to discuss why it is done. One may ask, "Why is it important to know about and use theory in OT practice?" Not applying theory to practice is similar to taking a trip without a road map. The trip will be disorganized and lack structure. The traveler may eventually find a way to the final destination but may not know exactly how he or she got from point A to point B. Consequently, it will be difficult to give directions to anyone else or to replicate the journey in the future. It is necessary to develop an appreciation for theory, because only when an individual knows the reason something is done can he or she do it well; only when a person knows the theory on which various practices and techniques are based will he or she be innovative and employ good clinical reasoning.

In an *American Journal of Occupational Therapy* article, Parham states the importance of theory. "Theory is a key element in problem setting and in problem solving. It is a tool that enables the practitioner to 'name it and frame it.' Both language and logic are needed to identify a problem (name it) and to plan a means for altering the situation (frame it). Theory provides these by giving us words or concepts for naming what we observe and by spelling out logical relationships between concepts."[19] Theory allows the OT practitioner to structure and organize his or her intervention.

Five additional reasons for using theory are identified[14]: (1) to validate and guide practice, (2) to justify reimbursement, (3) to clarify specialization issues, (4) to enhance the growth of the profession and the professionalism of its members, and (5) to educate competent practitioners. More importantly, however, a theoretical base serves as a unifying foundation for the profession and helps tie together its unique aspects.

Theories used in OT practice originated in science-based disciplines such as biology, chemistry, physics, psychology, and occupational science. The practitioner may use a number of theories during intervention and combine parts of theories. To do so, however, the practitioner must be knowledgeable of the theories that are in use to ensure that they are compatible with one another. Theories used in OT include those developed by Mosey, Kielhoefner, Ayres, Reilly, Llorens, and Fidler. It is beyond the scope of this introductory text to describe the various theories used. It is recommended that the reader refer to the text by Miller[14] for an overview of the work of each theorist.

How does the practitioner apply theory to practice? Theory is linked to clinical practice through frames of reference. These are the means by which theory relates to intervention.

FRAMES OF REFERENCE

Williamson states that, "**Frames of reference** are produced from the body of knowledge of the profession and address a specific aspect of the profession's domain of concern." A specific area of practice is the focus of a frame of reference, which describes a process for change in the client and identifies principles for moving a client along a continuum from dysfunction to function. Depending on the focus of intervention, the practitioner may use several frames of reference at one time or use them sequentially over time.[23]

There are four components of a frame of reference.[13,17] The first component is a statement of the theoretical base from which the frame of reference is derived. The second component is a continuum, which defines the behaviors that are characteristic of function and dysfunction. These behaviors, which vary according to the frame of reference, are evaluated by the therapist during the assessment process. The third component describes the process and methods for evaluating the person's status along a function-dysfunction continuum. The fourth component is prescriptive statements. These statements, which relate back to the theoretical base, describe how an individual is aided to make changes and progresses from a state of dysfunction to one of function. These statements provide a guide as to how the practitioner will interact with the client and the environment.

Several frames of reference can be found in OT, and they vary in breadth and depth. For illustration purposes, two different frames of reference are described using Mosey's four components. The first is the biomechanical frame of reference. This frame of reference is derived from theories in kinetics and kinematics (sciences that study the effects of forces and motion on material bodies).[22]

On the function-dysfunction continuum, the biomechanical frame of reference is used with individuals who have deficits in the peripheral nervous, musculoskeletal, integumentary (e.g., skin), or cardiopulmonary system. These individuals, however, have a central nervous system that is intact.[20,22] The deficits may cause posture and mobility problems, impairment in range of motion and strength, and decreased endurance. Disabling conditions that may benefit from this approach include rheumatoid arthritis and osteoarthritis, fractures, burns, hand traumas, amputations, and spinal cord injuries.

The practitioner evaluates the client's range of motion, muscle strength, and endurance through the use of a variety of tools. Through exercise, activity, and physical agent modalities (see Chapter 16), change in the person's range of motion, strength, and endurance can be demonstrated.[11]

Another frame of reference used for illustration purposes is the cognitive disability frame of reference proposed by Claudia Allen.[1,2] This frame of reference is based on the premise that cognitive disorders in those with mental health disabilities are caused by neurobiologic defects or defects related to the biologic functioning of the brain.[10] Its theoretical base is derived from research in neuroscience, cognitive psychology, information processing, and biologic psychiatry.[11]

Along the function-dysfunction continuum, function exists when an individual is able to process information to perform routine tasks demanded by the environment.[11] Dysfunction results when the person's ability to process information is restricted in such a way that carrying out routine tasks is impossible. Allen defines six cognitive levels, which are organized in a hierarchy along a continuum. Level 1 represents the individual who has a profound disability in information processing, whereas level 6 represents the normal ability to acquire and process information. Each cognitive level defines the information processing behaviors indicative of function-dysfunction. Two specific tools used by practitioners to evaluate an individual's level of functioning are the *Allen Cognitive Level (ACL) Test* and the *Routine Task Inventory Test*.[11]

The cognitive disability frame of reference proposes that change occurs because of (1) the capacity of the client and (2) the environment. Change in the capacity of the client may be influenced by medical intervention and psychotropic medications, as well as OT intervention, which teaches the client how to perform routine tasks (cognitive levels 4 and 5). OT intervention can also produce change in the environment through modification of task procedures, amount of assistance offered, directions, and setting.[10,11] Environmental changes may allow the client to experience greater success in performing activities.

These are only two of many frames of reference used in the field of OT. For

information on other frames of reference, the reader is referred to the section entitled, *Frames of Reference in Occupational Therapy: Introduction* in the text *Willard &
Spackman's Occupational Therapy.*[11]

Now that a basic understanding of the nature of theory and the frames of reference used in OT has been presented, it is important to focus on what is considered
the scope of practice, or the domain of concern in OT.

DOMAIN OF CONCERN IN OCCUPATIONAL THERAPY

Mosey describes a model of the occupational therapy profession as the way a profession perceives itself. One of the elements in a profession's model is the **domain of
concern.** "The domain of concern is the profession's area of expertise." It basically
provides an outline of the areas addressed by OT practitioners, which is **occupational performance.**[15] Occupational performance is the ability of a person to perform
functional activities in related occupational roles. **"Occupational roles** are the life
roles the individual holds in society."[20] For example, student, employee, parent, sis-
ter, and daughter are occupational roles. The principle underlying occupational
performance is that if activities or occupations are a basic fact of life, their interruption will cause problems and their restoration or development will promote health.
Interruption of person's life can be caused by an injury, an illness, or a developmental condition. It is the OT practitioner's responsibility to understand which activities, underlying abilities, and related contexts are affected by the interruption and
to provide intervention to restore the individual's occupational performance.

The evolution of occupational performance as the domain of concern has tak-
en place over the last 25 years through a series of American Occupational Therapy
Association (AOTA) task forces and committees.[20] AOTA published *The Roles
and Functions of Occupational Therapy Personnel* in 1973, which referred to occupational performance as a frame of reference.[3] This document included three performance skills (later changed to areas) and five performance components. In 1974
AOTA published the concept of the occupational performance frame of reference
in *A Curriculum Guide for Occupational Therapy Educators.*[4] The purpose of this
publication was to diagram OT practice and to identify areas of concern that can be
used to guide the content of curriculum. In the book, *Occupational Therapy:
Configuration of a Profession*, Mosey presents the occupational performance framework with some modifications, which she calls the "domain of concern for occupational therapy."[18]

AOTA has published three documents that define the terms related to occupational performance. The first document, *Occupational Therapy Product Output
Reporting System and Uniform Terminology for Reporting Occupational Therapy
Services*, was published in 1979 as part of a national project for reporting on hospital-
based OT services.[5] There have been two further revisions of this document,

Uniform Terminology for Occupational Therapy, 2nd edition,[6] published in 1989 and the most recent revision, *Uniform Terminology for Occupational Therapy*, 3rd edition,[7] published in 1994. The terminology has been standardized and used in several AOTA documents to describe the domains of concern of OT. The current version can be found in Appendix D. It is recommended that the student commit to memory the domain of concern of the profession profiled in this document.

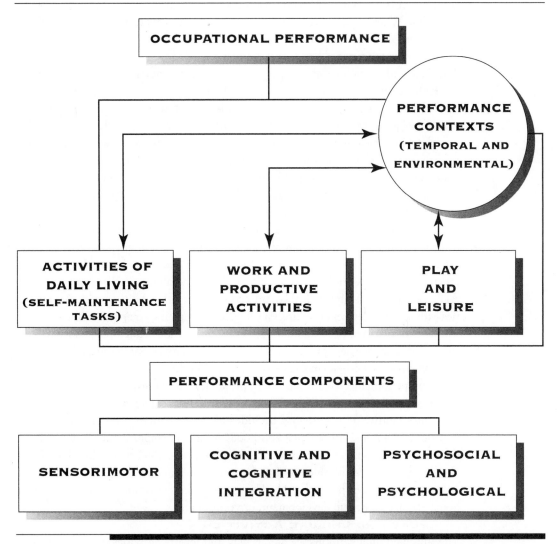

FIGURE 9-1. OCCUPATIONAL PERFORMANCE MODEL. (MODIFIED FROM UNIFORM TERMINOLOGY FOR OCCUPATIONAL THERAPY, ED 3, <u>AMER J OCCUP THER</u> 48:1047 AND AMERICAN OCCUPATIONAL THERAPY ASSOCIATION: A CURRICULUM GUIDE FOR OCCUPATIONAL THERAPY EDUCATORS, ROCKVILLE, MD, 1974, AOTA.)

Occupational performance (Figure 9-1) is characterized by three performance areas, three performance components, and two performance contexts.

PERFORMANCE AREAS

As discussed in Chapter 3, OT practitioners commonly categorize the occupations that individuals perform on a day-to-day basis into three **performance areas:** (1) activities of daily living, (2) work or productive activities, and (3) play or leisure activities. When each activity that humans perform in a typical day is examined, it fits into one of these domains.

ACTIVITIES OF DAILY LIVING

The first and most fundamental performance area is **activities of daily living** (ADLs), or self-care or self-maintenance. Different settings show different title preferences; by whatever label, however, this area of occupation focuses on that which is required of a person to take care of himself or herself. ADLs include feeding, dressing, grooming, hygiene, toileting, management of medications, health maintenance, social expression, functional mobility, functional communication, sexual expression, and emergency response.[7] Whereas some of the tasks are necessary for survival (i.e., eating and hygiene), others serve as a basis for existence in our social world (i.e., grooming, dressing).[9]

ADLs is an area in which the purpose of OT is most readily seen and demonstrated. Independence is the central concern of the field. All efforts in therapy are directed at helping the client achieve and maintain the highest possible degree of independence. Independence is seen as not only the ability of clients to perform ADLs on their own, but also it takes into consideration the ability to perform activities with assistive devices or to direct a caregiver through the completion of the activity. OT strives to maximize functioning. Every step toward greater independence is a step toward enhancement of human dignity and an improvement in the quality of life.

WORK AND PRODUCTIVE ACTIVITIES

The next performance area is **work and productive activities.** These activities are performed to develop oneself, make a contribution to society, and support oneself and one's family. This category includes all achievement-directed activities, whether in the home, school, neighborhood, or place of employment. Work activities usually have a direct effect on others through interaction between an individual and the culture or environment of family, peer group, or community. Work in some ways implies the pursuit of a goal. The goal can be educational, care of others, home management, skill development, or vocational.

PLAY AND LEISURE ACTIVITIES

The third and final performance area is **play and leisure activities,** which includes activities that refresh and bring pleasure and joy but are also nonthreatening ways to "rehearse" for life. Leisure activities include sports, games, hobbies, role play, music, and social activities. Play and leisure are those in which individuals engage because they want to, as opposed to work activities and ADLs in which there is an obligation. For this reason, it is through play and leisure activities that one truly expresses who he or she is as a person.[8]

For children, play is considered a necessary activity to development of motor, cognitive, and social skills. Bundy[8] describes play as being manifested in a style or in another way of being in the form of *playfulness*. Playfulness is seen as a way to approach problems in a flexible manner. Bundy maintains that a playful approach to situations may be more important than any play or leisure activity, in and of itself.[8] In any event, play and playfulness serve an important function in people's lives.

Using the categories of performance areas—ADLs, work, and leisure—the OT practitioner evaluates the client's ability to perform tasks in one or all of these areas. The practitioner then plans a way to allow for improved functioning in areas of need. The far-reaching concern is for the client to achieve a healthy balance among the three areas, and the therapeutic plans are aimed at any or all of them. The reality is that the practitioner's time with the client may not permit such an extensive focus, but the ultimate intent is to maintain this holistic perspective in seeking appropriate goals.

PERFORMANCE COMPONENTS

Performance components are the basic abilities that the person brings to the performance of activities. Components are required in varying degrees to successfully carry out the activities in a performance area and are grouped into one of these categories: sensorimotor components (sensory, neuromusculoskeletal, motor), cognitive and cognitive integration components, or psychosocial skills and psychological components. As a student progresses through OT studies, a refinement of knowledge evolves, enabling these concepts and terminology to become more meaningful. However, this introductory text calls for simplification; a brief examination of the performance components is provided.

The **sensorimotor components** involve the ability to receive sensory input and to process and respond to it by producing an output. There are three elements to the sensorimotor component. The *sensory* element concerns the awareness and the processing of stimuli. This includes the ability to receive different stimuli, such as sound, light, and touch, and to interpret these stimuli for what they are. The *neuromusculoskeletal* element includes reflexes, range of motion of joints, muscle tone, strength and endurance, and postural control and alignment. The *motor* element concerns gross and fine coordination, bilateral integration, motor planning and control, and eye-hand coordination.[7]

The **cognitive** and **cognitive integration components** involve the ability to use higher mental functions. These include factors related to the level of alertness, orientation, recognition, and attention; the ability to initiate and terminate an activity; memory, sequencing, and categorization; the ability to organize information to form thoughts and ideas; and to mentally manipulate the position of objects, problem solving, learning, and generalization.[7]

The last component, **psychosocial skills and psychological components,** is the management of relationships and the processing of emotions. The *psychological* element of this component concerns values, interests, and self-concept. The *psychosocial skills* relate to the ability to balance various roles, conduct oneself in social interactions, use various emotions to express oneself, and the ability to cope with stress, manage time, and modify behavior in response to the environment.

It is important to know and understand these components and examine activities in relation to them. To determine the needs of a client and to select helpful activities, the OT practitioner must complete a thorough analysis to determine what is missing and what is needed. This concept of performance components forms the foundation of a systematic approach to this analytic process. The components are the basis of activity analysis, which is a necessary skill for an OT practitioner and is discussed in Chapter 16.

PERFORMANCE CONTEXTS

An important influence on an individual's occupational performance is the **performance contexts** in which the individual's various roles and related activities are performed. The performance contexts encompass both temporal and environmental aspects. When determining whether a particular intervention is effective, the OT practitioner takes into consideration the performance context. The practitioner may decide to work within the context and choose interventions appropriate toward that end, or the practitioner may decide on an intervention that involves alteration of the context for the most effective performance.[7] This concept is described further in Chapter 16.

Temporal aspects include the individual's chronologic age, developmental stage or phase of maturation, place in important life phases (e.g., career cycle, parenting cycle, or educational process), and disability status. *Disability status* considers the nature of the individual's disability, such as whether it is acute, chronic, progressive, or terminal in nature.[7]

Environmental aspects encompass physical, social, and cultural environments. The *physical* environment considers the nonhuman aspects of contexts, such as accessibility to and performance in buildings, in and around furniture and objects, and on different types of outside terrains. The *social* environment involves the expectations and availability of significant others, as well as larger social groups that influence social norms, role expectations, and social routines. The *cultural* aspects include beliefs, customs, activity patterns, behavior standards, and expectations that are passed from one generation to another. Also part of the cultural environment are political factors and opportunities for education, employment, and economic support. The OT practitioner should have an awareness of different cultures and be sensitive to the beliefs and customs of individuals from other cultures.

In all choices made with and for the client, the OT practitioner must be aware of the individual's unique attributes and his or her environment or the one to which he or she will return. A person who lives in a nursing home has a different life space than one who lives alone in an apartment—the identified needs will differ, even if the disability and age are the same.

The following is a real-life illustration of what can happen when consideration of life space is ignored. An OT practitioner, who was a consultant to a day program for adults with developmental disabilities, attended a planning meeting with a female client's family and the staff at the center. The client had minimal physical deficits but very limited verbal skills. One goal had been to teach the client some homemaking skills so she could perform simple jobs at home. This was viewed as an opportunity to improve her self-esteem and, at the same time, offer a valuable service for the family. The staff worked with her for months to develop laundry skills—sorting colored clothes from white, measuring soap powder, loading the washing machine, and folding clothes as they were taken from the dryer. She practiced at the center and demonstrated independence in the tasks. An enthusiastic response was expected from the family; instead, the mother informed the practitioners that the client never performed laundry tasks at home. After further discussion, the embarrassed staff discovered the family did not own an automatic washer and dryer but used an old wringer washer and hung the clothing on a line to dry. The client was unable to generalize from the automatic appliance to the more basic technology. They had taught her a skill that was useless in her life space. The moral of this example—remember life space!

The relationship between the performance areas, performance components, and performance contexts is interactive.[7] The ultimate concern of OT is function in performance areas. Performance components need to be considered as they relate to a person's function in the performance area. An individual's performance areas and performance components are always viewed within performance contexts. For example, the practitioner does not evaluate the performance component of depth perception as an isolated entity. It is considered as it contributes to activities the individual needs or wishes to perform. The OT process, which is discussed in the next chapters, involves assessment of the performance areas, performance components, and performance contexts, and the intervention that is directed toward deficits in these elements.

SUMMARY

It is important that the OT practitioner understand the importance of theory in practice. Theories provide a road map for clinical assessment and intervention and consist of a set of concepts and principles that define a specific phenomenon. Theory is linked to practice through frames of reference. As discussed in Chapter 3, the **model of human occupation** is one theory upon which the profession is based.[12]

The domain of concern in OT is occupational performance. Occupational performance is the ability of the person to perform functional activities in related occupational roles. Occupational performance is characterized by performance areas, performance components, and performance contexts. The performance areas are ADLs, work and productive activities, and play and leisure activities. The abilities of the human being are called performance components and are categorized as sensorimotor (sensory, neuromusculoskeletal, motor), cognitive and cognitive integration, or psychosocial and psychological skills.

Occupational performance is considered in terms of the individual's performance contexts. This consideration includes assessing the temporal (person's chronologic and development ages, life cycle, and disability status) and environmental (physical, social, cultural) aspects. The occupational performance areas, performance components, and performance contexts interact with one another. One cannot be considered without the others. In evaluation and treatment, the OT practitioner considers all three.

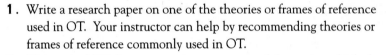

Activities

1. Write a research paper on one of the theories or frames of reference used in OT. Your instructor can help by recommending theories or frames of reference commonly used in OT.
2. Visit several OT departments in your area, and determine which theories and frames of reference are used at each setting. Ask to observe a practitioner during a treatment program that implements one of the frames of reference.
3. Working in small groups of two or three, select several games (or design one simple game) that emphasize one of the performance components.
4. Keep track of all the activities in which you engage during a recent week day and weekend day. For each day, classify the activities according to the three occupational performance areas, and make a chart that tracks the amount of time spent for each performance area.
5. Make a collage (using diagrams, pictures, etc.) that illustrate the performance contexts of three different individuals.
6. So often we get caught up in our work and productive or self-care activities that we forget activities that we enjoy and help us to relax. To come up with activities that you may consider "play or leisure," sit down with a blank piece of paper. Across the top write the words, "My Bliss List." Think of activities both small (watching the sunset) and large (planting a garden) that you enjoy. As you think of these activities, list them on your paper. Throughout the next week, select one of the activities to perform each day.

REFERENCES

1. Allen CK: *Occupational therapy for psychiatric diseases: measurement and management of cognitive disabilities*, Boston, 1985, Little, Brown.

2. Allen C: Activity, occupational therapy's treatment method, *Amer J Occup Ther* 41:563, 1987.

3. American Occupational Therapy Association: *The roles and functions of occupational therapy personnel*, Rockville, Md, 1973, AOTA.

4. American Occupational Therapy Association: *A curriculum guide for occupational therapy educators*, Rockville, Md, 1974, AOTA.

5. American Occupational Therapy Association: Occupational therapy product output reporting system and uniform terminology for reporting occupational therapy services. In *Reference manual of the official documents of the American Occupational Therapy Association*, Rockville, Md, 1989, AOTA.

6. American Occupational Therapy Association: Uniform terminology for occupational therapy, ed 2, *Amer J Occup Ther* 43:808, 1989.

7. American Occupational Therapy Association: Uniform terminology for occupational therapy, ed 3, *Amer J Occup Ther* 48:1047, 1994.

8. Bundy AC: Assessment of play and leisure: delineation of the problem, *Amer J Occup Ther* 47:217, 1993.

9. Christiansen C: Occupational therapy, intervention for life perspective. In Christiansen C, Baum C: *Occupational therapy, overcoming human performance deficits*, Thorofare, NJ, 1991, Slack.

10. Donahue MV: Claudia Allen. In Miller RJ, Walker KF, editors: *Perspectives on theory for the practice of occupational therapy*, Gaithersburg, Md, 1993, Aspen Publishers.

11. Dutton R, Levy LL, Simon CJ: Frames of reference in occupational therapy: introduction. In Hopkins HL, Smith HD: *Willard & Spackman's occupational therapy*, Philadelphia, 1993, JB Lippincott.

13. Ludwig FM: Anne Cronin Mosey. In Miller RJ, Walker KF, editors: *Perspectives on theory for the practice of occupational therapy*, Gaithersburg, Md, 1993, Aspen Publishers.

14. Miller RJ: What is theory, and why does it matter? In Miller RJ, Walker KF, editors: *Perspectives on theory for the practice of occupational therapy*, Gaithersburg, Md, 1993, Aspen Publishers.

15. Miller RJ, Walker KF, editors: *Perspectives on theory for the practice of occupational therapy*, Gaithersburg, Md, 1993, Aspen Publishers.

16. Mish F, editor: *Merriam-Webster's collegiate dictionary®*, ed 10, Springfield, Mass, 1994, Merriam-Webster.

17. Mosey AC: *Three frames of reference for mental health*, Thorofare, NJ, 1970, Slack.

18. Mosey AC: *Occupational therapy: configuration of a profession*, New York, 1981, Raven Press.

19. Parham D: Toward professionalism: the reflective therapist, *Amer J Occup Ther* 41:555, 1987.

20. Pedretti LW: Occupational performance: a model for practice in physical dysfunction. In Pedretti LW: *Occupational therapy practice skills for physical dysfunction*, ed 4, St Louis, 1996, Mosby.

21. Reed KL: Understanding theory: the first step in learning about research, *Amer J Occup Ther* 38:677, 1984.

22. Trombly CS, Scott AD: *Occupational therapy for physical dysfunction*, Baltimore, 1977, Williams & Wilkins.

23. Williamson GG: A heritage of activity: development of theory, *Amer J Occup Ther* 36:716, 1982.

On plucking thistles and planting flowers...

How one lives life or chooses an occupation can be simple and straightforward or a long journey. As an undergraduate student, I wanted to be in premed—convinced that my calling was to be a physician. During undergraduate school, I explored two directions. My first job was as a genetics technician in a university-based medical center. My days were spent centrifuging and fixing samples on slides, counting chromosomes, and photographing and creating karyotypes. When I closed my eyes each night, all I could visualize was chromosomes floating in emulsion. I would briefly meet people when they gave a sample in the laboratory, but I never got to know them or know what having the test meant to the greater scheme of their lives.

My second exploration was as a volunteer in an occupational therapy department in a psychiatric hospital. Suddenly I was fascinated by people and their stories—intrigued by what went wrong and how their lives could be reorganized, allowing them to return to some sense of normalcy in their day-to-day lives. Occupational therapy seemed less scientific yet so very meaningful—listening while we were doing. I found that change and growth can be found through doing. I was a potential "agent of change"—the very meaning of the word "therapist" directed me to choose occupational therapy. The process of occupational therapy reminds me of Abraham Lincoln's words, which I have embraced: "I want it said of me by those who knew me best that I always plucked a thistle and planted a flower where I knew one would grow." I chose occupational therapy and have been plucking and planting. What a garden has grown and continues to grow each and everyday! ■

Ann Burkhardt, MA, OTR/L, BCN
Assistant Director
Occupational Therapy, Department of
    Rehabilitation Medicine
Columbia—Presbyterian Medical Center
Clinical Instructor, Program in
    Occupational Therapy
College of Physicians and Surgeons
Columbia University
New York, New York

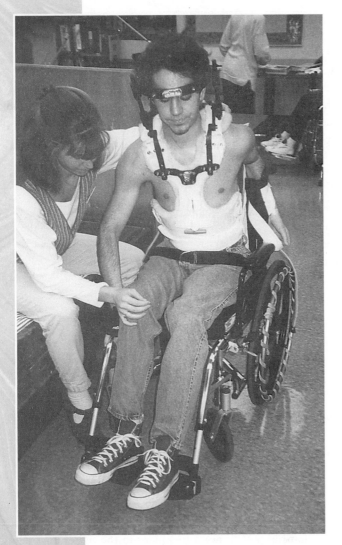

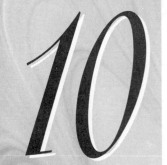

Overview of the
Occupational Therapy
Process

Objectives

After reading this chapter, the reader will be able to:

❖ Identify and describe the stages in the occupational therapy process

❖ Distinguish between direct service functions and indirect service functions

❖ Characterize the roles of the Registered Occupational Therapist (OTR) and the Certified Occupational Therapy Assistant (COTA) as they engage in the occupational therapy process

Key terms

Occupational therapy process
Service management
Indirect service functions
Direct service functions
Referral
Screening
Assessment
Evaluation
Evaluation procedures
Treatment plan
Treatment implementation
Re-evaluation
Transition services
Discharge plan
Discharge summary

When a practitioner is retained to provide services, the professional interaction is referred to as the **occupational therapy (OT) process** and includes all aspects of the professional relationship. OT is not a treatment in the sense of a prescribed "do-this-for-that-problem" approach. Rather, it is an evolving interaction with the client in the context of changing goals, thus it is referred to as the OT process.

It is significant that OT service delivery is referred to as a *process* because, according to *Merriam-Webster's Collegiate Dictionary*®,[6] the term is defined as "a natural phenomenon marked by gradual changes that lead toward a particular result." The OT process is the interaction between *two* active agents involved in the process—the therapist *and* the client. The interaction is not something *done to* the client, rather the interaction engages *with* the client, while problem solving to support an increase in independent functioning of the client.

Chapter 10 photo: Early MB: *Physical dysfunction practice skills for the occupational therapy assistant,* St Louis, 1998, Mosby.

Some disciplines define what they do in terms of treatment planning. The OT process includes a treatment plan but regards the plan as a step in the process, not an end in itself; the plan is always open to modification. The interactive process is primary. Development and change calls for many choices to be made along the way.

STAGES IN THE OCCUPATIONAL THERAPY PROCESS

The OT process can be formally defined by eight stages, which are based on the American Occupational Therapy Association's (AOTA) *Standards of Practice* (found in Appendix C). These stages set the guidelines for the delivery of services for all OT practitioners. The following eight stages are important because they delineate a minimum standard of service provision of OT practitioners for all populations. These stages are:

(1) Referral
(2) Screening
(3) Assessment
(4) Intervention plan
(5) Intervention
(6) Transition services
(7) Discontinuation of services
(8) Service management

Stages one through seven identify different decision-making stages in the therapeutic interaction with the client. Theoretically, a client is brought into the therapy process by a referral, and the completion of the process is marked by a discharge (Figure 10-1). In the "real world," however, some stages may overlap or be combined, but all therapeutic interactions can be understood in terms of these stages.

Stage eight, **service management,** includes the general tasks that are part of a practitioner's day-to-day existence, as required to keep the department or program operational and relevant. Also referred to as **indirect service functions,** service management includes functions such as ordering supplies, keeping equipment in working order, doing administrative paperwork (such as charting the number of treatments or making daily schedules), and performing quality assurance activities. Service management may also involve attending workshops to keep current on developments and new techniques in the field. In Chapter 13, these service management functions are discussed in greater detail.

These seven stages are also collectively referred to as **direct service functions.** As the name implies, these functions are performed directly with or for the benefit of a particular client. It therefore includes such functions as meeting with

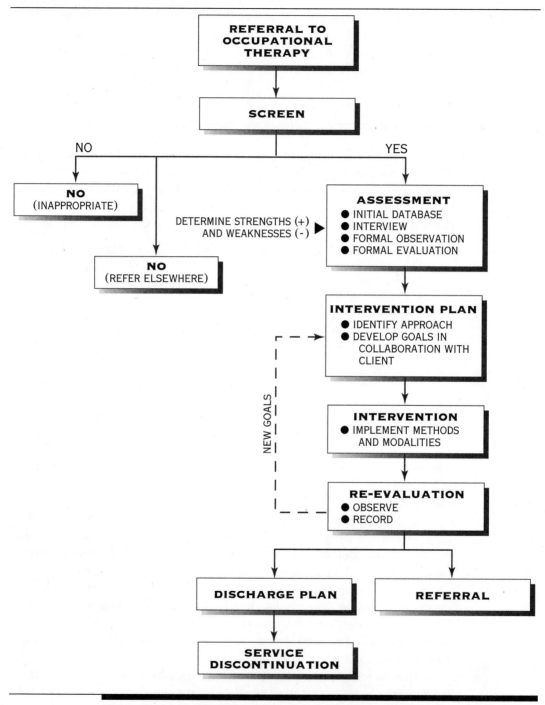

FIGURE 10-1. THE OCCUPATIONAL THERAPY PROCESS.

family members or researching a specific program need. Direct service functions also include the education of other staff members regarding OT treatment goals for the clients being served. An example of a direct service function is an explanation to a unit aide regarding the best positioning and adaptive equipment for the client whose therapy goals include feeding himself during meals. The following text provides an overview of these seven stages in the OT process and delineates the roles of both the OTR and the COTA for each stage.

REFERRAL

The first stage in the OT process is **referral.** Referral is the point at which the initial request for service for a particular client or a change in the degree and direction of service is made.[2] There are several ways in which a referral is made. The person may be a self-referral; he or she may be referred by a physician, another professional, or another agency; or the person may be automatically sent to OT because he or she is a client at the facility or a client in the program. Depending on the setting, a referral could be anything from a physician's prescription for upper-extremity strengthening, to a teacher's suggestion that a student "seems to have a problem," to a psychologist requesting that a client be given some assistance in structuring time. To provide OT services, the type of referral required (e.g., whether a physician's referral is necessary) is determined by federal, state, and local regulations and the policies of third-party payers. AOTA does not dictate whether a physician's referral is required.[2]

The OTR is responsible for overseeing the referral and determining the appropriateness of further evaluation and treatment for the client. The COTA can acknowledge requests for service and enter cases only under the supervision and collaboration of an OTR. COTAs cannot accept and enter cases at their own discretion.[1] In the situation where the COTA is given a referral, the COTA must relay this information to the supervising OTR so that the appropriate procedures can be followed. Furthermore, steps should be taken by both the OTR and COTA to educate others regarding the correct procedure for referring clients.[3]

SCREENING

Through **screening,** the OT practitioner gathers preliminary information about the client and determines whether further evaluation and OT intervention is warranted[1] (Figure 10-2). The questions asked at the time of screening are, "Is this person's problem appropriate for this setting?" "Can we offer helpful services?" "Shall we schedule this person for further assessment and treatment?"

Screening may involve a review of the client's records, the use of a screening test, an interview with the client or caregiver, observation of the client, or a discussion of the client with the referral source or at staff conferences. During the initial screening, the OT practitioner also shares information about OT with the client. By providing a little information about OT, its aims and the modes of treatment, the practitioner relieves the client's anxiety and sends the client the message, "You are a person who I care about." The client should also have the opportunity to ask questions and provide information. In this way the OT practitioner recognizes the client as a whole person and confirms that he or she is not a mere object that the practitioner expects to "work on." This interaction establishes a base for cooperation; the sharing of purpose and intent enlists the client as an active agent in the treatment process.

Screening is the first step in the process where a *yes* or *no* decision regarding intervention is made. The decision may be *no* for a particular client for a number of supporting reasons. The client may not have the kind of problem(s) that can be addressed by the facility, meaning that there is either no need for service or that the needs can be addressed more appropriately by another therapy or in a different

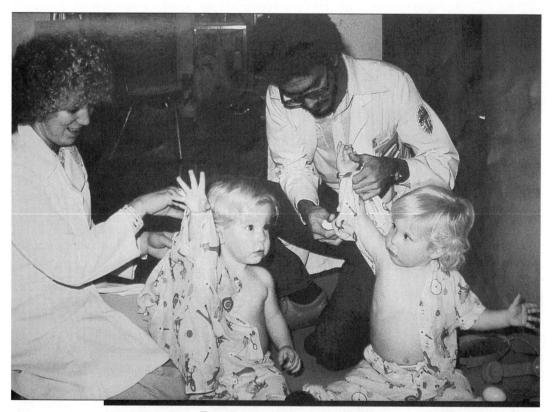

FIGURE 10-2. THE OCCUPATIONAL THERAPIST IS ASSESSING THE DEVELOPMENTAL SKILLS OF THESE TWINS. SCREENING FOR DEVELOPMENTAL PROBLEMS PERMITS TIMELY DELIVERY OF OCCUPATIONAL THERAPY SERVICES, IF NECESSARY. (COURTESY OF AOTA AND ST. JOHN'S IN CLEVELAND, OHIO, JOE ROSENDAUL.)

facility. It may be a *no* decision because the client is referred inappropriately or because the therapist judges that other services are needed first. In these types of cases, the OT practitioner makes a referral elsewhere. If the decision is *yes,* the OT process is scheduled. The results of the screening, regardless of a *yes* or *no* decision, are communicated to the appropriate individuals, including the party who made the referral.[1]

The OTR is responsible for carrying out the screening process using methods that are appropriate to the client's developmental level, gender, cultural background, and medical and functional status.[1] The COTA contributes to the screening process under the direction of an OTR; before the screening tasks are performed by an entry-level COTA, it should be determined whether he or she has service competency in the particular tasks being delegated (see Chapter 4).

ASSESSMENT AND EVALUATION

If it is determined during the screening process that the client is in need of services, the next stage in the OT process is a comprehensive **assessment.** It is through this assessment process that the data are gathered about the client, the problems are identified, a hypothesis is formulated, and the decisions are made for treatment intervention.[4] Often the terms *assessment* and *evaluation* are used interchangeably. For the purposes of this text, assessment is defined as the sum of the evaluation results, which provide a composite picture of the client's level of function. **Evaluation** is the series of tests used to measure an individual's skills and deficits.[4,5]

Although screening has been placed in an earlier stage, the assessment process actually begins with a screening of the client as described. After the screening, the therapist identifies a frame of reference that applies to the client's situation and selects **evaluation procedures** based on this frame of reference.[4] The evaluation procedures are the specific methods or techniques used to collect information during the evaluation stages.[4,5] These procedures take several forms and can be classified into four major types: medical records review, skilled observation, interview, and tests (standardized and nonstandardized). In Chapter 11, each of these procedures are described in detail. This step of the process calls for important judgments on the part of the therapist, who must select the most appropriate evaluation procedures to meet the needs and abilities of the individual being assessed.

After identifying a frame of reference and after the evaluation procedures are selected, the OT practitioner employs these procedures to gather information on the individual's abilities and deficits (also referred to as strengths and weaknesses) as related to performance areas, performance components, and performance contexts (see Chapter 9). The purpose of identifying the performance levels in these areas is to determine the strengths and weaknesses of the client. An evaluation may take place over several sessions; therefore, the OT practitioner should carefully and thoroughly identify and record data as they are accumulated.

Once the necessary data are obtained, the OTR compiles and analyzes the evaluation findings and formulates an assessment report of the individual's functional status. This report consists of the identification of the individual's life roles and role dysfunction and a list of the person's assets and problems, alternatively called strengths and weaknesses or abilities and deficits.[4] Results of the assessment are documented by the OTR in the client's records.[1] This assessment forms the basis for the initial treatment plan.

Assessment is seen as a critical decision-making role requiring a depth of understanding of many factors; as a result, the final responsibility of assessment rests with the OTR. The COTA, though not responsible for the complete assessment, may have certain evaluation procedures delegated as responsibilities and thus may contribute to an evaluation under an OTR's supervision. The COTA communicates the results of all evaluation procedures with the OTR. As with the screening process, service competency for tasks performed by an entry-level COTA needs to be established. Indeed, within any given setting a COTA may become very proficient in specific phases of evaluation. Self-care is a common example; often the COTA develops expert competency in this area. The overall assessment, or the process of compiling all of the information to form a composite picture of the client, however, is the responsibility of an OTR.

TREATMENT PLAN

The **treatment plan** is the recommendations made for OT intervention based on an analysis of the information accumulated during the assessment.[1] The treatment plan considers the strengths and weaknesses of the individual; interests of the client and caregivers; estimate of rehabilitation potential; expected outcomes (short- and long-term goals) along with frequency and duration of treatment; recommended methods and media; apparent environmental and time constraints; identification of a plan for re-evaluation; and discharge planning (Figure 10-3).[1]

The development of the treatment plan involves several steps. After the assessment, client information is analyzed. Based on the problems and the identified frame of reference and the input received from the client, the practitioner determines goals for treatment (expected outcomes). With these goals in mind, possible media and therapeutic activities are selected. When there are several goals, priorities are set and a sequence of activities is selected that will lead to improved functioning. The practitioner then determines the frequency and duration of services needed to reach the goals. In many instances the plan is formally entered in the client's records. In other cases it may be less formal—recorded only for the use of the therapist or the OT department.

Generally, it is expressed that the OTR formulates and documents the treatment plan.[1] In many settings, however, the COTA has active input and partici-

CASE

PERSONAL DATA

NAME

AGE

DIAGNOSIS

DISABILITY

TREATMENT GOALS STATED IN THE REFERRAL

OTHER SERVICES

FRAME OF REFERENCE AND TREATMENT APPROACH

OT EVALUATION

PERFORMANCE COMPONENTS

1. SENSORIMOTOR

2. COGNITIVE/COGNITIVE INTEGRATION

3. PSYCHOSOCIAL/PSYCHOLOGICAL SKILLS

PERFORMANCE AREAS

1. ACTIVITIES OF DAILY LIVING

2. WORK AND PRODUCTIVE ACTIVITIES

3. PLAY OR LEISURE ACTIVITIES

EVALUATION SUMMARY

ASSETS

PROBLEM LIST

OUTLINE TREATMENT PLAN

1. PROBLEM

2. OBJECTIVE

3. METHODS

4. GRADATION

FIGURE 10-3. TREATMENT PLAN MODEL. (ADAPTED FROM PEDRETTI LW: <u>OT: PRACTICE SKILLS FOR PHYSICAL DYSFUNCTION</u>, ED 4, ST LOUIS, 1996, MOSBY.

pates in program planning (i.e., develops goals, selects techniques and media) for those clients specifically assigned to him or her. In Chapter 12 the treatment planning process is discussed in further detail.

IMPLEMENTATION OF TREATMENT AND RE-EVALUATION

Treatment implementation is putting the treatment plan in place, working with the client through therapy to reach treatment goals. An important part of implementation is educating the client, family, and caregiver in activities that support the intervention plan. It is often the caregivers who are responsible for ensuring that the client performs the activities and strategies learned in therapy. When caregivers are responsible for implementing treatment, they need to be aware of the risks and benefits of intervention as well.[1]

As treatment is implemented, the OT practitioner continually performs a process known as **re-evaluation.** This part of the process is ongoing in that the OT practitioner must always keep up to date on changes, remain aware of circumstances or needs that arise, and change the direction of treatment, either temporarily or permanently, if needed. Re-evaluation may mean changing activities, retesting, writing a new plan, or making needed referrals; in other words, re-evaluation asks that the practitioner use observational skills to remain attuned to the client with the readiness to meet emerging needs. The client's program is modified on the basis of the individual's response to the intervention.

The implementation stage includes necessary reporting, both oral and written. In this age of accountability, documentation is critically important. All treatment must be recorded. When a therapist works with a client, he or she is expected to keep an accurate record of the treatment. In addition to a record for each treatment session, the OT practitioner writes regular progress notes (based on the results of the ongoing re-evaluation), reports at client conferences, and communicates with other professionals and with the families of the clients regarding therapy.

Implementation is the most visible stage of the OT process; it is the day-to-day treatment that can be seen when entering the OT department. If the first four stages in the OT process receive adequate attention and the activities are consistent with the treatment goals, implementation can be a mutually satisfying interaction. Although the implementation is the responsibility of both OTRs and COTAs, it is the *central* responsibility of the COTA. Similarly, re-evaluation is a responsibility shared by both the OTR and COTA. Educational programs are designed to ensure that COTAs develop an understanding of the philosophy and skills of OT to enable them to interpret and implement treatment plans. Treatment implementation by the COTA is done under the supervision of the OTR. The more complex the treatment setting and the more frequent the program changes, the more necessary it becomes for the COTA to have close OTR supervision.

TRANSITION SERVICES

Transition services is the coordination or facilitation of services for the purpose of preparing the client for a change. Transition services may involve a change to a new functional level, life stage, program, or environment. The OT practitioner is involved in identifying services and preparing an individualized transition plan to facilitate the client's change from one place to another.[1] In other words, the transition plan needs to be individualized to meet the goals, needs, and environmental considerations of the individual client. For example, Mrs. G has been hospitalized for a total hip replacement but is married and able to return home with little support because her spouse can provide support for cooking and cleaning and can assist with her self-care. Her transition service plan includes training Mr. G to safely and easily assist Mrs. G in her care when she goes home. On the other hand, Ms. W has undergone the same procedure but is widowed and lives alone. The transition plan for Ms. W requires more consideration for the provision of outside support before returning home. As Ms. W's case illustrates, some clients need more outside support than is available; it may be necessary to develop a plan in which the client is transferred to a lower level of care (i.e., a skilled nursing facility) before returning home. Regardless, careful planning is the key to preparing the client for the transition.

Ideally, planning for transition should be a part of the initial treatment plan and considered throughout the OT process. The OT practitioner should always be asking questions such as, "Where is this client likely to go next?" "What type of program is most suitable and into what type of environment is this client returning?" "How can I best prepare this individual for the transition to the new program or environment?" Planning for transition should be done in collaboration with the client, family members, other disciplines involved in treating the client, and community support services, if available.[1]

SERVICE DISCONTINUATION

The last stage of the OT process is the discontinuation of the client from OT services. The client is discharged from OT when he or she has reached the goals delineated in the treatment plan or when it is determined that he or she has realized the maximum benefit of OT services.[1] Just before discontinuation, a **discharge plan** is developed and implemented. The discharge plan conforms to the individual's therapy and personal goals and addresses the resources available in the community that may be appropriate for the client upon discharge. The OTR prepares and implements the discharge plan with input from the COTA.[1]

The OTR also documents what is called a **discharge summary.** In this summary the status of the client's functional level at the time of discharge is recorded, as well as changes that were made throughout the course of OT intervention. The discharge summary also contains the plans for discharge and the equipment and services that are recommended after discharge, including follow up OT services, if needed. The COTA contributes to the formulation of the discharge summary.[1]

SUMMARY

The OT process is interactive, consisting of eight distinguishable stages: referral, screening, assessment, treatment planning, treatment implementation, transition services, discontinuation of services, and, in a broad sense, service management. The first seven stages are referred to as direct service functions in which the client typically enters at the referral stage and proceeds through to the discontinuation stage. Service management functions are those that are not directly related to the provision of services to a specific client but are necessary for the overall operation of an OT department or program. These functions include scheduling, equipment maintenance, ordering supplies, quality assurance, and practitioner education.

Although there are many OTR duties that are indistinguishable from those of the experienced COTA (i.e., implementing treatment on a one-to-one basis), other responsibilities (i.e., interpreting evaluation results) highlight the differences. The OTR is responsible for the assessment process and for the development of the initial treatment plan, although the COTA can contribute to both of these stages. The COTA contributes to each phase of the OT process under supervision of the OTR.

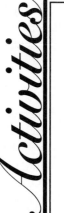

1. Outline the steps of the OT process. Interview a therapist regarding his or her professional duties. Under each heading of the OT process, list some specific duties a therapist may be called on to do.
2. Design a diagram of the OT process that includes the decisions that are needed at each stage.
3. Make a color-coded chart to indicate standard responsibilities for the roles of the OTR and COTA (i.e., color A for COTA responsibilities, color B for OTR responsibilities, color C for shared responsibilities.)
4. Interview therapists in OT departments that employ both OTRs and COTAs to determine how "supervision" is interpreted in the facilities. Document your findings.

REFERENCES

1. American Occupational Therapy Association: Standards of practice for occupational therapy, *Amer J Occup Ther* 48:1039, 1994.

2. American Occupational Therapy Association: Statement of occupational therapy referral, *Amer J Occup Ther* 48:1034, 1994.

3. Hiramu H: *Occupational therapy assistant: a primer,* Baltimore, 1996, CHESS Publications.

4. Pedretti LW: Occupational therapy evaluation and assessment of physical dysfunction. In Pedretti LW, editor: *Occupational therapy: practice skills for physical dysfunction,* ed 4, St Louis, 1996, Mosby.

5. Smith HD: Assessment and evaluation: an overview. In Hopkins HL, Smith HD, editors: *Willard & Spackman's occupational therapy,* ed 8, Philadelphia, 1993, JB Lippincott.

6. Mish F, editor: *Merriam-Webster's collegiate dictionary®,* ed 10, Springfield, Mass, 1994, Merriam-Webster.

I remember my first months in practice as an occupational therapist. I simply could not believe that anyone would pay me for doing what was pure fun and enjoyment. Today, some 17 years later, I no longer mind being paid for my services as a pediatric therapist. However, I continue to love the practice of occupational therapy with children and marvel that something as fun as therapy is considered to be a "job." Perhaps we should keep it a secret!

Why does occupational therapy with children continue to be personally exciting and stimulating? First, it forces me to critically analyze and solve problems. Simultaneously, I must be concerned about (1) the child's behavior and performance; (2) the parent's perceptions, desires, and concerns; (3) the conditions in the environment that seem to relate to my first two concerns; and (4) the interests and concerns of other adults invested in the child (e.g., a physical therapist, teacher, speech therapist). While analyzing all of the variables that influence the child's functional performance and behavior, I must select interaction styles, therapeutic activities, and recommendations that will optimally benefit the child and promote development. What a challenge! Understanding the child-family-environment interaction, solving problems related to the child's function and behavior, and implementing the steps that will lead to a mutually agreed-upon vision for the child is just the right challenge for me. ■

Jane Case-Smith, EdD, OTR/L, BCP, FAOTA
Associate Professor
Division of Occupational Therapy
Ohio State University
Columbus, Ohio

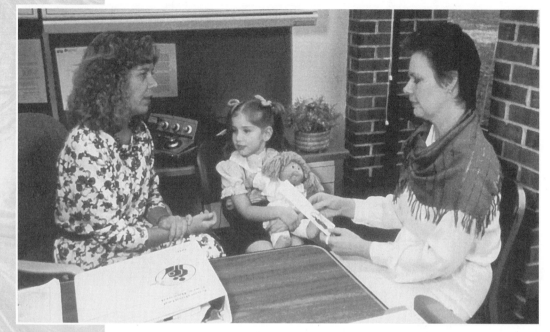

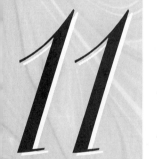

Occupational Therapy
Assessment

Objectives

After reading this chapter, the reader will be able to:

✤ Identify the steps in the assessment process and the four methods that are used for gathering assessment data
✤ Recognize the type and value of the information collected for the initial database
✤ Understand the importance of observation skills in the evaluation process
✤ Implement techniques to develop observation skills
✤ Identify the three stages of an interview
✤ Understand the need to blend formal and informal elements in the interview process
✤ Understand how to create a desirable atmosphere for interviewing
✤ Understand the factors that affect the decision to use particular formal evaluation procedures

Key terms

Initial database
Interview
Interest checklist
Activity configuration
Interview schedule
Observation
Structured observation
Activity battery
Formal evaluation procedures
Validity
Reliability
Test-retest reliability
Interrater reliability
Standardized test
Normative data
Nonstandardized tests

In Chapter 10 an overview of the occupational therapy (OT) process is provided. One of the most critical steps in the OT process is the assessment phase, during which accurate and useful information must be gathered. This information is used by the Registered Occupational Therapist (OTR) to identify the needs and problems of the client and to plan treatment intervention. The evaluation procedures used during the assessment process to gather information regarding the client can be

Chapter 11 photo: Wallace HM, Biehl RF, MacQueen JC, Blackman JA: *Mosby's resource guide to children with disabilities and chronic illness*, St Louis, 1997, Mosby.

classified into four basic procedures: (1) collection of the initial database; (2) interview; (3) skilled observation; and (4) formal evaluation procedures.[8,12]

The sphere of practice will set some of the criteria for the assessment. However, every setting usually uses more than one type of evaluation procedure; therefore the OTR determines which specific procedures to use, based on the client's age, developmental level, education, socioeconomic status, cultural background, and functional abilities. In this chapter the steps in the assessment process are reviewed, and the various methods that are used to gather information during the assessment are described in detail.

STEPS IN THE ASSESSMENT PROCESS

The assessment process begins with screening the client to determine whether to continue with further OT evaluation and intervention. If a decision is made to continue, the next step is to identify a frame of reference (see Chapter 9) from which the evaluation is based. This frame of reference may be one used by the facility or one preferred by the OTR. Evaluation instruments that are consistent with the frame of reference are then selected.

The process continues with the administration of the selected evaluation instruments. Through the use of these evaluation procedures, the OT practitioner collects data that provide information regarding the individual's functional status as it relates to performance areas, performance components, and performance contexts. Once the necessary data have been collected, they are compiled and analyzed to form a composite picture of the client. This information is then used to develop goals and a plan for treatment.

COLLECTION OF THE INITIAL DATABASE

The first procedure typically executed by the OT practitioner is to develop the **initial database** of information about the client. It is helpful if most of the information for the database is gathered *before* evaluating the client. Then the OTR has some familiarity with the client and is not "going in cold" to the evaluation.

Information collected for the initial database may include the client's age and sex; reason and need for referral; medical diagnosis and medical history (including date of onset); prior living situation and level of function (e.g., independent at home or in a care home); and social, educational, and vocational background. The initial database will also provide information regarding precautions that need to be adhered to during the OT process. The information for the initial database is usually recorded in the client's OT chart and on the evaluation form. In Figure 11-1, which illustrates an example of an evaluation form used in an OT setting geared toward physical disabilities, the first section labeled *Information* is considered the initial database.

SANTA CLARA VALLEY MEDICAL CENTER
OCCUPATIONAL THERAPY DEPARTMENT
Page 1 of 2

Service _____ ❑ Inpatient ❑ Outpatient
❑ Initial ❑ Interim ❑ Discharge
(Rating scales on back of form)

OCCUPATIONAL THERAPY

INFORMATION

Onset Date: _____ Referral Date: _____ Sex: M F Language: _____
Diagnosis

Medical History:

Precautions/Diet:

Living Situation:

A/Vocational History:

UPPER EXTREMITY

Range of Motion
❑ Refer to range of motion form

Muscle Picture
❑ Refer to muscle test form

Sensation
(Light touch, pain, kinesthesia, other)

Hand Function
Dominance: ❑ Right ❑ Left

	Right			Left		
	Grip	3 point	Lateral	Grip	3 point	Lateral
Initial						
Interim/DC						
Norm						

Splinting

OTHER MOTOR
(Endurance, head/trunk posture and control, sitting/standing balance, reflexes, LE picture, functional ambulation)

VISUAL PERCEPTUAL SKILLS

VISUAL	Initial	Interim/DC	PERCEPTUAL	Initial	Interim/DC
Visual Attention			Motor planning		
Near Acuity			Graphic praxis		
Distance Acuity			Body scheme		
Pursuits			R/L discrimination		
Saccades			Form		
Ocular Alignment			Size		
Stereopsis			Part/whole		
Visual Fields			Figure ground		
Visual Neglect			Position in space		

SCALE: 0 = intact; 1 = impaired; 2 = severely impaired;
3 = unable to perform

COMMENTS:

Wears corrective lenses ❑Y ❑N Testing not indicated ❑

COGNITION AND BEHAVIOR
(Orientation, initiation, direction following, memory, judgment, organization, problem solving, impulsivity, attention span)

DISPOSITION – White – MEDICAL RECORD   Yellow – O.T. Chart   Therapist's Signature: _____

FIGURE 11-1. SAMPLE OCCUPATIONAL THERAPY EVALUATION FORM. (COURTESY OF OCCUPATIONAL THERAPY DEPARTMENT, SANTA CLARA VALLEY MEDICAL CENTER, SAN JOSE, CALIFORNIA.)

SANTA CLARA VALLEY MEDICAL CENTER
OCCUPATIONAL THERAPY DEPARTMENT
Page 2 of 2

Service _____ ☐ Inpatient   ☐ Outpatient

☐ Initial   ☐ Interim   ☐ Discharge
(Rating scales on back of form)

OCCUPATIONAL THERAPY

BED MOBILITY

ACTIVITY	Initial	Interim/DC	Goal	
Rolling R				Bed:
Rolling L				Positioning:
Bridging				Caregiver Training:
Scooting				
Long Sit				Comments:
Sidelying to Sit				

TRANSFERS

Bed				Type: Equipment:
Toilet				Caregiver Training:
Tub/Shower				
Car/Van Seat				Comments:
Furniture				

WHEELCHAIR

Management				Type: Weight Shift Type:
Weight Shift				Positioning/Cushion:
Home				Caregiver Training:
Community				
In/Out of Car				Comments:

DAILY LIVING SKILLS

Eating				Equipment:
Upper Body Dressing				
Lower Body Dressing				Home Environment:
Hygiene/Grooming				
Bathing				A/Vocational/Driving Skills:
Toileting				
Kitchen				Caregiver Training:
Homemaking				
Community				Comments:
Communication Tasks				

Problems:

Goals/Recommendations: ☐ Patient/Caregiver participated in goal setting

___X___ / Frequency / Session Length / Duration of Treatment

Therapist's Signature   Date   Physician's Signature

DISPOSITION – White – MEDICAL RECORD   Yellow – O.T. Chart

FIGURE 11-1. (CONT'D)

INTERVIEW

The **interview,** with both the client and his or her significant others, provides another method of gathering data. The interview is simply a planned and organized way to collect pertinent information. Since the focus of OT is *occupation* and the activities in which a person engages throughout the course of his or her day, gathering information related to the individual's occupations and activities is a primary concern of the OT practitioner. The practitioner usually asks questions regarding the client's function in daily activities before the onset of the problem that resulted in his or her referral to OT. Besides gathering information, the interview is also used as a means of developing trust and rapport with the client.[13]

In some instances the client is asked to fill out a checklist or questionnaire before the interview. Again, this checklist or questionnaire focuses on a person's interests and activities. The **interest checklist** (Figure 11-2) was developed by Matsutsuyu[10] and has served as a model for many others. These interest checklists are used to enable the client to self-report on hobbies and interests. Another technique for addressing a client's interests and activities is the **activity configuration**. First, the person is asked to chart how his or her time is spent each day during a given period of time—a week or a few days. The chart shows what portion of the day is given to each activity. After completing the chart, the client uses it to compile a list of all the different activities in which he or she has participated during the designated time period. Each activity is classified according to which function it serves (e.g., work, rest, chore, etc.) and is rated according to whether the activity is one he or she *has* to do or *wants* to do and how adequately the activity is performed. From the chart the OTpractitioner can determine how the person spends his or her day, in what types of activities he or she is involved, and whether the person leads a balanced life.

The interview should take place in a setting that is quiet and allows for privacy.[13] Ideally, the interview should be relaxed and comfortable for both the interviewer and the client, never a rigid sequence of questions and answers. The skill of interviewing is a blending of the formal and informal—the formal accumulation of information and the informal person-to-person communication. Three stages of an interview can be identified: initial contact, information gathering, and closure.

INITIAL CONTACT

The skilled interviewer will spend the first few minutes of the interview putting the subject at ease. Often a person is worried and anxious at a therapy interview. They may be suffering from the shock of the illness or trauma, or they may feel threatened by the prospect of entering into therapy because it is new and unfamiliar. Even the client who has experienced therapy in the past may feel ill at ease about changes that a new therapy experience promises.

Rather than beginning to immediately gather information, it is better to tell the person a little about the clinic and the program: "We often have four to five

NAME   **UNIT**   **DATE**

Please check each item below according to your interest.

ACTIVITY	INTEREST CASUAL	STRONG	NO	ACTIVITY	INTEREST CASUAL	STRONG	NO
1. Gardening				41. Exercise			
2. Sewing				42. Volleyball			
3. Poker				43. Woodworking			
4. Languages				44. Billiards			
5. Social clubs				45. Driving			
6. Radio				46. Dusting			
7. Bridge				47. Jewelry making			
8. Car repair				48. Tennis			
9. Writing				49. Cooking			
10. Dancing				50. Basketball			
11. Needlework				51. History			
12. Golf				52. Guitar			
13. Football				53. Science			
14. Popular music				54. Collecting			
15. Puzzles				55. Ping pong			
16. Holidays				56. Leather work			
17. Solitaire				57. Shopping			
18. Movies				58. Photography			
19. Lectures				59. Painting			
20. Swimming				60. Television			
21. Bowling				61. Concerts			
22. Visiting				62. Ceramics			
23. Mending				63. Camping			
24. Chess				64. Laundry			
25. Barbeques				65. Dating			
26. Reading				66. Mosaics			
27. Traveling				67. Politics			
28. Manual arts				68. Scrabble			
29. Parties				69. Decorating			
30. Dramatics				70. Math			
31. Shuffleboard				71. Service groups			
32. Ironing				72. Piano			
33. Social studies				73. Scouting			
34. Classical music				74. Plays			
35. Floor mopping				75. Clothes			
36. Model building				76. Knitting			
37. Baseball				77. Hair styling			
38. Checkers				78. Religion			
39. Singing				79. Drums			
40. Home repairs				80. Conversation			

FIGURE 11-2. NPI INTEREST CHECKLIST. (REPRINTED WITH PERMISSION OF THE UNIVERSITY OF CALIFORNIA AT LOS ANGELES, FROM FIG. 1 IN MATSUTSUYU JS: THE INTEREST CHECK LIST, AMER J OCCUP THER 23:323, 1969.)

clients working with three or four OT practitioners." "We do a variety of things from craft activities to cooking groups." "We usually see people in half-hour time blocks." "Our group activities usually last an hour and a half." These statements convey some general information but do not burden the anxious person with specific details that he or she may be afraid of forgetting.

An OT practitioner develops his or her own interviewing style. Regardless, taking the time to create a relaxed and unthreatening atmosphere is beneficial to future therapy. The interview creates the "first impression" of the therapy process. The client who is made to feel welcome and who feels that the OT practitioner is interested in her or him as a person will begin therapy prepared to become a partner in the therapy process.

INFORMATION GATHERING

After a few relaxing minutes of informative discussion about the center or therapy process, the OT practitioner changes the focus with a request like, "Tell me a little about yourself." As the interview session moves into information gathering, the skilled interviewer guides the conversation in a way that yields the desired data yet keeps the flow conversational, rather than cold and rote. It is the interviewer's responsibility to regulate the flow of conversation and to direct it to address the client's concerns. If the OT practitioner is sensitive to the client's responses, these responses can help determine when to stay with a topic or when to change to a new one. Such a modulation of topic emphasis also signals to the client that he or she is important to the practitioner.

The OT practitioner writes brief notes, such as dates. To avoid alarming the interviewee with note-taking, the practitioner explains before beginning that a few notes will be taken during the interview. The questions are asked conversationally, while making eye contact, and are never directly read from a sheet of paper.

An unskilled interviewer may find himself or herself spending a great deal of time talking only to discover the needed information has not been gathered. To assure that the desired information is secured, the OT practitioner works from an **interview schedule**—a list of words or phrases that reminds the interviewer of needed data. An interview schedule differs from a list of questions in that it is a guide to conversation rather than a highly structured mechanism. An OT practitioner may have some standard items she or he wishes to cover, but there are often specific things to ask a client; therefore it is wise to prepare the interview schedule just before the interview.

CLOSURE

The interviewer must keep the time frame of the interview in mind. Whatever is allotted, the OT practitioner must remain aware of the time in order not to get lost in conversation and fail to cover the necessary details. Practice and skill are required to guide the interview in a way that allows for the collection of needed data and yet results in a pleasant, conversational experience. The interviewer should give some signal when the interview is about to end, such as summarizing the information gathered. This technique avoids the discomfort of an abrupt "time is up" ending. A good way to bring closure is to stand and say, "Thank you for your time...." and walk the person to the door or, in the case of a hospital patient who cannot move about freely, accompany the words with a touch on the arm or a hand on the shoulder before leaving the room.

OBSERVATION

Observation is the means of gathering information about a person or an environment by simply being present and noticing. Observation may be through a structured series of steps introduced by the OT practitioner, or it may be intentionally left unstructured to see what takes place.[6] Even through informal observation, such as the initial meeting, the OT practitioner is able to obtain a wealth of information about the client. The OT practitioner can observe the person's posture, dress, social skills, tone of voice, and physical abilities (i.e., use of the limbs and ambulation).[13]

Keen observation is valuable to the practitioner whenever there is client interaction, but it is especially valuable during assessment procedures. In *Willard & Spackman's Occupational Therapy,* 8th edition,[14] it is stated, "A key to successful evaluation lies in the therapist's skills in observation. The abilities to see and listen well must be accompanied by the abilities to sort through the mass of perceptual and conceptual data that may be presented and to focus on what is relevant to the process."

DEVELOPING OBSERVATION SKILLS

Professionally speaking, the importance of observation cannot be over-emphasized. The skill of observation is the enhancement of what each person already possesses. It is not a skill that is acquired through explicit technical training, like driving a car; it is an ability that each person already possesses and uses in day-to-day living. However, observation becomes a "skill" by consciously working to further develop it and to refine and improve it. Focusing on observation makes a person become aware of things that would otherwise escape notice. Like most skills, some people are naturally better at it than others. Whatever the degree of natural ability, the skill can be improved.

The best way to improve the powers of observation is to practice using them, which can be done almost any time. The key to good observation is focused attention. It can be as simple as saying while waiting for the bus, "Now let me see how many things I notice about this place." While watching and listening to people in line at the movies, the powers of observation can make a person aware of the feelings that are actually being transmitted or communicated between people.

Practicing observation with a goal in mind helps to further develop the skills; that is, to know what to look for. If the long-range goal is to describe a person's appearance as completely as possible, then gather the information systematically. Concentrate on each aspect of dress separately, and try to notice as much as possible. Go beyond the general (i.e., wearing a blue shirt) to identify the detail (with a pointed collar and tiny white buttons down the front and opened at the neck; long sleeves rolled up to the elbows; tucked in neatly at the waist). Then go to another aspect.

The next level of observation skill development is to employ thought and discrimination before making the observation, in order to gather information about what is needed. Preselect needed or desired information, and structure the observation to gather this necessary information.

STRUCTURED OBSERVATION

A **structured observation** consists of watching the client perform a predetermined activity. OT practitioners frequently use structured observation to gain knowledge of what the person can or cannot do in relation to the demands of the task. The activity can be simulated or carried out in the real environment. If, for example, the OT practitioner wishes to evaluate a self-care activity like shaving, the client is asked to shave the way he usually does. While observing, the practitioner learns what is needed to improve function in this task. The client's performance may range from complete inability to merely a limited problem with one phase. With information that identifies the extent of the limitation, the OT practitioner can make a plan for correction or improvement.

Another method to carry out a structured observation is through the use of an **activity battery,** or simply a battery. Many OT clinics, especially in psychosocial settings, use different versions of an activity battery. Much can be learned by observing a person engaging in an activity. By putting together several activities in a standardized format, an activity battery is constructed, which can be used to evaluate a person's performance.

In using an activity battery, not only is the end result examined but also how the person responds to directions, approaches the activity, and engages in the task, as well as how he or she relates to the one giving the battery. To standardize the format of the battery, (1) select the activities to be used, (2) choose the exact media (always using the same items), (3) state the time allotment for each activity, and (4) decide upon the verbalizations permitted by the tester. Box 11-1 shows an observation guide for a simple activity battery. A battery should contain a guide for the tester to enable him or her to focus on the desired information being sought. The tester takes notes while the client engages in the activity; from these notes, the tester later writes a summary of the observations. Box 11-2 shows a sample activity battery.

Box 11-1

OBSERVATION GUIDE FOR ACTIVITY BATTERY

There are many types of information that can be gathered from an activity battery, depending on what the evaluator wants to know. Here are three approaches to gathering information:

(1) Analyze the client involvement in terms of the components of the activity:

- Sensorimotor
- Psychological and psychosocial
- Cognitive and cognitive integrative

(2) Assess the client in terms of an overall impression during activities:

- Physical appearance
- Reaction to testing situation
- Response to examiner
- Approach to tasks
- Quality of production
- Verbalizations

(3) Gather information related to specific qualities:

- Attentiveness
- Independence
- Ability to follow verbal instructions
- Ability to follow written instructions
- Cooperativeness
- Initiative
- Response to authority
- Ability to read and write
- Timidity or aggressiveness
- Neatness
- Accuracy
- Distractibility
- Passive or active involvement

Box 11-2

SAMPLE ACTIVITY BATTERY

THIS SAMPLE ACTIVITY BATTERY CONSISTS OF THREE BRIEF ACTIVITIES TO BE COMPLETED WITHIN ONE-HALF HOUR.

ACTIVITY 1: ASK THE CLIENT TO DRAW A SIMPLE PICTURE. THE CLIENT WILL BE ASKED TO DESCRIBE WHAT THEY HAVE DRAWN. THIS IS A FREE-FORM ACTIVITY—IT IS UNSTRUCTURED. THE CLIENT SHOULD NOT BE OFFERED DIRECTION AS TO WHAT TO DRAW.

MATERIALS NEEDED ARE:
PAPER, 8$\frac{1}{2}$" X 11"
SET OF COLORED PENCILS

ACTIVITY 2: ASK THE CLIENT TO COMPLETE A PEG BOARD ACTIVITY, PROVIDING HIM OR HER WITH STANDARDIZED VERBAL STEP-BY-STEP DIRECTIONS. ANY TYPE OF PATTERN CAN BE SET UP (I.E., STAR, LINE, SIMPLE HOUSE). ASK THE CLIENT TO ATTEMPT TO REPRODUCE THE VISUAL PATTERN.

MATERIALS NEEDED ARE:
PEG BOARD
COLORED PEGS
  RED
  BLUE
  GREEN

ACTIVITY 3: ASK THE CLIENT TO WRITE A CHECK, PROVIDING HIM OR HER WITH STANDARDIZED WRITTEN AND VERBAL STEP-BY-STEP DIRECTIONS.

MATERIALS NEEDED ARE:
BLANK CHECK
PEN
DESK CALENDAR
PRINTED INSTRUCTIONS

NOTE: THE OT PRACTITIONER CAN SET UP THESE ACTIVITIES IN A NUMBER OF WAYS; THE ACTUAL ACTIVITIES CAN BE DIFFERENT THAN THOSE SUGGESTED. THE BATTERY IS A GUIDE. IT IS MORE IMPORTANT TO STANDARDIZE THE INSTRUCTIONS TO ENSURE THAT EACH ACTIVITY IS THE SAME FOR ALL CLIENTS.

AFTER EACH ACTIVITY HAS BEEN COMPLETED, THE TESTER (OT PRACTITIONER) SAYS THE FOLLOWING:

"WHAT HAVE YOU LEARNED ABOUT YOURSELF AFTER COMPLETING THESE ACTIVITIES?"

"ARE THERE ANY QUESTIONS YOU WOULD LIKE TO ASK ME ABOUT THE ACTIVITIES YOU HAVE COMPLETED TODAY?"

"THANK YOU FOR YOUR COOPERATION."

A battery is useful in enabling the OT practitioner to quickly learn how the client functions and his or her strengths and weaknesses, as well as gives an indication of his or her response patterns. This information also allows the practitioner to plan future activities that are appropriate and helpful.

With focused attention and refinement of ability as an observer, an OT practitioner begins to observe more subtle pieces of information. The truly skilled observer knows exactly what it is that he or she wants or needs to know from a given person or situation.

FORMAL EVALUATION PROCEDURES

Before meaningful treatment planning can begin, it is necessary to determine the existing performance level of the clients through **formal evaluation procedures.** Formal evaluation procedures include test strategies or instruments that provide specific guidelines for what is to be examined, how it is to be examined, how data are to be communicated, and how the information is to be applied in clinical problem-solving. Because they have specific guidelines, formal evaluation procedures can be duplicated and critically analyzed[12] but may or may not have reliability or validity.

A test is said to have **validity** if it has been demonstrated through research testing to be a true measure of what it claims to measure. Test **reliability** is a measure of how accurately the scores obtained from the test reflect the true performance of the client. There are several different types of reliability with which the OT practitioner must be familiar. **Test-retest reliability** is an indicator of the consistency of the results of a given test from one administration to another. **Interrater reliability** is an indicator of the likelihood that test scores will be the same no matter who is the examiner.[12] The degree of confidence the OT practitioner can place in a particular instrument relates to both its validity and reliability.

Not all formal evaluation procedures are valid or reliable. A **standardized test** has gone through a rigorous process of scientific inquiry to determine its validity and reliability. There is a carefully established manner in which standardized tests must be administered. A test protocol is not just a "nice way to do it." Test reliability and validity rests on following set procedures for its administration and scoring, including the exact words used when administering the test. If standard protocol is not followed, a person may be unduly influenced by the manner of presentation. In addition, standardized tests provide **normative data,** often called *norms,* collected from a representative sample that can then be used by the examiner to make comparisons with his or her subjects. Normative data are compiled by administering the test to a large sample of subjects and determining the scores that are expected of a normal group.[3]

Although there are many standardized tests used by OT practitioners, there are few standardized tests that have been developed by OT practitioners.[12] Two such instruments are the *Miller Assessment for Preschoolers* (MAP)[11] and the *Sensory Integration and Praxis Tests* (SIPT).[4]

OT practitioners also use **nonstandardized tests** for measuring function. These tests often have a set of guidelines for administering and scoring the test; however, some have not gone through the rigorous process of determining test reliability and validity and do not have normative data. The administration and scoring of nonstandardized tests are more subjective and rely on the clinical skill, judgment, and experience of the therapist.[2] Examples of such evaluation procedures are the manual muscle test, which evaluates strength in a muscle or muscle group, and the various sensory tests, which evaluate superficial pain, light touch, proprioception, and hot or cold sensation.

The range of evaluation instruments available to OT practitioners is extremely broad, and the tests named in this section represent only a few sample possibilities. So how does the OTR select the test to use? The frame of reference used at the setting or by the OTR is the first criterion that guides the selection of a test instrument. The selection of a frame of reference (and ultimately the testing instrument used) should consider the background, diagnosis, and needs of the client.

The *Uniform Terminology for Occupational Therapy*, 3rd edition,[1] also is a useful guide in test selection by helping the OTR identify the performance components and performance areas that need to be evaluated for a particular client. There are a number of formal test procedures that may be used to test each of the occupational performance components, areas, and contexts. For example, the performance component of "fine motor coordination and dexterity" can be evaluated using the *Crawford Small Parts Dexterity Test*,[7] the *Purdue Pegboard Test*,[15] or the *Minnesota Rate of Manipulation Test*[16] (Figure 11-3). In Christiansen and Baum's *Occupational Therapy: Overcoming Human Performance Deficits*,[5] several chapters address assessment procedures for a particular performance area, context, or component. The book, *Occupational Therapy Assessment Tools: An Annotated Index*[3] provides information on test instruments used in OT and is also organized according to the *Uniform Terminology*, 3rd edition (see Appendix D). Another resource is the chapter on "Assessment and Evaluation" in *Willard & Spackman's Occupational Therapy*.[14]

Administering any test instrument requires that the OT practitioner be properly prepared.[3] A therapist is expected to know some principles of testing. Any test should be carefully reviewed and practiced before being used to collect actual evaluation data. Before administering a test, the OT practitioner must become familiar with the procedures and know the correct way to score the test and how to interpret the data. (Most standardized tests have booklets with full explanations.) Comfort with any testing procedure is acquired through practice. Some tests even require special training or certification before they can be administered.

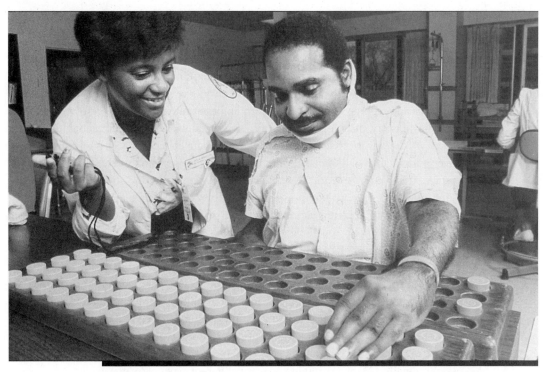

FIGURE 11-3. THIS CLIENT IS BEING EVALUATED USING THE MINNESOTA RATE OF MANIPULATION TEST. (COURTESY OF AOTA, BETHESDA, MD.)

DOCUMENTING THE ASSESSMENT

The findings and summary of the assessment are documented by the OTR. The format of the assessment documentation varies depending on the setting. In some settings, a preprinted form (see Figure 11-1) is all that is used to record evaluation data and summarize the findings. In other settings, the data from the evaluation are summarized in the format of a narrative report.

Regardless of the format used, the initial assessment report should include the following: (1) general information regarding the client (e.g., diagnosis, prior level of function); (2) results of the evaluation and interpretation; (3) status of the client's functional level; and (4) summary of the evaluation, including a problem list, goals, and plan for treatment.[9]

With practice and experience in all of the evaluation procedures described, the OT practitioner becomes effective at gathering the appropriate information during the assessment. The better the information collected during the initial assessment, the easier it is to develop a goal-directed treatment intervention for the client. The next chapter examines how this information is used to develop treatment goals and a plan for intervention.

SUMMARY

The assessment process involves several different approaches for gathering information about a client. These approaches include collection of the initial database, skilled observation, interview, and formal evaluation procedures.

Collection of the initial database entails reviewing the person's medical records and reports, as well as gathering information regarding his or her diagnosis, medical history, prior level of function, and social, work, and educational history.

A therapy interview is a blend of formal data collection with an informal conversational approach aimed toward establishing rapport and trust. There are three stages to an interview: initial contact, information gathering, and closure. During the initial contact, it is important to put the client at ease. Actual information gathered in the interview varies according to the setting. However, the needs of the client are best met through careful planning before client contact is made and then by guiding the interview with the use of an interview schedule. When it is time to end the interview, a pleasant closure impacts favorably on future therapy sessions.

The ability to gather useful information about a client simply through observation is a critical OT skill. By focusing attention on this ability and making a conscious effort to improve it, the natural ability becomes a tool of therapy that is useful in all service delivery—but especially for the purposes of assessment. It is the responsibility of the OT practitioner to develop this skill.

Finally, OT practitioners use many different types of formal evaluation procedures, which have prescribed methods for gathering and recording assessment data. Those formal evaluation procedures that have undergone a thorough scientific inquiry and have measures of reliability and validity, as well as normative data, are referred to as standardized tests. Nonstandardized tests have not undergone this process and, although they may have specific procedures for administration and data recording, do not have data related to norms, reliability, and validity. It is the OT practitioner's responsibility to understand the principles of testing, which will assist in the selection and use of test instruments. It is also necessary that the OT practitioner become familiar with the various tests available and practice using them or attend a training session before administering tests to clients.

GUIDE A: OBSERVATION EXERCISE (from Suggested Activities)

PHYSICAL CHARACTERISTICS

Describe a person and the special qualities that make them an individual. Start with sex, age, and race. Notice face (hair, eyes, mouth, teeth, skin); physique (height, weight, build, posture); arms and legs (scars and defects, marks), and also note hands and fingernails.

MOVEMENTS

Distinguish quality and frequency (e.g., slow, fast, fidgety, rigid, sedentary).

COMMUNICATIONS

Note manner of speaking, quality of voice, content of speech, and nonverbal messages.

ATTITUDE

Observe tone and manner, mood, response to others, qualities or characteristics.

HOW HE OR SHE MAKES YOU FEEL

Be aware of your own emotions (e.g., relaxed, nervous, happy, frustrated, annoyed, want or do not want further contact).

OTHER

GUIDE B: VIDEOTAPE (from Suggested Activities)

VIDEOTAPE TITLE:

SUBJECT MATTER:

GOAL (WHAT YOU WANT TO LEARN):

IMPORTANT POINTS:

OTHER POINTS (REQUIRING RESEARCH):

NAMES AND VOCABULARY TO BE AWARE OF:

PERSONAL OBSERVATIONS:

SUMMARY OF CONTENT:

MY CONCLUSIONS (INCLUDE EVALUATION):

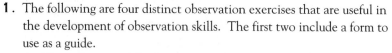

1. The following are four distinct observation exercises that are useful in the development of observation skills. The first two include a form to use as a guide.

   A. The intention of the first exercise (Guide A) is to seek out people's physical descriptions, the object of which is to make the description so complete that the person can be "seen" by the reader. (Keep the focus on the person, not the clothing.)

   B. The next exercise (Guide B) is to be used for videotape viewing so the student can glean the most important points and become aware of things not specifically pointed out. This is fun to do as a class. After watching a videotape, each person notes his or her observations and shares them with the class. The class then watches the videotape again, noticing how much more can be observed the second time when attention is directed to specific points.

   C. Work in twos or threes to design an observation guide for a specific situation that members of the class will experience. Different situations call for changes in focus. Design one for a visit to a clinic. Ask yourself, "What do I want to learn here?" "What do I want to see?" "What are the things I'd like to know about this place?" Then use it for the clinical visit. Discuss it with group members and with the class as a whole if time permits. See if you learn more of what is useful when you develop questions beforehand to help you focus.

   D. A group exercise that demonstrates the power of observation when attention is focused and directed is a "lemon find" (of course, apples and limes can be used). From a bag of randomly selected lemons, equal in amount to the number of participants, each person takes one. Everyone then studies his or her lemon carefully for a few minutes, examining every detail of it. The lemons are then returned to the pile and the participants are asked if they can identify "their" lemons.

2. In groups of two or three, select one of the tests used in OT. Study how to administer it, practice on each other, and demonstrate it to the class.

3. Working in groups of three, choose an interview situation to role play. Identify an interviewer, interviewee, and an observer. Keep the interviewee unaware of the specific content while the other two develop the interview schedule. Then role play an interview in the designated time frame. The observer gives feedback on the interaction. If available, have the observer make a videotape of the interview. Together, assess the results.

Activities—cont'd

> **4.** Select an article from occupational therapy literature that describes a case study. Compile an initial database from the information in the article.

REFERENCES

1. American Occupational Therapy Association: Uniform terminology for occupational therapy, ed 3, *Amer J Occup Ther* 48:1047, 1994.

2. Atchison B: Selecting appropriate assessments. In *Physical disabilities special interest section newsletter,* Bethesda, Md, 1987, AOTA.

3. Asher IE: *Occupational therapy assessment tools: an annotated index,* ed 2, Bethesda, Md, 1996, AOTA.

4. Ayres AJ: *Sensory integration and praxis tests (SIPT),* Los Angeles, 1988, Western Psychological Services.

5. Christiansen C, Baum C: *Occupational therapy: overcoming human performance deficits,* Thorofare, NJ, 1991, Slack.

6. Cook AM, Hussey SM: *Assistive technologies: principles and practice,* St Louis, 1995, Mosby.

7. Crawford JE, Crawford DM: *Crawford small parts dexterity test,* San Antonio, 1956 (rev 1981), Psychological Corporation.

8. Dunn W: Assessing sensory performance enablers. In Christiansen C, Baum C, editors: *Occupational therapy: overcoming performance deficits,* Thorofare, NJ, 1991, Slack.

9. Jabri J: Documentation of OT services. In Pedretti LW, editor: *Occupational therapy: practice skills for physical dysfunction,* ed 4, St Louis, 1996, Mosby.

10. Matsutsuyu J: The interest checklist, *Amer J Occup Ther* 23:323, 1969.

11. Miller L: *Miller assessment for preschoolers (MAP),* San Antonio, 1982, Psychological Corporation.

12. Opacich KJ: Assessment and informed decision-making. In Christiansen C, Braum C, editors: *Occupational therapy: overcoming human performance deficits,* Thorofare, NJ, 1991, Slack.

13. Pedretti LW: Occupational therapy evaluation and assessment of physical dysfunction. In Pedretti LW, editor: *Occupational therapy: practice skills for physical dysfunction,* ed 4, St Louis, 1996, Mosby.

14. Smith HD: Assessment and evaluation: an overview. In Hopkins HL, Smith HD, editors: *Willard & Spackman's occupational therapy,* ed 8, Philadelphia, 1993, JB Lippincott.

15. Tiffin J: *Purdue pegboard test,* 1948 (rev 1960), Lafayette, Ind, Lafayette Instrument Company.

16. University of Minnesota Employment Stabilization Research Institute: *Minnesota rate of manipulation test (MRMT),* Circle Pines, Minn, 1969, American Guidance Service.

17. Watanabe S: Regional Institute on the evaluation process, *New York Report* RAS-123-T-68, Rockville, Md, 1968, AOTA.

I was attracted to the profession when I realized the power of its medium—occupation. Life is, essentially, a chain of occupations. Occupation gives the context in which people build their skills, discover their interests, and reveal their hopes. Purposes in life are worked out through occupation. At the same time, occupation can influence and transform these purposes. The power of occupation lies in its intertwining of the person's body, mind, soul, and world. The work of the occupational therapist is to be an expert on the complexity of occupation and to use that knowledge artfully to help others achieve a life that is purposeful and meaningful. It is within this process where the therapist finds purpose and meaning; it is within this process where curiosity and wonder about how people create occupation grows. ■

René Padilla, MS, OTR/L
Assistant Professor
Department of Occupational Therapy
Creighton University
Omaha, Nebraska

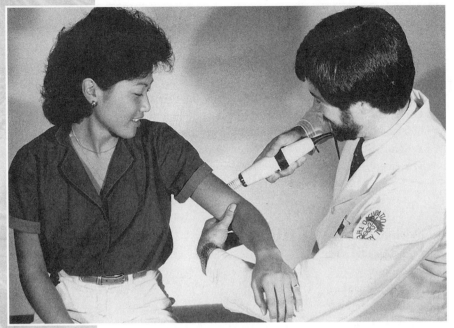

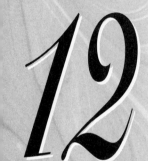

Treatment Planning and Implementation

Objectives

After reading this chapter, the reader will be able to:

❖ Identify the steps in a generic problem-solving approach and recognize the relevance to the occupational therapy (OT) process
❖ Become familiar with specific techniques to improve problem-solving skills
❖ Identify the five general treatment approaches used in OT
❖ Understand the difference between long-term and short-term goals
❖ Recognize the importance of documentation throughout the OT process and the elements that comprise effective documentation

Key terms

Critical thinking
Functional fixedness
Brainstorming
Problem identification
Solution development
General OT goals
Rehabilitative and educational approach
Compensatory approach
Assistive technology approach
Activity or environmental accommodation approach
Personal assistance approach
Individual client goals
Long-term goals
Short-term goals
Plan of action
Treatment implementation
Re-evaluation
RUMBA
Problem-Oriented Medical Record
SOAP note

The introductory chapter of this text begins with the definition, "Occupational therapy is goal-directed activity to promote independence in function." The aim of the OT practitioner is to enable the person with a disability to function more independently in his or her environment. This goal requires finding solutions to problems; therefore OT can be further defined as "problem solving to develop a plan that improves function in those whose occupational performance is impaired." Throughout OT's differing

Chapter 12 photo: Pedretti LW: *Occupational therapy: practice skills for physical dysfunction*, ed 4, St Louis, 1996, Mosby.

approaches and considering the enormous range of the clients it serves, problem solving to improve function is the unifying theme that identifies OT.

Accordingly, the role of an OT practitioner is that of a problem solver. It is necessary for the practitioner to call upon problem solving and clinical reasoning skills to set goals and build a program that is both functional and purposeful, as well as meaningful to the client. To grasp the OT process more fully, it is important to have an understanding of how the practitioner plans the client's program, selects his or her activities, and directs treatment that then guides the client to learn ways of improving occupational performance.

PROBLEM-SOLVING APPROACH

Problem solving means identifying problems and setting goals, then taking the needed steps—adapting what is at hand—to accomplish these goals. This approach is fundamentally different from mechanically applying a prescribed technique. Skill in problem solving is important to the successful practice of OT. The practitioner who clearly realizes that problem solving promotes independence and better function will not lose the sense of purpose of the therapy. The practitioner who regards himself or herself as engaged in a problem-solving process is seeking ever higher levels of client performance. He or she is less likely to allow clinical involvement to become repetitive and boring.

Problem solving has received much attention in recent years with a new focus in psychology called *cognitive psychology*. This focus, which has grown with the use of computers, attempts to understand and explain human thought processes. One unique human ability is solving problems—gathering many pieces of information and putting them together in such a way as to accomplish what otherwise may seem an impossible task.

Cognitive psychologists identify the following generic components of the problem-solving process: (1) *preparation* (or formulating the problem; also called *exploration*), (2) *production* (or generating possible solutions), and (3) *evaluation* (or evaluating solutions). Some authorities prefer to divide the first step into two: (a) identify and (b) prepare—thus yielding a four-step process.[7] This process of gathering information in search of a solution to a problem requires critical thinking, a process that has received emphasis within the educational community. Since 1980, Sonoma State University's Center for Critical Thinking has sponsored conferences on "Critical Thinking and Educational Reform." The same principles that underlie critical thinking apply to the steps of the OT process, because clinical practice demands a high degree of reasoning.

Critical thinking is the ability and willingness to examine information and circumstances in such a way as to assess what is presented, look for the flaws, and make objective judgments based on well-supported reasons. It is the ability to be creative and constructive by generating possible explanations for findings, identifying possible implications, and applying new knowledge from a broad range of sources, while remaining open to new possibilities. Among essential critical thinking skills are information gathering, organizing, analyzing, generating, integrating, and evaluating.[3] The OT process plainly fits with what cognitive psychologists and educators teach about efficient and effective problem solving (Figure 12-1).

DEVELOPMENT OF PROBLEM-SOLVING SKILLS

Since clients are needed to apply the OT process, it cannot be readily accomplished in the classroom. However, it is possible to lay the foundation by becoming thoroughly familiar with and gaining practice in general problem-solving techniques.

UNDERSTANDING THE PROBLEM

In problem solving the emphasis is on clarity of thinking. To do this, one must separate the steps of thinking when seeking solutions. Often effectiveness is

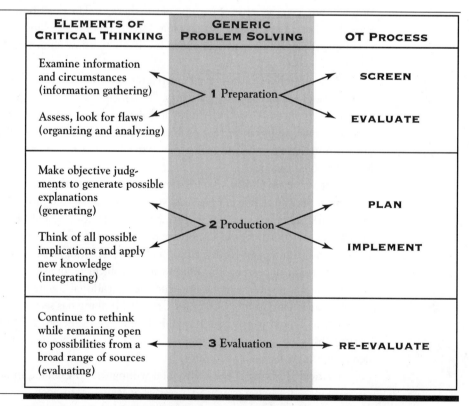

ELEMENTS OF CRITICAL THINKING	GENERIC PROBLEM SOLVING	OT PROCESS
Examine information and circumstances (information gathering)	1 Preparation	SCREEN
Assess, look for flaws (organizing and analyzing)		EVALUATE
Make objective judgments to generate possible explanations (generating)	2 Production	PLAN
Think of all possible implications and apply new knowledge (integrating)		IMPLEMENT
Continue to rethink while remaining open to possibilities from a broad range of sources (evaluating)	3 Evaluation	RE-EVALUATE

FIGURE 12-1. OPERATING FROM A PROBLEM-SOLVING FRAME OF REFERENCE.

confused by jumping to an answer too soon. An answer should be delayed until the problem is clearly understood.

In a book entitled *Psychology*, Spencer Rathus tells us, "We prepare ourselves to solve a problem by familiarizing ourselves with its elements and clearly defining our goals." He continues, "One of the difficulties in solving the problems of daily life is that they tend to be ill defined. The elements in the problems are not clearly laid out, and the goals or desired outcomes are also cloudy."[7] These should be words of caution to OT practitioners, who must learn to define the problem clearly before trying to develop solutions. If the problem is not clearly defined, it is likely that the solutions that are proposed and implemented will not be effective.

FUNCTIONAL FIXEDNESS

A block to good problem solving is "getting locked into standard ways of thinking so that you fail to see other possibilities." This is termed **functional fixedness.** If asked to list uses for a paper clip—beyond holding papers together—the length of the list will bear an inverse relationship to one's functional fixedness. The more that things are viewed in terms of their familiar usage, the more "fixed" the thinking. Breaking out of fixed patterns of thinking enables OT practitioners to identify good adaptations and solutions to problems.

It would be a good skill-building practice to identify common items and make lists of uses—as long as possible—adding to the list as new ideas occur. To expand on this concept, the reader is referred to Roger von Oech's book, *A Whack on the Side of the Head.*[11]

Brainstorming is a technique used by people to come up with numerous possibilities for solving a problem. This technique is familiar to many people and has become a commonly used word to describe any production of ideas by a group of people. However, it is actually the name of a specific technique with rules of operation (Box 12-1). The concept behind brainstorming is that the ideas generated by the individuals in the group are not to be criticized or judged. This allows individuals to feel comfortable presenting whatever ideas come to mind without being fearful of being "wrong." Many real-life problems can be solved in this manner, and it is fun! It is a good way to practice group problem solving.

The student, in preparation to becoming a future practitioner, must learn by reason, not rote memorization of someone else's thought. Understanding will not just "happen"; it requires disciplined reasoning and practice at problem solving. In the journal, *Educational Vision*, it is stated, "Students must think their way in and through content: creating understanding, making connections, and mastering applications."[4] Furthermore, as Arthur Schopenhauer wrote in 1851, "Thinking has to be kindled, as a fire is by a drought, and kept going by some kind of interest in its object."[9] Whatever the methods or techniques, the more skilled the practitioner becomes at problem solving, the more effective he or she will be.

Box 12-1

BRAINSTORMING

A GROUP OF EIGHT TO TWELVE PEOPLE ARE ASSEMBLED. ONE MEMBER TAKES THE ROLE OF "FACILITATOR," AND ONE OR TWO MEMBERS ACT AS "RECORDERS." LARGE PIECES OF PAPER ARE PLACED ON THE WALL, AND MARKERS ARE AVAILABLE. BLACKBOARD AND CHALK MAY ALSO BE USED.

THE GROUP IS GIVEN A SPECIFIC PROBLEM AND A TIME FRAME. IN THE FIRST PHASE THE TASK OF THE GROUP IS TO GENERATE AS MANY DIFFERENT SOLUTIONS AS POSSIBLE, COMPLETELY FREE OF CRITICISM (NO JUDGMENTS ABOUT GOOD OR BAD, IF IT WILL WORK, HOW MUCH IT COSTS, ETC.). THE OBJECTIVE IS TO COME UP WITH SOLUTIONS—NO MATTER HOW FAR-FETCHED. THE FACILITATOR POINTS TO EACH GROUP MEMBER IN TURN AND REPEATS THEIR SOLUTION TO THE RECORDER, WHO WRITES THE SOLUTION DOWN AS FAST AS POSSIBLE. IDEAS TEND TO GENERATE IDEAS, AND MEMBERS ARE ENCOURAGED TO "SPARK OFF" OF EACH OTHER.

AT THE END OF THE IDEA-GENERATING PHASE, THE GROUP EVALUATES AND PRIORITIZES—USELESS IDEAS ARE ELIMINATED, SOME ARE COMBINED, AND EVENTUALLY THE GROUP IDENTIFIES A SOLUTION OR THE SOLUTIONS OF CHOICE.

PROBLEM SOLVING IN OCCUPATIONAL THERAPY

Whereas all problem-solving methods are useful for the OT practitioner, the attention of this text now turns toward a specific problem-solving method that is used in OT and described by many authors.[1,2,5] Specifically, Hopkins describes one problem-solving approach that includes the following five steps[2]:

1. Problem identification
2. Solution development
3. Development of a plan of action
4. Implementation of the plan
5. Assessment of results

One can easily see the similarities between this approach and that of cognitive psychology and critical thinking.

IDENTIFICATION OF THE PROBLEM

Problem identification is the initial step in the treatment planning process. The OT practitioner gathers all the information from the evaluation. It is analyzed and summarized to delineate the client's deficits in occupational performance areas and performance components. The problems identified are ones that require OT intervention.

The first step is to review the results of the OT evaluation. The OT practitioner examines the person's total output in terms of strengths (skills) and weaknesses (deficits) and compares this information with what the person desires or what is required by the environment. From this, a list of the individual's problems and assets is compiled. (A case study showing an example of such a list is shown in Box 12-2.)

Problem identification also includes determining, as much as one is able at this point, the cause of the problem. Understanding the root of the problem will help the OT practitioner select the most appropriate approach to treatment.[1]

DEVELOPING SOLUTIONS

After the examination of the OT evaluation and the identification of the problems, **solution development** begins. At this juncture, alternatives for treatment are investigated, and goals and objectives are formed. The OT practitioner then makes recommendations for solving the performance problems.

FRAMES OF REFERENCE

Selecting a frame of reference from which the OT practitioner operates is the first step in solution development. There are several frames of reference that are available for use in treatment. As discussed in Chapter 9, each frame of reference is based on a body of knowledge and identifies principles and processes of change. The frame of reference selected influences the problem-solving process and provides guidelines for the practitioner's clinical reasoning and treatment planning.[5] Referring again to the case study in Box 12-2, the rehabilitative and biomechanical frames of reference are used.

GENERAL OCCUPATIONAL THERAPY GOALS

It is also important to take into consideration the general goals of OT during the solution development phase. **General OT goals** apply to service delivery in a broad sense; they identify the general intent of OT services and, as such, represent "the big picture." To manage the diversity of possibilities, an OT practitioner frames the individual treatment plan within the general goals of OT.

Is it possible to make general statements about the goals of OT that will apply to all unique situations? Yes, by defining OT's purpose and framing the fundamental concepts—concepts that form the base from which many unique applications are generated. For the OT practitioner, these concepts must be internalized; they become part of the practitioner's "alphabet."

Perhaps an analogy will make this point more clear. To become literate, a person first learns the alphabet and practices the characters until they become second nature. Once a person reaches literacy, he or she rarely thinks of the alphabet. As the person reads or writes, he or she merely considers the words before thinking of the ones to use for expression. The words are the focus.

The analogy is appropriate, since OT practitioners are not technicians who perform specific sets of tasks. They employ fundamental concepts to new and ever-changing situations, never knowing ahead of time what will be needed in the next situation. An OT practitioner must have the "OT alphabet" so ingrained that there is no need to give attention to it but rather focus on the problems and solu-

Continued on page 164

Box 12-2

CASE STUDY

PERSONAL DATA

NAME: Dale Horton

AGE: 19

DIAGNOSIS: Spinal cord injury, C7, C8 secondary to motor vehicle accident

REASON FOR REFERRAL: OT evaluation and treatment for increased functioning in activities of daily living, upper extremity strengthening, community re-entry

OTHER SERVICES: Physician, physical therapy, social services

FRAMES OF REFERENCE

REHABILITATIVE AND BIOMECHANICAL

OT EVALUATION SUMMARY

Muscle testing reveals that the client has normal strength for all shoulder movements; good strength for elbow extension, radial wrist flexion, ulnar wrist extension, and forearm pronation; fair strength for flexion of the elbow, PIP, DIP, and MCP extension; poor strength for extension of the PIP and DIP joints and MCP flexion. Trunk muscles are poor, and trunk control impaired.

Range of motion is within normal limits for all joints. Coordination and dexterity are impaired in both hands as a result of reduced strength. Grasp and release are limited. Endurance is fair, and he is able to tolerate OT treatment 2 hours per day but needs periodic rest breaks.

Sensory modalities of touch, pain, temperature, and proprioception are intact in both upper extremities. The client has no feeling below his navel. No cognitive or perceptual deficits are observed.

Before his injury, Dale lived with his parents and attended the local community college. He was enrolled in computer science courses. He was independent in all ADLs. He was very active, played football, and enjoyed going to rock music concerts. He was also employed as a part-time cashier at a video store.

The injury has brought about the loss of Dale's independence in ADLs. He is able to feed himself independently. He is independent with upper body dressing but requires moderate assistance for lower extremity dressing. He requires moderate assistance to transfer in and out of his wheelchair and minimal assistance to roll side to side and come from a supine to a sitting position. He has a manual wheelchair for mobility and propels using both upper extremities. His endurance for wheelchair mobility is decreasing and limited to smooth, even surfaces. He requires assistance for getting through doors, going up ramps, and

ADLs, Activities of daily living; DIP, distal interphalangeal; MCP, metacarpophalangeal; OT, occupational therapy; PIP, proximal interphalangeal.

Box 12-2—cont'd

maneuvering over rough terrain. A lightweight wheelchair will need to be prescribed and purchased for his use after discharge. Evaluation for driving also needs to be considered.

After his injury, Dale has been depressed. He does not see how he can return to school and to his former job as a cashier. Furthermore, he realizes that he will not be able to play football; he was a good football player and loved the sport, spending most of his free time on the practice field.

ASSETS

1. In excellent health and fitness before injury; good residual upper body strength
2. Good joint mobility
3. Supportive family and friends
4. Home is on ground level, single story, and accessible
5. Cognitive and perceptual skills intact

PROBLEMS IDENTIFIED

1. Dependence in wheelchair mobility
2. Dependence in lower extremity dressing
3. Assistance required for transfers from wheelchair to various surfaces
4. Assistance required for rolling and sitting to and from supine position
5. Low physical endurance
6. Apparent depression; does not realize his own potential for rehabilitation
7. Interruption in leisure and play and in education and work activities

PROBLEM 1: DEPENDENCE IN WHEELCHAIR MOBILITY*

Long-term goal

Dale will be independent in wheelchair mobility over all surfaces and in all situations.

Short-term goals	**Methods and modalities**
1. Within 3 days, Dale will propel his wheelchair over a smooth surface (e.g., linoleum) for 50 feet with supervision.	1. Progressive resistive exercises and activities for increasing upper extremity strength for wheelchair mobility are prescribed.
2. Within 5 days, Dale will independently propel his wheelchair 100 feet over a smooth surface.	2. Instruct and demonstrate proper techniques for wheelchair mobility.

*Only one problem is listed. In actual practice the OT practitioner writes goals and treatment plans (methods and modalities, gradation and assistive devices) for each problem identified.

Continued

Box 12-2—cont'd

Short-term goals—cont'd

3. Within 7 days, Dale will independently maneuver his wheelchair in and out of doors.
4. Within 9 days, Dale will independently propel his wheelchair over varied terrain, including carpet, grass, dirt, and asphalt.
5. Within 14 days, Dale will independently propel his wheelchair up a standard ramp.

Methods and modalities—cont'd

3. Instruct and demonstrate access in and out of doorways, up and down ramps, and over curbs.
4. Training is provided for teaching wheelchair management over varied terrain including linoleum, carpet, grass, dirt, and asphalt.
5. Assistance is provided in obtaining appropriate wheelchair and related adaptations as needed.

GRADATION AND ASSISTIVE DEVICES

Grade by increasing resistance and repetitions for exercises; progressing from smooth and level terrain to rough and uneven terrain. Grade by increasing amount of time and distance propelling wheelchair as endurance improves. Provide lightweight wheelchair, friction tape for wheelchair hand rims, and appropriate cushion.

tions at hand. As with the literate person who does not focus on the letters but mentally manipulates the internalized alphabet to read or express, so the practitioner develops goals or selects activities.

As stated previously, the overall aim of OT is to help the client with a disability to function as independently as possible in his or her environment. This focus is the same, no matter the sphere of practice in which the OT practitioner works. There are five basic approaches, or general goals, that the OT discipline uses to reach this aim.[10] These approaches, which may apply to any general type of client population, are: (1) the **rehabilitative and educational approach,** which aims to improve the intrinsic abilities and functional skills of the individual; (2) the **compensatory approach,** wherein the person gains other skills to help him or her adapt in spite of the impairment or disability; (3) the **assistive technology approach,** wherein the individual is provided devices to help function in the presence of a disability; (4) the **activity or environmental accommodation approach,** wherein the environment or the expectations of the tasks required are adapted; and (5) the **personal assistance approach,** in which the individual is assisted by another person (e.g., spouse, caregiver, parent) to perform a task or tasks.[10]

This approach can be applied to a situation in which an individual has had a cerebral vascular accident, also referred to as a stroke. He has lost the use of the right side of his body and, among other things, is now unable to tie his shoes. Figure 12-2

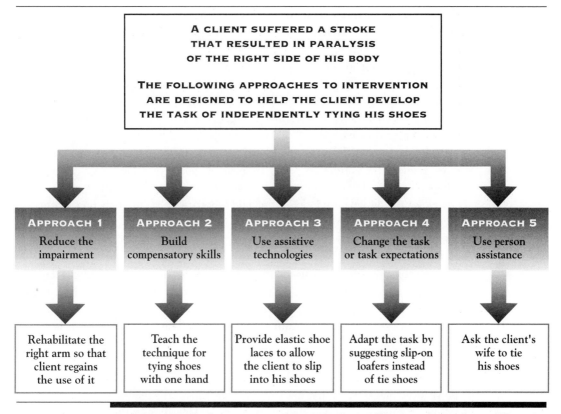

FIGURE 12-2. APPROACHES TO INTERVENTION. (MODIFIED FROM SMITH RO: MEASURING THE OUTCOMES OF ASSISTIVE TECHNOLOGY: CHALLENGE AND INNOVATION, <u>ASSISTIVE TECHNOLOGY</u>, 8(2):71, 1996.)

shows the five approaches previously described and the ways OT could be applied in this situation. Possible options for the OT practitioner include: (1) rehabilitating the right arm so that the client regains the use of this extremity, (2) teaching the person a compensatory technique for tying his shoes wherein only one hand is used, (3) providing the person with elastic shoe laces (assistive technology) that will allow him to simply slip his foot into the shoes, (4) changing the expectations of the environment (making it acceptable to go barefoot) or adapting the task by suggesting he wear slip-on loafers instead of tie shoes, and (5) asking his wife to tie his shoes.

As this example demonstrates, problems confronting OT practitioners can be addressed in a number of ways. Although this may seem overwhelming to the student, the approaches described are examples of the "OT alphabet," and thinking through theses options becomes automatic for the experienced OT practitioner. These general OT goals identify parameters within which practitioners can work as they develop the goals for any individual's treatment plan.

INDIVIDUAL CLIENT GOALS

The **individual client goals** are those within the person's treatment plan that delineate specific accomplishments toward which he or she is aiming. A good treatment plan is based on very specific and individualized goals. The individualized goals identify a target for treatment and the means for reaching it. The best idea can be lost without an approach that enables it to be realized. The goals of the individual treatment plan are the means for turning a good idea into a realistic outcome. Stating goals enables the practitioner to organize his or her thinking in a way that will support progressive movement toward improved functioning.

Goals developed for the individual's treatment plan are labeled in different ways. Some OT practitioners prefer to speak of "goals" and "objectives," whereas others prefer "goals" and "subgoals" or "general goals" and "specific goals." Still others use the designation "long-term" and "short-term" goals. Labeling is a matter of personal choice; the important thing is to learn to clearly identify expected outcomes. For purposes of this text, the terms "long-term goals" and "short-term goals" are used.

At this point it is best to identify what goals mean in therapy. Goals developed for the individual's treatment plan provide both a long-term and short-term focus. A **long-term goal** is a broad view that identifies the general changes in the individual's function over a certain period of time. The long-term goal is broken down into smaller bits, which are steps on the way to the long-term goals. These steps are called **short-term goals.**

The long-term goal is a broad statement of individual program intent and answers the question, "What am I trying to achieve?" Examples are: "The client will be independent in wheelchair mobility." "The client will verbally express feelings." "The client will transfer hand dominance." All of these could be appropriate long-term goals for different clients in different settings. The short-term goals are an enumeration of the smaller steps that lead to the ultimate accomplishment of the long-term goal. The case study presented in Box 12-2 illustrates an example of a long-term goal and short-term goals related to the problem of dependence in wheelchair mobility.

Writing goals forces the practitioner to clarify what needs to be accomplished. The elements of the problem are clearly laid out, and the solution is defined, assuring better therapy. Goal writing is a professional responsibility, and it is another element of the "OT alphabet." The efficient writing of goals requires time, practice, and continual refinement of work selection. Later in this chapter the writing of goals and other forms of written documentation are addressed.

PRACTICE IN GOAL SETTING

Setting goals is not reserved for therapy programs; the principle of setting goals can always apply to day-to-day living. To prepare for future goal writing, begin to *think* in terms of goals. The following example from everyday life illustrates how this concept can be practiced.

A person taking a psychology class wants to get a good grade. She sets a long-term goal: "To get an A on the next examination." She sets four short-term goals to enable her to achieve the main goal: (1) attend all classes and take good notes; (2) read and highlight assigned chapters 4, 5, and 6; (3) correlate class notes to text reading to identify emphasized points; and (4) complete the exercises in the study guide the day before the test. If this plan is followed, she will achieve the goal.

Goal setting is a plan of action—establish the goal of what is wanted or needed, then identify the steps to ensure achievement of that goal. The argument, "Everyone decides what they want and takes steps to get it," misses the point. Actions *are* (or should be) goal directed. Formal goal setting keeps an individual focused on the goal and ensures accomplishment without getting side-tracked.

DEVELOPING A PLAN OF ACTION

Once long- and short-term goals have been developed, the next step is to identify treatment methods and modalities that will help the client fulfill the goals. This step becomes the **plan of action.** The plan details the activities that will be used to achieve the goals, as well as the tools or equipment needed and special positioning, where the activity will take place, how it will be structured and graded, and whether it is to be performed in a group or individually.[2] (Refer to Box 12-2 for an example of treatment methods and modalities for the client in the case study.)

The OT practitioner selects treatment methods based on the frames of reference or treatment principles, which are related to the underlying problems.[1] The practitioner uses his or her knowledge of the disability and the treatment principles and activities to predict which methods will likely achieve the desired results (e.g., as stated in the goals). In Chapter 16 the types of therapeutic activities that are used in OT are discussed.

IMPLEMENTING THE TREATMENT PLAN

Treatment implementation is, as the term suggests, the implementation of the treatment plan developed for the client. The OT practitioner keeps the plan in mind and ensures that the correct sequence of activities is supporting a graded program of activity. In some cases this will be the time to discuss what the client is doing outside the treatment time to support his or her goals; the practitioner will often give "homework" assignments. The program must be in agreement with the tolerance level of the client. It is also necessary to remember that outside stresses may affect a person's ability to perform or engage in an activity on any given day. The OT practitioner must always be ready to adapt to unexpected needs or demands.

It is important to note that interaction between the practitioner and client is an essential element of therapy and requires decision making. A therapeutic relationship should always have the interest of the client as its central concern. The practitioner's role is to choose the interaction style that best supports the goals of the treatment plan and to help the client move toward independence. Setting the tone of interaction will be a decision made on the basis of the overall cognitive ability and attitude of the client. An adolescent with a history of substance abuse, an older person who has had a stroke, or a child with cerebral palsy will call for different approaches. The OT practitioner must decide which approach will be the most therapeutic and beneficial to the client. Although it does not usually happen immediately, a "therapeutic climate" emerges. In Chapter 15 the development of a therapeutic relationship is described in detail.

ASSESSMENT OF THE RESULTS

Once the treatment plan has been implemented, it is important to monitor or assess the results. This assessment is accomplished through an on-going process of **re-evaluation.** If the goals for the client have been clearly written, it should not be difficult to determine if progress toward them is being made. Re-evaluation can be done formally or informally.

The OT practitioner automatically performs an informal assessment of the client during each treatment session. As the practitioner's decisions are implemented, he or she continuously monitors the impact and evaluates whether the activity being performed by the client is having the desired therapeutic effect. For example, if the activity becomes too easy for the client, the OT practitioner may increase the level of difficulty by adding resistance or by asking the client to sit rather than stand. Schon refers to this informal assessment as "reflection-in-action,"[8] or informal re-evaluation; it is an extremely important aspect of the therapeutic process. As an OT practitioner becomes more experienced, the ability to monitor, evaluate, and revise will improve.

Formal assessment, or formal re-evaluation, of the client can also take place. This means re-administering one of the evaluation procedures described in Chapter 11 to determine whether the client has improved. Through on-going re-evaluation, the OT practitioner determines whether the goals need to be changed (as a result of the client not making progress), or it may be determined that the client has met all of the goals outlined and is ready for discharge.

DISCONTINUATION OF SERVICES

At some point the client is discharged from OT. A number of factors determine the appropriate time to terminate an individual's treatment. The best situation is one in which the client meets all goals delineated in therapy and functions independently in the occupational performance areas. In another instance the initial treatment goals are met and new goals are identified on which services can focus. Finally, in another instance the client is not making any significant progress toward the goals even though several adjustments have been tried. Sometimes progress slows or stops altogether; in such cases, continuation of OT services can no longer be justified.

It is important that the client is prepared for the discontinuation of services and that a discharge plan is developed before actual discontinuation. As discussed in an earlier chapter, the discharge plan includes recommendations for continued services (including OT, if necessary), equipment recommendations, and any program of therapy the client is to follow after discharge. In addition, if training of family members and caregivers has not already taken place, it should be carried out before the client's discharge.

DOCUMENTATION

In today's world it is extremely important to keep accurate records on all the aspects of care giving. There are evaluation reports, daily progress notes, summary reports, and discharge plans, as well as the need to give constant attention to the treatment plan to determine whether identified goals require revision. It is necessary to communicate to others, orally and in writing, the status of the clients in treatment. A system of checks and balances requires that all treatment remains on target.

Documentation will vary from facility to facility. Many ways to document evaluations and treatment plans are available for use by the OT practitioner. The evaluation and treatment plan depends on the record system used in the employment setting.

Documentation that is correctly written is **R**elevant, **U**nderstandable, **M**easurable, **B**ehavioral, and **A**chievable. To determine whether documentation satisfies this criteria, recall the mnemonic code, **RUMBA.**

A *relevant* goal is one that reflects the needs and wishes of the person and family. Independence is not fostered by improving function in something about which the person cares little. A goal that is relevant relates to function. Increasing an individual's grip strength from 10 pounds to 80 pounds is not relevant unless it is related to a functional goal (e.g., returning to a line of work as a grocery checker).

Documentation that is *understandable* is legible, easy to read, and void of jargon. The OT practitioner should remember that others will be reading his or her documentation, and they may not understand the jargon familiar in OT. Documentation that is concise and free of spelling and grammatical errors is understandable.[6]

Writing goals that are *measureable* means that a type of criterion in which success will be measured is included. For example, the statement, "Mary will propel her wheelchair," cannot be easily measured. "Mary will propel her wheelchair independently from her room to therapy at least once a day for a week," more precisely indicates what is expected of Mary and when she has met the stated goal.

A goal or statement that is *behavioral* focuses on "occurrences that are seen and can be measured."[6] For example, sitting straight in a wheelchair is a behavior that can be observed and measured. The phrase "tolerated treatment well" is not an observable behavior.

Finally, a goal that is *achievable* can be realistically met by the client within given time constraints (e.g., imposed by insurance or regulatory bodies).[6]

Another aspect of documentation worthy of discussion is the progress note. The type of progress reporting varies from facility to facility. In some cases a progress note is required each time the client is seen (also called a treatment note); in other cases it is required on a daily or weekly basis. Progress notes can be as brief as a checklist, in which the OT practitioner places a check mark by the activities that were performed in treatment, to a daily narrative note describing the treatment session (Box 12-3), to a weekly progress note (Box 12-4).

A common method of progress note writing that is used in medical settings is the **Problem-Oriented Medical Record** (POMR). This format, developed by Dr. Lawrence Weed,[12] is a way of providing a structure to note writing. As the name suggests, this system is based on a list of problems identified by the treatment team during the assessment of the client. Subsequent progress notes relate to the problem(s) identified in the list. The format used for writing the progress note is referred to as the **SOAP note. S** is *subjective* (information reported by the client); **O** is *objective* (clinical findings or measurable, observable data); **A** is *assessment* (OT practitioner's professional judgment or opinion); **P** is *plan* (specific plan of action to be followed).[6] In Box 12-5 a sample SOAP note documents a treatment session for the client in the case study (see Box 12-2).

𝓑𝓸𝔁 12-3

SAMPLE NARRATIVE DAILY NOTE

CLIENT ACTIVELY PARTICIPATED IN EATING RETRAINING AND RIGHT UPPER EXTREMITY STRENGTHENING PROGRAM. CLIENT ATE 75% OF MEAL WITH ADAPTED UTENSILS AND REQUIRED MINIMAL ASSISTANCE FOR CUTTING MEAT. ESTABLISHED TREATMENT PLAN TO CONTINUE.

Modified from Early MB: *Physical dysfunction practice skills for the occupational therapy assistant*, St Louis, 1998, Mosby.

𝓑𝓸𝔁 12-4

SAMPLE WEEKLY PROGRESS NOTE

CLIENT HAS BEEN SEEN DAILY FOR EATING RETRAINING AND RIGHT UPPER EXTREMITY FUNCTIONAL STRENGTHENING PROGRAM. USING ADAPTED UTENSILS, CLIENT ATE 75% OF MEAL WITH MINIMAL ASSISTANCE FOR CUTTING MEAT. PREVIOUSLY, CLIENT ATE 50% OF MEAL AND REQUIRED MODERATE ASSISTANCE FOR CUTTING MEAT. CLIENT WILL EAT INDEPENDENTLY WITH NO ASSISTIVE DEVICES IN 1 WEEK.

Modified from Early MB: *Physical dysfunction practice skills for the occupational therapy assistant*, St Louis, 1998, Mosby.

ℬox 12-5

SAMPLE SOAP NOTE

PROBLEM 1: DEPENDENCE IN WHEELCHAIR MOBILITY

S: CLIENT STATED THAT HIS HANDS OFTEN SLIP ON METAL HAND RIMS WHEN PROPELLING WHEELCHAIR.

O: FRICTION TAPE PLACED ON RIMS OF WHEELCHAIR TO IMPROVE CLIENT'S ABILITY TO GRASP AND PROPEL CHAIR. WHEELCHAIR MOBILITY TRAINING OUTSIDE OVER GRASS AND ASPHALT WAS PROVIDED. CLIENT PARTICIPATED FOR 30 MINUTES IN WHEELCHAIR TRAINING WITH ONLY 5-MINUTE REST PERIOD. NO DIFFICULTY PROPELLING WHEELCHAIR OVER VARIED TERRAIN.

A: FRICTION TAPE ON RIMS HELPED IMPROVE CLIENT'S ABILITY TO PROPEL WHEELCHAIR. CLIENT'S ENDURANCE FOR WHEELCHAIR MOBILITY IMPROVED OVER YESTERDAY.

P: CONTINUE OT TRAINING IN WHEELCHAIR MOBILITY. INCREASE TIME AND DISTANCE FOR WHEELCHAIR MOBILITY. TEACH CLIENT HOW TO MANEUVER WHEELCHAIR IN AND OUT OF DOORS AND UP AND DOWN RAMPS.

The individual philosophy of the employment setting is the final determinant of the what, where, and how of record keeping, but the habit of good planning and regular charting makes record keeping easier, whatever the demands. Good planning and record keeping lead to better quality treatments.

SUMMARY

Critical-thinking skills are essential to becoming a competent OT practitioner. These skills include information gathering, organizing, analyzing, generating, integrating, and evaluating. It is therefore essential that the student become a self-determining, independent thinker. The task of therapy is to find solutions to existing problems and to teach clients to apply them.

The OT process involves a problem-solving approach that includes five steps. Identifying and understanding the nature of the problem is the first step to a solution. Consideration of the available frames of reference, the general OT goals, and the needs of the client is the second step to a solution. The development of solutions leads to the specification of a plan of action. This plan includes the delineation of individualized long-term and short-term goals that are relevant to the person's situation.

With a plan in mind, the OT practitioner proceeds with its implementation through the appropriate treatment methods. Once the plan has been implemented, the astute practitioner begins assessing the results, continuously re-evaluating (formally or informally) the client and making adjustments to the treatment plan as needed. The OT practitioner determines whether the client is progressing toward the identified goals.

The client is discharged from therapy when it is determined that all OT goals have been met or when insufficient progress is being made to justify continued treatment. It is important that all OT evaluation and treatment is documented in the form of a report, progress note, or discharge summary. The type and frequency of documentation varies, depending on the facility.

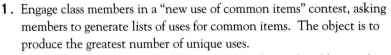

1. Engage class members in a "new use of common items" contest, asking members to generate lists of uses for common items. The object is to produce the greatest number of unique uses.
2. Conduct a class brainstorming session. Identify a real problem in the school or club. Lead the class in brainstorming the problem.
3. Research functional fixedness (psychology textbooks are one source), and present to the class several simple exercises or problems that encourage breaking out of functional fixedness.
4. Seek out a published problem-solving method. Present it to the class through visual aids, and then have the class engage in the method, if appropriate.
5. For an specific time period, select and set several goals for yourself. Write long-term and short-term goals that will direct you toward achievement. Follow your progress with a checklist or chart.
6. Visit a local OT department, and discuss with the staff OT practitioners the type of documentation used by his or her facility. If the facility allows it, ask to see examples of documentation (e.g., assessment reports, progress notes, treatment plans, and discharge summaries).

REFERENCES

1. Early MB: *Mental health concepts and techniques for the occupational therapy assistant,* ed 2, New York, 1993, Raven Press.

2. Hopkins HL: Tools of practice: section 4, problem solving. In Hopkins HL, Smith HD, editors: *Willard & Spackman's occupational therapy,* ed 8, Philadelphia, 1993, JB Lippincott.

3. Paul R: *Critical thinking,* ed 3, Santa Rosa, Calif, 1994, Foundation for Critical Thinking.

4. Paul R, editor-in-chief: Practical workshops revitalize teaching. In *Educational vision: the magazine for critical thinking,* 2(2):28, 1994.

5. Pedretti LW: Treatment planning. In Pedretti LW, editor: *Occupational therapy: practice skills for physical dysfunction,* ed 4, St Louis, 1996, Mosby.

6. Perinchief JM: Service management: section 2, documentation. In Hopkins HL, Smith HD, editors: *Willard & Spackman's occupational therapy,* ed 8, Philadelphia, 1993, JB Lippincott.

7. Rathus S: *Psychology,* Austin, Tex, 1987, Holt, Rinehart & Winston.

8. Schon DA: *The reflective practitioner: how professionals think in action,* New York, 1983, Basic Books.

9. Schopenhauer A: On thinking for yourself. In *Educational vision: the magazine for critical thinking,* 2(2):33, 1994.

10. Smith RO, Benge M, Hall M: Technology for self-care. In Christiansen C, editor: *Ways of living: self-care strategies for special needs,* Rockville, Md, 1994, AOTA.

11. von Oech R: *A whack on the side of the head,* New York, 1990, Warner Books.

12. Weed LL: *Medical records, medical education and patient care,* Chicago, 1971, Year Book Medical Publishers.

Being a recipient of occupational therapy and a person with a disability who has to function in society, I believe occupational therapists play a major role in a person's rehabilitation process, assisting them with functioning and, at times, with the success of the goals they want to accomplish in life.

Whenever I meet one of my former patients in the supermarket or pass them on the road (he or she is the driver), it makes me feel good that I was instrumental in getting them back to this level of function. These experiences always reinforce the fact that I selected the right profession. ■

Charles W. Gray, OTR/L
Coler/Goldwater Memorial Hospital
Roosevelt Island, New York

When you see clients with Alzheimer's disease smile because they have dressed themselves or brushed their teeth, and you are the one who has made these achievements possible, you realize the satisfaction of being an occupational therapist. ■

Coralie H. Glantz, OTR/L, FAOTA
Co-owner
Glantz/Richman Rehabilitation Associates, LTD
Riverwoods, Illinois

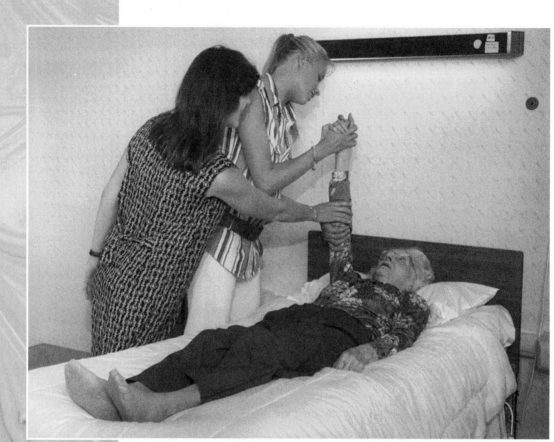

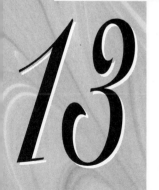

13 Service Management Functions

Objectives

After reading this chapter, the reader will be able to:

✤ Explain the various service management functions

✤ Identify the factors that lead to a safe and efficient clinical environment

✤ Describe how the spread of infection is prevented in the workplace

✤ Explain the factors taken into consideration for the scheduling of staff appointments

✤ Define the three major categories of funding sources that reimburse for occupational therapy (OT) services

✤ Understand the importance of educational activities for professional development

✤ State the importance of marketing and public relations as a professional responsibility

Key terms

Service management functions

Emergency procedures

Centers for Disease Control and Prevention

Universal Precautions

Public funding sources

Private funding sources

Worker's compensation benefits

Program evaluation

Program structure

Program process

Outcome measures

Inservice presentations

Public relations

Marketing

Having discussed the steps involved in direct client care, it is time to examine the functions that are not a part of direct client care but are equally important in the operation of an OT department. These indirect service functions are referred to as **service management functions** and include maintaining a safe and efficient workplace, ordering supplies, keeping equipment in working order, charting the number of treatments or making daily schedules, billing for services, and performing quality assurance activities. Service management functions may also involve remaining current on developments in the field by attending workshops on new techniques. (Documentation is considered to be related to the direct care for a client and is discussed in Chapters 11 and 12.)

Chapter 13 photo: Lohman H, Padilla R, Byers-Connon S: *Occupational therapy with elders: strategies for the COTA*, St Louis, 1998, Mosby.

MAINTAINING A SAFE AND EFFICIENT WORKPLACE

Maintaining an orderly and safe environment for the provision of OT services is important for the OT practitioner and for the well-being of the clients who are seen in this environment. Because the clients have disabilities, a safe and efficient clinic has great significance. It is imperative that all areas in the clinic be free of clutter and wheelchair accessible, have good lighting and ventilation, and have equipment that is properly stored and maintained.

Each person who works in the clinic setting should assume the responsibility for maintaining a safe and efficient work environment. This does not necessarily imply that each practitioner is directly responsible for the maintenance itself; rather, it means each should take responsibility for reporting problems to the OT administrator or to the maintenance department. However, each OT practitioner *is directly responsible* for putting away equipment and supplies that have been in use during a treatment session and for cleaning the work area. When everyone participates and cooperates in maintaining a safe and efficient work environment, the department will operate more effectively and with less stress. The following text examines in greater detail the many factors that contribute to a safe and efficient work environment.

SAFE ENVIRONMENT

Each setting should have written policies and procedures relating to the functions of maintaining a safe work environment. Many safety procedures are actually mandated by the various accrediting bodies.[5] It is the responsibility of the OT practitioner to be familiar with these policies and procedures.

The clinical setting should provide plenty of room in which staff and consumers can move without running into equipment or objects. Items that represent a potential safety hazard should be properly stored and, in some instances, placed in locked cabinets. This precaution is particularly important in psychiatric settings where scissors, knives, and other sharp objects could be potentially used by a client to harm themselves or someone else. Other items that require careful storage consideration are toxic chemicals and flammable substances.

Many OT departments have kitchen facilities; safety in this area needs to be carefully considered. In particular, food used in the kitchen needs to be handled and stored safely. In addition, all staff should be trained in the proper of use equipment and supplies that are found in the OT clinic, including the use of protective goggles when using power equipment and face masks when using toxic chemicals.[5]

Another important safety aspect in the clinic is the prevention of injury to the OT practitioners. Settings in which lifting and moving of clients from bed to wheelchair is required, the practitioner may be injured if proper body mechanics are not used. Injuries to the back are the most common and may force the practitioner to take a leave from work to allow the back to heal. Clinical employers should provide training in the proper use of body mechanics to lift and transfer clients. OT practitioners should attend these training sessions at all times and make a concerted effort to be aware of his or her body mechanics.

All staff should be familiar with **emergency procedures** in the case of an injury or accident in the clinic. These procedures should name the person to contact for help in the case of an emergency. OT practitioners should maintain a current certification in cardiopulmonary resuscitation (CPR) and training in first aid. In addition, the OT practitioner should know how to determine blood pressure and pulse rate, manage a seizure, and know what to do if someone is choking.[5] After an injury or accident in the clinic, the practitioner must complete a report that documents what occurred, filing it in accordance with the procedures of the facility. Box 13-1 summarizes safety considerations in the OT clinic.

INFECTION CONTROL

Controlling the spread of infections is an important safety consideration in health care settings. Health care workers, including OT practitioners, are at risk for contracting infectious diseases that are transferred from person to person (i.e., hepatitis B virus [HBV], human immunodeficiency virus [HIV], and tuberculosis [TB]). Clients are also susceptible to infection from the health care worker.

Box 13-1

SAFETY CONSIDERATIONS IN THE OCCUPATIONAL THERAPY SETTING

1. SHARP OBJECTS SHOULD BE PROPERLY STORED IN A LOCKED CABINET OR DRAWER.

2. THE CLINICAL ENVIRONMENT SHOULD BE FREE OF CLUTTER SO THAT STAFF AND CLIENTS CAN MOVE SAFELY. SHARP CORNERS ON CABINETS SHOULD NOT PROTRUDE INTO TRAFFIC AREAS, AND EQUIPMENT AND FURNITURE SHOULD BE KEPT OUT OF TRAFFIC AREAS.

3. BATHROOM AREAS THAT ARE USED BY CLIENTS SHOULD HAVE SECURELY ANCHORED GRAB BARS.

4. THE EMERGENCY CALL SYSTEM SHOULD BE READILY AVAILABLE, AND ALL STAFF SHOULD BE AWARE OF EMERGENCY PROCEDURES.

5. FLOORING SHOULD BE NONSLIP, AND THE STAFF SHOULD BE ALERT TO ANYTHING THAT MAY CHANGE THIS CONDITION (I.E., WATER).

6. ALL STAFF SHOULD HAVE PROPER TRAINING IN THE SAFE USE OF EQUIPMENT AND SUPPLIES FOUND IN THE OT CLINIC.

7. IN KITCHEN AREAS, FOODS SHOULD BE SAFELY STORED AND HANDLED.

8. STAFF SHOULD BE TRAINED IN THE USE OF PROPER BODY MECHANICS WHEN LIFTING OR MOVING CLIENTS, EQUIPMENT, AND SUPPLIES.

The **Centers for Disease Control and Prevention** (CDC), which is a federal agency established to record disease epidemics, conducts research to eliminate diseases through education and the development of vaccinations. In 1987 the CDC developed **Universal Precautions,** a set of guidelines designed to prevent the transmission of HIV, HBV, and other blood-borne pathogens to health care providers. Under Universal Precautions, blood and certain body fluids of all clients are considered potentially infectious. These guidelines change as new research becomes available; therefore it is recommended that OT practitioners remain up-to-date on the guidelines.

Universal Precautions recommend the use of protective barriers such as gloves, gowns, aprons, masks, or protective eyewear to reduce the risk of exposure to blood and other body fluids that are potentially infectious. It is recommended that OT practitioners wear protective gloves whenever working with a client during his or her activities for daily living (ADLs), such as grooming, personal hygiene, toileting, and dressing. When it is necessary for the health care worker to wear one of the other protective barriers, a notice should be placed in the client's medical record and a sign should be posted outside the client's room to indicate the needed precautions.

The most effective method for preventing the transfer of disease is hand washing. The OT practitioner should wash his or her hands before and after each treatment, after using the toilet, and after sneezing, coughing, or coming in contact with oral and nasal areas, and before and after eating.[7] Procedures for hand washing are provided in Box 13-2.

The responsibility for controlling the spread of infection rests with federal agencies, employers, and employees.[8] The regulations are established and monitored by the CDC and by the Occupational Safety and Health Administration (OSHA). OSHA monitors compliance of employers and fines those settings that do not follow the regulations, whereas CDC monitors exposure to any diseases of individuals while in the workplace.

OSHA standards define the responsibilities of the employer, which include providing education on the Universal Precautions and on the use of protective barriers. The employer is also responsible for providing the necessary protective barriers and hand washing facilities and supplies needed by the employees. Employers are also required to provide employee health services for the purposes of mandatory annual test for TB, optional HBV vaccine, and maintenance of employee health records (i.e., tests and vaccines given and any exposure to infectious disease).[8]

It is the employees' responsibilities to attend the educational programs that are offered and to follow the Universal Precautions guidelines. Employees are also required to have an annual TB test and to report any exposures to the employee health services department. It is the prerogative of the employee to decide whether

---

Box 13-2

TECHNIQUES FOR EFFECTIVE HAND WASHING

1. REMOVE ALL JEWELRY, EXCEPT PLAIN BAND RINGS. REMOVE WATCH OR MOVE IT UP THE ARM. PROVIDE COMPLETE ACCESS TO AREA TO BE WASHED.

2. APPROACH THE SINK, AND AVOID TOUCHING THE SINK OR NEARBY OBJECTS.

3. TURN ON THE WATER, AND ADJUST IT TO A LUKEWARM TEMPERATURE AND A MODERATE FLOW TO AVOID SPLASHING.

4. WET WRISTS AND HANDS WITH FINGERS DIRECTED DOWNWARD, AND APPLY APPROXIMATELY 1 TEASPOON OF LIQUID SOAP OR GRANULES.

5. BEGIN TO WASH ALL AREAS OF HANDS (PALMS, SIDES, BACKS), FINGERS, KNUCKLES, AND BETWEEN EACH FINGER USING VIGOROUS RUBBING AND CIRCULAR MOTIONS. IF WEARING A BAND, SLIDE IT UP OR DOWN THE FINGER AND SCRUB SKIN UNDERNEATH IT. INTERLACE FINGERS AND SCRUB BETWEEN EACH FINGER.

6. WASH FOR AT LEAST 30 SECONDS, KEEPING HANDS AND FOREARMS AT ELBOW LEVEL OR BELOW AND HANDS POINTED DOWN. WASH LONGER IF A PATIENT KNOWN TO HAVE AN INFECTION WAS TREATED.

7. RINSE HANDS WELL UNDER RUNNING WATER.

8. WASH AS HIGH UP WRISTS AND FOREARMS AS CONTAMINATION IS LIKELY.

9. RINSE HANDS, WRISTS, AND FOREARMS UNDER RUNNING WATER.

10. THOROUGHLY DRY HANDS, WRISTS, AND FOREARMS WITH PAPER TOWELS. USE A DRY TOWEL FOR EACH HAND. WATER SHOULD CONTINUE TO FLOW FROM TAP AS HANDS ARE DRIED.

11. USE ANOTHER DRY PAPER TOWEL TO TURN WATER FAUCET OFF. DISCARD ALL TOWELS IN AN APPROPRIATE CONTAINER.

Modified from Zakus SM: *Clinical procedures for medical assistants*, ed 3, St Louis, 1995, Mosby.

to take the HBV vaccine and sign a waiver, if this option is declined.[8] Since these procedures have been established after much research and are for the safety of the health care worker, it is beneficial to the OT practitioner to comply.

ORDERING AND STORING SUPPLIES

An important part of maintaining an efficient therapy setting is having appropriate equipment and supplies on hand when needed. The amount of supplies ordered and stored at any one time varies among facilities, depending on the size of the OT department, its storage capacity, and the policies of the administration.[5]

It is necessary for effective operations to predict the supplies that may be needed over a particular period of time and to order an adequate amount to ensure that supplies do not run out. Using an inventory system will help the staff manage this information. Usually, one individual is responsible for tracking the supply inventory and ordering supplies as needed. In those facilities that employ a Certified Occupational Therapist Assistant (COTA), this responsibility is often part of his or her job. However, this may vary from facility to facility.

SCHEDULING

To keep things flowing smoothly in the clinic, a schedule of the appointments for each practitioner needs to be maintained and displayed where it is visible by all staff members. A schedule is a useful tool for time management; it helps the therapist prioritize what needs to be accomplished and serves as a plan.[4,5]

The first priority for scheduling is to identify the clients who need to be seen each day. After client treatment, the schedule should take into account the time needed to complete the indirect functions described in this chapter. The schedule should reflect the time needed for each OT practitioner to attend meetings or client conferences and to complete paperwork, scheduling, and billing.

Scheduling clients will vary depending on the type of facility and caseload seen in each setting. In a mental health outpatient program, treatment may be performed by the therapist in groups that meet only once a week. In another outpatient setting in which clients with hand injuries are seen, it may be necessary to schedule individuals two or three times a week and sometimes even daily. Scheduling in outpatient settings may also vary because of family schedules, other appointments that the client may have, and the availability of transportation to and from the clinic.

Third-party payers also have a significant influence over the duration and frequency in which clients are seen. Medicare requires clients who are in acute rehabilitation to be seen twice a day. If the client cannot tolerate two daily treatments, he or she should be transferred to a setting that provides a lower level of care (e.g., skilled nursing facility). Many health maintenance organizations (HMOs) limit the number of outpatient visits to the OT practitioner; typically twelve visits are the maximum. All these factors need to be considered during the development of the schedule.

The supervising Registered Occupational Therapist (OTR) usually decides which staff person to schedule with which client and communicates the schedule to the staff.[5] This decision-making step involves consideration of client needs, staff expertise, and cost-effectiveness. Today, productivity in OT departments is highly scrutinized, as it is for all health care services. If a client can be treated by a COTA instead of a OTR, this assignment will be more cost-effective for the department. If there are not enough clients to complete a staff person's schedule for a day, the manager may decide to reduce the practitioner's hours. Once the schedule is in place, it is important that the practitioner manages his or her time wisely and adheres to the schedule to ensure that everything is completed as planned and the schedules of others are not affected.

GETTING REIMBURSED

OT departments need to produce revenue to stay in business. Revenue is produced through the collection of fees for services provided. Each OT practitioner is responsible for submitting accurate charges that are reflected in either units based on the amount of time spent with the client or the fee based on services provided.[5] Determining the fees involves a complex process usually performed by the administration of the facility and the department. Briefly, third-party payers each have different amounts that they will pay in "allowable charges" for a particular client. In essence, the fees set by the facility do not reflect what is actually paid by the third-party payer for an individual client but rather the client population as a whole.

OT services are reimbursed from a number of sources, which can be categorized into three groups. They are: (1) public sources that include federal, state, and local government agencies; (2) private payers that include insurance companies; and (3) other sources that include service agencies and volunteer organizations. Each source of payment has different regulations and guidelines that identify the services for which it will pay (number of visits and equipment) and how much. Since these regulations and guidelines often change, it is the responsibility of the OT practitioner to remain current. The administration of the facility and the department should also keep current on funding regulations and inform staff members of any changes.

PUBLIC FUNDING SOURCES

Public funding sources come from the federal, state, and local levels. These sources include funds provided by Medicare, Veteran's Administration, Medicaid, Maternal and Child Health programs, Department of Education, vocational rehabilitation services, and Social Security benefits. Typically, Congress authorizes funding through a specific legislation and designates a federal agency to determine the scope and criteria for the program. In each state an agency is designated to receive the federal funds and ensure compliance with the programs mandated by the federal government.[3] The funds are then distributed to the local agencies or programs, which are responsible for ensuring that mandated services are provided. In Chapter 2, federal legislation that has mandated OT as a reimbursable service is discussed.

PRIVATE SOURCES OF FUNDING

Private funding sources include the individual's health insurance policy, worker's compensation, casualty insurance, and disability insurance. In some cases, private funding may come from the client. Most individuals are provided with the details of their health insurance policies, which stipulate whether OT services are covered and whether there are any limitations on those services (e.g., maximum number of visits, maximum amount of dollars). Funding by private health insurance companies is based on a medical diagnosis and justification that the treatment is medically necessary.

Under **worker's compensation benefits,** expenses incurred from work-related injuries are covered. Worker's compensation benefits are regulated by state agencies and managed by private insurance companies. For that reason, allowable OT services vary from state to state.

OTHER SOURCES OF FUNDING

Sources of funding that do not fall under the categories of public or private agencies include service clubs, private foundations, and volunteer organizations. In many communities there are various service clubs (e.g., Kiwanis, Rotary Club) that may be a source of funding for individuals without other means. In some cases, private foundations, which are usually related to a specific disability group, will provide funding for an individual with that disability.[3] Finally, there are some volunteer agencies that provide funding.

OT practitioners need to educate third-party payers on a continual basis regarding the benefits of OT services, as well as be an advocate for the inclusion of OT as a reimbursable service under the various policies and regulations. It is important to keep abreast of proposed changes in state and federal legislation and regulations that have the potential to affect the payment for OT services. This can be done on an individual basis and by supporting local and national OT associations that provide lobbying efforts for the purpose of influencing legislation that may affect the profession.

PROGRAM PLANNING AND EVALUATION

Program planning and evaluation are primarily the responsibilities of the administrator, although the staff provides input into both processes. In an OT department, the administrator is involved in planning such things as space utilization, equipment needs, staff levels and how to use staff members effectively, the annual budget, department policies and procedures, and new programs and services.

It is important as a health care profession that the effectiveness of the programs are measured. This is referred to as **program evaluation** and involves "determining the extent to which programs are achieving the goals and objectives established for them and using that information as necessary to modify activities."[1]

Program evaluation examines three different aspects of the services provided. The first aspect is the **program structure** of the system in which the services are delivered; for example, the staff levels and expertise, the equipment, the budget, and the range of services provided are examined. In evaluating this aspect of a program, the types of questions asked include, "Is there adequate staff to provide services?" "Are staff members competent in their area of service delivery, and are they current with the latest approaches?" "Do we have an adequate budget and equipment on hand to provide services?"

The **program process** in which the services are delivered includes all of the stages described in Section II of this text: referral, assessment, and implementation. In evaluating this aspect of a program, individual client records are examined to determine whether certain stages occurred as they were intended and whether the procedures were acceptable. For example, "Did the client have the appropriate referral for occupational therapy?" "Was the assessment completed in a timely manner and performed accurately?" Usually several clients' records are randomly selected for review to determine whether the process was appropriately followed.

The last consideration in program evaluation is **outcome measures,** an aspect that evaluates the results of the intervention after the service has been provided.[10] There are a number of tools that are used to measure outcomes. One of the more popular tools is the Functional Independence Measure (FIM). The FIM measures the client's performance on eighteen factors under the categories of self-care, sphincter control, mobility locomotion, communication, and social cognition.[2] The person is given a score for each item and a total score. The FIM and similar measures are used to score a client at different points in the rehabilitation process (e.g., at time of referral and at discharge), and they provide a fairly objective measure of how the individual is progressing.

By examining these three aspects as a part of program evaluation, specific problem areas can be addressed. After identifying the problem areas, corrective measures can be taken. Program evaluation is an ongoing process that helps ensure quality services are provided by the OT program. The conclusions made from a program evaluation provide valuable information to the practitioner, the consumer, and the third-party payer, each of whom has an interest in the quality of the services provided.

EDUCATIONAL ACTIVITIES

There are a number of ways in which both the OTR and COTA can be involved in educational activities. The first responsibility for OT practitioners is to participate in educational programs to further their professional development. This is accomplished through continuing education activities, which are available throughout the country and in many different types of formats.

Another way that OT practitioners can be involved in education is through the fieldwork educational process and supervision of fieldwork students. OTRs and COTAs with a minimum of 1 year of work experience are eligible to supervise students. Clinical internships are critical to the continuation of the profession.

Practitioners who mentor the next generation of OT practitioners provide a valuable service to their profession. Not only is fieldwork an important component of the student's training, it is also a valuable and rewarding experience for the student supervisor, who learns and grows professionally from the mentoring experience.

OT practitioners also participate in educational opportunities in their departments or facilities through **inservice presentations,** which vary depending on what is needed. For example, an OT practitioner working in the school district may provide an inservice presentation to teachers and aides on how to properly feed a child with swallowing difficulties, or an OT practitioner who has attended a workshop on special treatments technique may spend an hour presenting the information he or she learned to the OT staff. Inservice presentations are an effective way to train staff members, both internally and externally, as well as a good public relations tool for the OT department.

PUBLIC RELATIONS AND MARKETING

Participation in **public relations** programs to increase the visibility of OT should be considered a part of one's professional responsibilities. The average person is not likely to be familiar with what OT is, and any opportunity to educate people regarding the value of OT services is important. Many departments plan and implement public relations activities during the month of April, which is designated as National Occupational Therapy Month. For example, a booth set up in the facility's cafeteria that demonstrates adaptive equipment will attract a lot of attention. The American Occupational Therapy Association (AOTA) is involved in many efforts to increase the visibility of OT and has materials available for members to promote the profession. These materials include a booklet that describes ways to promote OT, along with brochures, videotapes, banners, and posters.

Today, competition in the health care market is strong; therefore practitioners need to be involved in marketing OT services more than ever. **Marketing** is slightly different from public relations efforts in that it involves the development and implementation of a marketing plan, which is typically the responsibility of the administrator of the department. However, it is important for the practitioner to have at least a basic awareness of what is involved in marketing OT services.

The development of a marketing plan requires consideration of four target groups: (1) the clients who are served, (2) the physicians who refer or have the potential to refer clients to OT, (3) the administration (or internal source of funding for the department) of the facility, and (4) the third-party payers who reimburse (or have the potential to reimburse) for OT services.[9]

In addition, Olson and Urban describe five key concepts of marketing that need to be addressed when developing a marketing plan. The first concept is *product,* and the questions asked are, "What is the product or service that we are providing?" "Is this product or service needed by the community?" The second concept is *price,* and it asks whether the pricing of the service is fair and within reason for the market. The third concept is *place,* and it addresses the how, when, and where the services will be offered and who will be eligible to receive them. *Promotion* is the fourth concept, and it strives to make the product visible to the target market and considers how to promote and advertise the services that are provided. Finally, *position* is the relative place of the product among similar products in the marketplace. For example, "What unique attributes set our product apart from other similar products?" From these five key concepts, a marketing plan can be developed to promote the services that appeal to the consumer.[9]

SUMMARY

Service management functions are performed by the OT practitioner and do not relate to direct care of the client. These functions include maintaining a safe and orderly work environment, scheduling, reimbursement, program planning and evaluation, educational activities, and public relations and marketing. For an OT department to operate effectively, it is important that each practitioner take the responsibility for being involved in these activities.

Activities

1. Practice time management by making a weekly schedule for yourself and adhering to it. Note whether you seem to get more accomplished when using the schedule.
2. Visit any occupational therapy department. After leaving the facility ask yourself, "How would I feel about working in this setting?" Prepare written notes about the environment of the department. Is the storage adequate? Does there appear to be an adequate amount of equipment and supplies? Does the clinic appear cluttered, or is it neat with everything safely put away? Are there any obvious safety hazards that you noticed during your visit?
3. Interview either a COTA and an OTR about the types of service management functions they perform. Compare notes with your classmates. Is there a significant difference between what OTRs and COTAs do? Is there any difference across the spheres of practice?
4. In a group of two or three students, come up with several public relations activities that you could use to promote National Occupational Therapy Month. Select one of the activities and perform the activity at your school or the local mall.

REFERENCES

1. Bair J, Gray M, editors: *The occupational therapy manager*, Rockville, Md, 1985, AOTA.

2. Christiansen C: Occupational therapy intervention for life performance. In Christiansen C, Baum C, editors: *Occupational therapy: overcoming performance deficits*, Thorofare, NJ, 1991, Slack.

3. Cook AM, Hussey SM: *Assistive technologies: principles and practice*, St Louis, 1995, Mosby.

4. Early MB: *Mental health concepts and techniques for the occupational therapy assistant*, ed 2, New York, 1993, Raven Press.

5. Jones RA: Service operations. In Ryan SE, editor: *Practice issues in occupational therapy: intraprofessional team building*, Thorofare, NJ, 1993, Slack.

6. Marcil WM: The adult with AIDS. In Ryan SE, editor: *Practice issues in occupational therapy: intraprofessional team building*, Thorofare, NJ, 1993, Slack.

7. Leiter P: Facility planning. In Bair J, Gray M, editors: *The occupational therapy manager*, Rockville, Md, 1985, AOTA.

8. Meriano C: Universal precautions. In Sladyk K, editor: *OT student primer: a guide to college success*, Thorofare, NJ, 1997, Slack.

9. Olson TS, Urban C: Marketing. In Bair J, Gray M, editors: *The occupational therapy manager*, Rockville, Md, 1985, AOTA.

10. Perinchief JM: Service management. In Hopkins HL, Smith HD, editors: *Willard & Spackman's occupational therapy*, ed 8, Philadelphia, 1993, JB Lippincott.

IN THIS FINAL SECTION THE FOCUS CHANGES FROM THE PRACTICE OF OCCUPATIONAL THERAPY TO THE SPECIFIC SKILLS THAT ARE NEEDED OF THE PRACTITIONER. FIRST, TWO GENERAL SKILLS ARE EXPLORED: TERMINOLOGY AND HUMAN INTERACTION SKILLS. IN CHAPTER 16, THE SPECIFIC THERAPEUTIC MODALITIES USED IN OT ARE EXAMINED, INCLUDING THE USE OF PURPOSEFUL ACTIVITY AND ACTIVITY ANALYSIS.

THE LAST CHAPTER IN THIS SECTION DISCUSSES SOUND CLINICAL REASONING, THE DEVELOPMENT OF WHICH IS THE ULTIMATE AIM OF ALL THEORY AND PRACTICE SKILLS. IN THE APPLICATION OF CLINICAL REASONING A CONNECTING STRUCTURE IS PRESENTED, ENABLING ONE TO SEE HOW OT ALLOWS FOR A GREAT VARIETY OF PRACTICE MODELS AND SPECIALTY FOCUSES, YET FITS TOGETHER AS ONE UNIQUE, IDENTIFIABLE HEALTH CARE SERVICE. WITH THIS CONCEPT OF CLINICAL REASONING, THE OVERVIEW OF THIS PROFESSION IS COMPLETE.

THREE

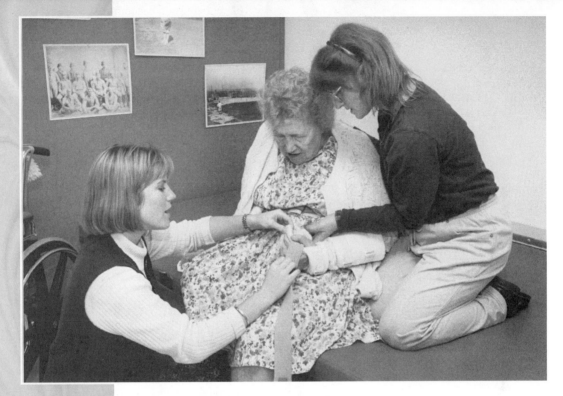

Specific Skills of the Occupational Therapy Practitioner

Occupational therapy, by its very nature, facilitates a holistic way of being and becoming in the world. The therapist allows a natural unfolding of the human being with whom he or she interacts and thereby encourages the patient to develop skills that will nurture them and sustain them through daily life. Skill building includes physical, emotional, and psychosocial skills, and with the holistic approach the therapist empowers the therapy process, with the end result being a more capable, responsible, and self-sufficient client. Responsibility for one's health—one's physical, emotional, and spiritual health—is facilitated and taught by the occupational therapist. It is through this interaction that people grow, become empowered, cope, and achieve what is needed to carry out daily tasks that are meaningful to a person and a person's lifestyle. It is a privilege to share in the lives of others so that we, too, can grow and learn and help, in our very small way, to change the world—one person at a time! ■

Michael Pizzi, MS, OTR/L, CHES, FAOTA
Executive Director, National Center for Wellness and Health Promotion
CEO, Positive Images and Wellness, Inc.
Silver Spring, Maryland

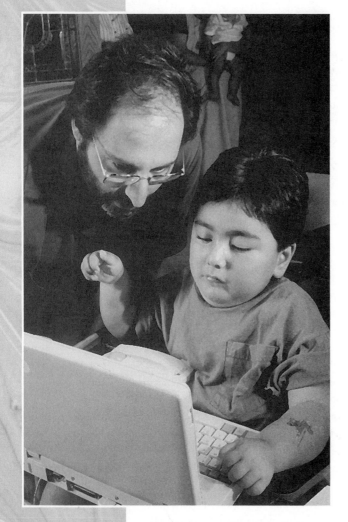

14

Terminology

Objectives

After reading this chapter, the reader will be able to:
- ✤ Recognize the need to develop proficiency in the use of professional terminology
- ✤ Understand the basic word-building system that is used in medical terminology
- ✤ Employ a self-paced study program including the use of a checklist as a tool for completing the learning processes
- ✤ Recognize the basic terminology regarding the human body

Key terms

Terminology
Root
Prefix
Suffix
Self-paced study programs

Since people in a particular field rely on an agreed-upon vocabulary for all work-related communications, it is important that everyone entering the field master its unique terminology. One of the surest ways to distinguish a novice from a master in any field is to listen to how information is conveyed about his or her work. The novice gropes his or her way through awkward descriptions, whereas the master efficiently selects the precise words.

Before efficient word selection occurs, there must come the sometimes tedious task of simply learning the vocabulary. This task can be made easier by adding understanding to rote memorization and by employing study aids and games.

Using correct terminology is particularly important in the written documentation that occupational therapy (OT) practitioners use to communicate with other members of the health care team and third-party payers. The words used to identify and describe carry a special quality when used in formal reports. Language may be shared, but there can be differences between the way two people use a word. It is important that there is agreed-upon vocabulary and agreed-upon meaning of the terms used, if vital information is to be conveyed correctly. The study of terminology assures shared meaning.

APPROACHING TERMINOLOGY COMPETENCE

In OT, mastering the **terminology** involves learning two new *languages*. First, there is the terminology that is unique to the field of OT. Second, because the OT practitioner frequently works in and with the medical profession, it is also necessary to under-

Section III photo: Lohman H, Padilla R, Byer-Connon S: *Occupational therapy with elders: strategies for the COTA*, St Louis, 1998, Mosby.

Chapter 14 photo: Ratliffe KT: *Clinical pediatric physical therapy: a guide for the physical therapy team*, St Louis, 1998, Mosby.

stand and speak the medical language—therefore there is a need to study and understand medical terminology, as well. To the student, most of the medical terminology will be new. Most OT terminology is more familiar in everyday language; however, it is important to develop professional awareness of the specific concepts conveyed.

There are many ways to approach the development of terminology competence. One way is to simply be around it long enough and hope it happens. That, however, is not recommended! What is recommended is that the student immediately begin using one of the self-paced medical terminology books available.[2-7] These texts are designed to simplify the task by teaching the student word parts and by progressively building words using those parts. Computer programs are available that accomplish the same thing.

Medical terminology includes words that relate to anatomic structures, body systems, diseases, and medical processes or procedures. It is a language created to streamline communications and for the convenience and efficiency of people in and around the medical profession.

In studying medical terminology, it is helpful to recognize the importance of breaking complex words into component parts. The vocabulary of the medical field is systematically built. Time spent learning to recognize word parts and to simply break them into their component parts will pay dividends to understand new, unfamiliar medical terms. Although there are exceptions to the rules, understanding the system upon which the terminology is built will greatly speed the learning process.

BASIC COMPONENTS OF MEDICAL TERMINOLOGY

Most medical terminology is based on Greek or Latin word roots. The **root** is the foundation of a word or its main part—also called the *stem*. Two or more word roots may be combined to form a compound word. A **prefix** and/or **suffix** may be added to a word root. To mesh the parts smoothly, a combination form (usually an *o*) is often added to the stem (Figure 14-1).

ELEMENTS OF THE WORD-BUILDING SYSTEM:

PARTS:

WORD ROOT (from Greek or Latin)
COMPOUND WORD (combine two word roots)

never alone {
+ COMBINING FORM (usually an *o*)
+ PREFIX (at the beginning of the word; modifies the word)
    and/or
+ SUFFIX (at the end; forms new meaning, which would otherwise take a phrase to convey)

FIGURE 14-1. THE BUILDING BLOCKS OF MEDICAL TERMINOLOGY.

SELF-PACED STUDY PROGRAMS

In using **self-paced study programs,** it is important to remember that the key to success is setting a daily routine of review. Short intervals of study on a daily basis will both ensure success and reinforce taking the responsibility for the learning process. As an OT practitioner, taking responsibility for learning is fundamental.

Using a self-paced study program also provides the student with an opportunity to experience a technique that can be used in treatment as a therapeutic tool. The tool is a checklist, a helpful device to assist with on-task behavior (continuing to do the intended activity). A checklist can be designed in many ways, but basically it is simply a grid or chart that is divided by time or date and task, which the user checks off each day as the activity is completed (Figure 14-2). A checklist provides great psychological support for regularly continuing the activity.

HOMEWORK COMPLETED

SUN	MON	TUE	WED	THU	FRI	SAT
✔	✔					

FIGURE 14-2. SAMPLE CHECKLIST STUDY TOOL.

BASIC TERMINOLOGY

To begin studying medical terminology, a list of words with skeletal definitions is provided in Box 14-1. This basic terminology, commonly found in OT practice, is used to discuss the human body. Some terms refer to direction, some to position, and some to surfaces.

Figure 14-3 illustrates some of the terms listed in Box 14-1. Each term has a specific use; there are subtle differences that prohibit interchanging similar terms. For example, *superior* and *inferior* are terms of direction (toward); therefore these are not the same as the upper and lower portions of the body. *Prone* and *supine* are spe-

Box 14-1

BASIC TERMINOLOGY USED TO REFER TO THE HUMAN BODY

ABDUCTION Movement away from midline

ADDUCTION Movement toward midline

ANATOMIC POSITION Erect, arms at sides, palms facing forward

ANTERIOR Front or belly surface (*also* ventral)

CAUDAL Tail (*or* tail end of body)

CEPHALO Head (*or* head end of body)

DISTAL Away from point of origin (*or* attachment)

DORSAL Body's back surface or posterior

ERECT Standing upright

EXTENSION Straightening (*or* increase angle of bones)

FLEXION Bending (*or* decrease angle of bones)

INFERIOR Toward feet (*or* lower part)

LATERAL Outward or away from midline

MEDIAL Toward midline of body

MIDLINE Imaginary line down middle of front of body

PALMAR Inner surface of hand (palm)

PERIPHERAL At or near surface of body

PLANTAR Sole of foot

POSTERIOR Back surface (*also* dorsal)

PRONE Lying face down

PROXIMAL Nearest to point of origin (*or* attachment)

RECUMBENT Lying down

ROTATION Turning motion

SAGITTAL Plane through midline dividing into left and right

SUPERIOR Toward head (*or* upper part)

SUPINE Lying flat on back

VENTRAL Body's front surface or anterior

cific body positions, whereas *proximal* and *distal* are relative positions that need to be given a reference point. *Abduction* and *adduction* are directions with the midline as the identified reference point. Studying medical terminology requires accuracy and careful understanding of the subtle differences. The use of correct terminology is a measure of the skilled professional.

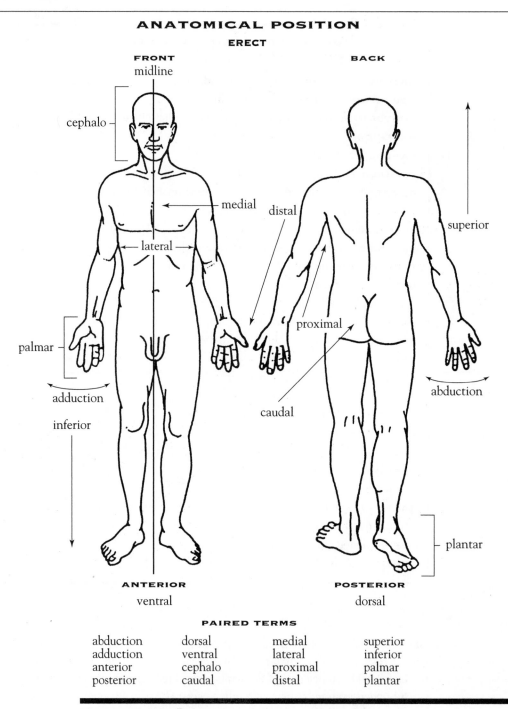

FIGURE 14-3. BASIC TERMINOLOGY ILLUSTRATED.

SUMMARY

One important quality to any professional is the appropriate use of the language relevant to their field. The OT student should familiarize himself or herself with professional terminology. Since OT works closely with the medical field, medical terminology must become part of the *language* of OT. Attention to the system upon which medical terminology is built will aid the learning process, as will the employment of a system of study that uses a checklist. With these tools a student can pursue self-study to better develop the needed skills.

Activities

1. Design a simple checklist to be used at home to help stay on task with the study of medical terminology.
2. Look up each of the terms listed in Box 14-1 in a medical dictionary for a more expanded definition.
3. Design a word game for the study of medical terminology. Television shows such as "Jeopardy" can serve as models. When played by a group, add enjoyment by having the losing team serve refreshments (and clean up, of course) for the winners. This approach not only helps bring fun to what might otherwise be tedious, but it also builds other skills—designing ways to bring enjoyment to some of the tedium in which clients must engage during therapy.
4. Use outside resources to find the meaning of terminology that you do not yet understand in *Uniform Terminology*, 3rd edition. The uniform terminology can be found in Appendix D.

REFERENCES

1. Anderson KN, Anderson LE, Glanze WD, editors: *Mosby's medical, nursing, and allied health dictionary*, ed 4, St Louis, 1994, Mosby.

2. Austrin MG, Austrin HR: *Learning medical terminology: a worktext*, ed 8, St Louis, 1995, Mosby.

3. Birmingham JJ: *Medical terminology: a self-learning text*, ed 2, St Louis, 1990, Mosby.

4. Campbell JB, Campbell JM: *Mosby's survival guide to medical abbreviations and acronyms, prefixes and suffixes, symbols, Greek alphabet*, St Louis, 1995, Mosby.

5. LaFleur-Brooks M, Starr MK: *Exploring medical language: a student-directed approach*, ed 3, St Louis, 1994, Mosby.

6. Mosby: *Body parts: Mosby's medical terminology flash cards*, St Louis, 1996, Mosby.

7. Williams RW: *Basic health care terminology with anatomy coloring exercises*, St Louis, 1995, Mosby.

I am fortunate to have chosen occupational therapy as my profession and have found it very rewarding to be a Certified Occupational Therapy Assistant (COTA) for 23 years. My work has been rewarding because of the opportunity to work with Registered Occupational Therapists (OTRs) who have encouraged me to expand my skills as a COTA. I have developed a self-confidence and the ability to establish trust with OTRs and have become of value to the rehabilitation teams. I strive to demonstrate competence in performing assigned tasks so that I learn more, widen my base of knowledge, and remain resourceful to patients, peers, and students.

As a COTA, I welcome the responsibility of tracking the daily progress of the patients under my care. Effective communication is the key, not only between the COTA and OTR, but it is equally important among the other rehabilitation disciplines that enhance the delivery of quality treatment to the patient. In addition to good communication, developing accurate observational skills is also essential to know when to move on and when to explore other alternatives.

Although I have been a COTA for 23 years, each day is a new and welcome challenge. Patients depend on the rehabilitation team to help them achieve their highest levels of independence. My "creative juices" flow when I help the patient reach these goals. The on-going problem-solving challenges and the need to be creative, develop strategies, and offer alternatives stimulate me to take charge. It is difficult for patients to accept their limitations and to learn basic skills over again. As a COTA, I accept patients for who they are—creating a nonthreatening atmosphere that promotes the desire to strive to reach their highest potential.

For me, a client's smile as he or she reaches the highest level of independence or function is worth one hundred "thank yous." Do I ask a lot from the patients and from myself? I sure do! ▪

Patricia L. Shiokari, AA, COTA
Vocational Specialist
Transitional Living Program for Head
　　Injured Adults
Orange, California

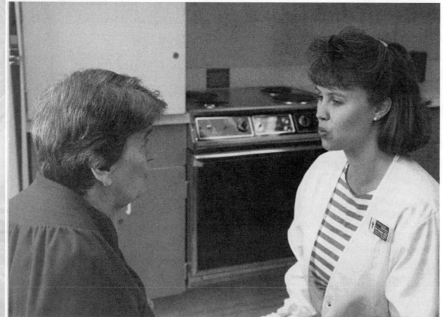

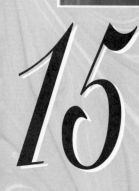

15 Therapeutic Relationships

Objectives

After reading this chapter, the reader will be able to:

✤ Explain the uniqueness of the therapeutic relationship
✤ Identify the stages of loss
✤ Describe how the "use of self" is used as one of the tools of therapy
✤ Understand the importance of self-awareness for effective therapeutic relationships
✤ Identify the three "selves" recognized in self-awareness
✤ Explain the skills needed for developing effective therapeutic relationships
✤ Demonstrate the necessary skills for "taking charge" of a group

Key terms

Therapeutic relationship
Universal stages of loss
Therapeutic use of self
Group
Self-awareness
Ideal self
Perceived self
Real self
Nonverbal communication
Empathy
Active listening
Restatement
Reflection
Clarification

People interact with one another on a daily basis without thinking much about it; but, what is human interaction? At the simplest level of understanding, the term means an exchange among people—an interaction with one another. This exchange is complex since each person lives in two worlds—an outer world of objects, actions, and situations, and an inner world of thoughts, feelings, and desires. Each world affects and is affected by the other. In therapy when the focus is on the person's outer world, technical skills are employed. When the focus is on the person's inner world, human interaction skills are used.

Human communication is complex, in and of itself, and the interaction between an occupational therapy (OT) practitioner and a client requires more than the skills used in everyday human interactions. The interaction between a practitioner and a client is the **therapeutic relationship** in which the OT practitioner is

Chapter 15 photo: Lohman H, Padilla R, Byers-Connon S: *Occupational therapy with elders: strategies for the COTA*, St Louis, 1998, Mosby.

responsible for facilitating the healing and rehabilitation process. The effective practitioner knows that the relationship established with each client is an important element of therapy. Regardless of the individual's cognitive, physical, or psychosocial deficits, the OT practitioner needs to have proficient communication skills to develop rapport with each person, ensuring that the client will actively participate in reaching his or her maximum potential.

PSYCHOLOGY OF REHABILITATION

From the beginning of one's study of the field of OT, the psychology of rehabilitation must be embraced. People who have suffered catastrophic trauma or illness have great emotional and physical needs. Usually the physical needs receive attention from many areas of treatment, but the emotional needs are frequently overlooked. Because of the intent of the profession and the nature of treatment, OT practitioners are in a unique position to give attention to these needs. Historically all OT literature emphasizes treating the whole person, and most treatment is individualized and personal with close body contact and ongoing practitioner-client interaction.

In psychology classes, OT students will likely study the stages of death and dying, first identified by Elizabeth Kübler-Ross.[4] These **universal stages of loss** are recognized as *denial, anger, bargaining, depression*, and *acceptance*. The majority of people in therapy, at various times, experience each. The OT practitioner's ability and willingness to recognize these stages will provide the client the opportunity to work through them.

Daniel Goleman's book, *Emotional Intelligence* is a groundbreaking study of the critical role emotions play in a person's life. He states, "...the design of the brain means we very often have little or no control over *when* we are swept by emotions, nor over *what* emotion it will be. But we can have some say in *how long* an emotion will last."[3] He continues, "...a universal trigger for anger is the sense of being endangered...not just an outright physical threat, but also, as is more often the case, by a symbolic threat to self-esteem or dignity."[3] Therefore anger is so often a part of a client's experience, and so too is depression. "The sadness that loss brings has certain invariable effects: it closes down our interest in diversions and pleasures, fixes attention on what has been lost, and saps our energy for starting new endeavors."[3] The OT practitioner's sensitivity to the emotional impact of the stages of loss will highlight the differences between a merely adequate and a truly competent practitioner.

THERAPEUTIC RELATIONSHIP

It is in light of the psychology of rehabilitation that the importance of the therapeutic relationship is recognized. Although some aspects of therapeutic interaction may appear like a friendship, the relationship is, by design, distinctly different.

Friendships are expected to be reciprocal; that is, each person contributes to and receives from the relationship in more or less equal measure. Each expects a balance of rewards and responsibilities. The therapeutic relationship is, however, unique and designed to benefit the one being served. The OT practitioner is fully aware that the purpose of the interaction is to meet the needs of the client. Yet, it is often true that the practitioner receives "reward," albeit not by intention or design.

In every therapy session the OT practitioner is expected to be aware of the client's needs and, using technical and interaction skills, to select responses or courses of action that benefit the one being served. Although technical skills employed by the OT practitioner are important, his or her interaction skills in the therapeutic relationship often make the difference between a successful and an unsuccessful therapy experience. As with any other therapeutic tool, an OT practitioner must constantly assess interaction skills and make judgments about when to use what, and to what degree. Just as technical skills can become mechanical and rob therapy of its value and purpose, so too can a "professional personality" develop and rob a relationship of its usefulness and meaning.

In *Patient-Practitioner Interaction*, Davis states, "Superior skill in the technology of the profession must be balanced with the art of relating to those who request our services in such a way that healing is facilitated rather than interfered with." Davis' reference to "the art of relating" is also termed the **therapeutic use of self,** which entails being aware of oneself and of the client and being in command of what is communicated.[1]

The OT practitioner must be aware of what is said and what is not said and keep both in proper balance in order for the client-practitioner relationship to be truly useful. In her book, *Mental Health Concepts and Techniques,*[2] Early lists ten qualities that must be developed by the practitioner who employs *therapeutic use of self* as a tool. These are active listening, empathy, genuineness, immediacy, respect, self-disclosure, sensitivity, specificity, trust, and warmth. These qualities are needed to establish and sustain a therapeutic relationship. (Later in this chapter these qualities are described in detail.)

The context in which a therapeutic relationship takes place may be a one-on-one interaction or a group treatment setting. A **group** is defined as more than two people interacting with a common purpose. OT treatment often occurs in groups, particularly in mental health settings. Other examples in which group treatment occurs are children's groups for diagnostic categories, geriatric groups, family support groups, and life-skill groups for the developmentally delayed, just to name a few. The establishment of a therapeutic relationship needs to be a consideration in both didactic (one-on-one) and group-treatment situations.

SELF-AWARENESS

OT regards *therapeutic use of self* as an important element in therapy. Through the *use of self*, the OT practitioner consciously builds a relationship with the client to promote treatment goals and pursue a higher level of function. To facilitate another person's healing and to develop an effective therapeutic relationship, the OT practitioner must have **self-awareness.** Self-awareness is knowing one's own true nature; it is the ability to recognize one's own behavior, emotional responses, and effect created on others. Throughout recorded history, some form of the admonition, "Know thyself," can be found. All wisdom begins with self-knowledge.

Self-awareness may appear so obvious that one may expect it to happen automatically, often disregarding the fact that it takes effort. Of course, experience does yield some measure of self-awareness, just as some knowledge about trees comes from just having them around. However, when trees are the *focus* and are systematically studied, greater knowledge is gained. True knowledge requires disciplined pursuit of specific awareness.

People often have the mistaken fear that too much focus on oneself will foster egoism. Egoism is seeing all things only from one's own point of view, only considering one's own wants and needs in all circumstances and situations. Most people have been correctly taught that egoism is a character trait to avoid. Although an appropriate development stage of early childhood, egoism is inappropriate for mature adults. Self-awareness, however, is very different than egoism.

The contrast between egoism and self awareness can be illustrated by the following simple example: A 3-year-old boy walks into a room of people watching television and stands in front of the screen without regard for the fact that he is blocking everyone's view. This behavior displays egoism. The child is aware only of what he wants. Conversely, self-awareness enables an adult to be conscious of the relative nature of self and others. Self-awareness causes an adult to look around, to become aware of blocking the view of others, and to adapt his or her behavior.

Self-awareness is essential for mature, healthy interaction and is often poorly developed because of the defenses erected to protect against unpleasant truths. To develop better self-awareness, consider the nature of the self.

Each person is composed of three selves: the ideal self, the perceived self, and the real self. Each is an aspect of the total self. The **ideal self** is what an individual would like to be if free of the demands of mundane reality. This aspect is the "perfect self," with only desirable qualities and with all wants and wishes fulfilled. The ideal self is an unrealistic goal, not an obtainable reality. The ideal self that resides in the inner world has access to all intention, feeling, and desire but remains little known to others. Each person feels the need to defend the ideal self (though not necessarily is it revealed) when it is not acknowledged by others.

The **perceived self** is the aspect that others see; it is what they perceive without the benefit of knowing a person's intentions, motivations, and limitations (i.e., as defined only by outward behavior). This perceived self is not the true self, however, since it comes from the perspective (and also the biases) of the one perceiving. The behavioral or perceived self exists in the outer world. Reports from others regarding the perceived self (comments on behavior) are often received as criticism. The reports are not in agreement with the ideal self's perceptions; consequently, there is denial of what others report as a person's behavior or his or her effect.

The **real self** is a blending of the internal and external worlds involving intention and action plus environmental awareness. The real self includes the feelings, strengths, and limitations of the person, as well as the reality in which the person exists (his or her environment). The inclusion of the perceived self, along with recognition of the limits of the ideal self, allows the emergence of the real self. The real self processes awareness and determines what behavioral adjustments are needed.

It is possible to be unaware of any or all of these aspects of self. Such a lack of awareness is the result of building defenses against unpleasant truths and denying that behavioral changes are needed. The results are distorted self-perceptions that are destructive to "real" relationships. When busy defending the ideal self and denying the perceived self, the real self is kept from emerging. The process of gaining self-awareness involves making a effort to realistically acknowledge shortcomings of both the internal and external worlds so a person can live from the real self. A self-aware person is able to distinguish among the three aspects and is able to realistically acknowledge his or her own shortcomings and limitations without self-condemnation.

Self-awareness is the process of opening up to the real self—the blend of all aspects. Individuals working on self-awareness examine both how they see themselves and how they are seen by others. The self-aware individual can contrast the ideal self with the perceived self and know they are, of necessity, different. There are many ways to develop self-awareness. Simply being aware of the multifaceted self is a step toward self-understanding. Keeping a journal—writing down feelings and reactions—is a rich source of self-knowledge. By opening up oneself to how he or she is seen by others, an individual can gain access to information not normally known. Participation in group interaction is another way to develop self-awareness, since the central purpose of a group is to give and receive feedback about the perceived self.

When a person lives predominately in the real self, he or she is ready to reach out and help others find their real selves, balancing strengths and weaknesses to embrace his or her humanness realistically. Self-respect is gained by being aware of and making conscious choices about behavior and by accepting the range of emotional responses experienced in the unexpected turns of life—by living in reality. A person relates successfully to others in proportion to her or his self-knowledge. Developing self-awareness is a lifelong undertaking that will reap rich rewards in all relationships but especially in the therapeutic relationships encountered as an OT practitioner.

SKILLS FOR EFFECTIVE THERAPEUTIC RELATIONSHIPS

Sustaining the therapeutic relationship is a skill. Warmth, caring, and empathy must be balanced with analysis, judgment, and a demand for performance. When the OT practitioner is too detached, technical, or critical, his or her relationship with the client may be damaged by coldness and alienation. When the practitioner is too friendly and "chummy," the therapy may be clouded by the failure to use clinical judgment to select the most beneficial course of action.

In addition to self-awareness, there are a number of skills and qualities needed to establish and maintain therapeutic relationships. The most essential are the abilities to develop trust, demonstrate empathy, understand verbal and nonverbal communication, and perform active listening.[1,2,5,7] The OT practitioner must also be skilled in leading a group.

TRUST

Foremost to establishing a therapeutic relationship is the ability to develop the trust of the client. The client needs to have confidence in the OT practitioner for a therapeutic relationship to be effective. Trust and acceptance will facilitate the relationship and motivate the client to be interested in the therapy and treatment.

As a part of gaining an individual's trust, the OT practitioner must be genuine about who he or she is. Sincerity and honesty without pretense will facilitate the development of trust between the practitioner and client. Opening up to the client in treatment and disclosing personal information is beneficial. In the therapeutic relationship the OT practitioner asks the client to divulge personal facts; the relationship can become more even if the practitioner discloses some personal information to the client.[2] However, self-disclosure needs to be done with care and consideration; as always, the timing needs to be appropriate. Self-disclosure is most appropriate when the client asks for it; it should never be offered when the client is in the middle of a crisis or expressing thoughts.[2] The amount and type of information disclosed also needs to be considered. It is not advisable for the OT practitioner to give his or her address or phone number to a client. Additionally, it is not appropriate for the practitioner to transfer all his or her problems and emotions onto the client.

UNDERSTANDING VERBAL AND NONVERBAL COMMUNICATIONS

Interaction between the OT practitioner and client requires that the OT practitioner understand not only what is expressed verbally but also what is expressed nonverbally by the client.

Not all communication is verbal. Frequently, nonverbal communication is used to express thoughts. **Nonverbal communication** includes facial expressions, eye contact, tone of voice, touch, and body language. The effective practitioner is aware of nonverbal forms of communication and is continually watchful of his or her client for this type of communication.

In many instances the client will verbally express one thought while communicating an entirely different message with facial expressions or body language. An example of this is the client, Mr. B, who is in therapy working to increase his shoulder range of motion after an injury. The OT practitioner is moving Mr. B's arm through its available range of motion and asks him if it hurts. Mr. B responds with a "no" answer to the OT practitioner, while expressing a nonverbal wincing of his face. The facial expression, which communicates that Mr. B is experiencing pain, should not be ignored by the OT practitioner. He or she needs to choose whether to confront the discrepancy between the client's verbal and nonverbal responses. This confrontation will depend on the nature of the relationship and the degree of trust.[5]

Because of the nature of his or her disability, in some instances the client may not be able to verbally communicate or understand verbal communication. In these situations both the OT practitioner and client rely on nonverbal forms of communication. Being attuned to the client's facial expressions and body language is extremely important.

The OT practitioner must also be aware of the nonverbal behavior that he or she uses. In therapeutic relationships it is usually desirable for the OT practitioner to convey friendliness and interest. This can be demonstrated by nonverbal behaviors such as smiling, touching, leaning toward the client, and making eye contact. The OT practitioner needs to use body language carefully, however, and match it to the particular needs of the client.[2] Obviously, it is not appropriate to smile when the individual is sharing feelings of how life has changed for the worse. Touching the person may also indicate that the practitioner cares and is there to help. However, some people may be uncomfortable being touched.[2] Different cultures, societies, and age groups vary in terms of the boundaries they have for being touched. In addition, individuals with central nervous system dysfunction may not tolerate being touched. The OT practitioner needs to be alert and sensitive to these possibilities and respect each person's individual differences regarding touch.

DEVELOPING EMPATHY

Empathy toward the client is another quality that needs to be developed. **Empathy** in the therapeutic relationship is the ability of the OT practitioner to place himself or herself in the client's position and understand what they are experiencing. Empathy is not to be confused with pity or identification. To express pity for the client is to feel sympathy with condescension. Pity is demeaning to the individual and conveys the attitude the practitioner is better than the client.[1] Equally as undesirable is identification with the client, which means the OT practitioner feels at one with him or her and, as a result, loses sight of the differences.[1] In identifying with a client, the practitioner may forget that the individual has different values and feelings; the values and needs of the practitioner may become confused with those of the client's in such a way that they become less important to the therapy process.[1]

Empathy toward another individual does not mean that therapeutic objectivity is lost.[1] When empathetic, the practitioner understands and is sensitive to the thoughts, feelings, and experiences of the client without losing objectivity.

Empathy is important to the development of trust in the therapeutic relationship. The client who sees that the OT practitioner empathizes with his or her experience is more willing to communicate and participate in treatment.[2]

ACTIVE LISTENING

A critical skill for conducting an effective therapeutic relationship is the ability of **active listening.** The practitioner actively listens to the client without making judgments, jumping in with advice, or providing defensive replies. With active listening, the receiver paraphrases the speaker's words to ensure that he or she understand the intended meaning. Active listening should not only be used with the client, but also in the practitioner's interactions with family and friends. Caution must be taken, however, against allowing active listening to become no more than a repetition of the client's words (also known as "parroting.")

Davis[1] describes active listening as having three processes: restatement, reflection, and clarification. Using **restatement** in the therapeutic relationship, the receiver of the message (the practitioner) repeats the words of the speaker (the client) as they are heard. To illustrate restatement, the client says, "I am angry that I had this stroke. I just retired, and my wife and I planned to travel and see the world." A restatement would be, "You are angry because your stroke may prevent you from traveling with your wife?" Restatement is used only in the initial phases of active listening. Its primary purpose is to encourage the person to continue talking.[1]

Reflection is a response wherein the purpose is to "express in words the feelings and attitudes sensed behind the words of the sender."[1] Using reflection in the therapeutic relationship, the OT practitioner verbalizes both the content *and* the feelings that are implied by the client. An example of the use of reflection is the client saying, "I've been trying to dress myself for weeks now; I just can't do it." A reply from the practitioner may be, "You're frustrated and feeling defeated because you can't dress yourself?" Using reflection, the OT practitioner demonstrates to the client that he or she is hearing the emotions behind the words, not just the words.[1] If the practitioner has not correctly identified the emotions, reflection is posed as a question, which gives the client an opportunity to clarify what he or she is really feeling.

During **clarification** in the therapeutic relationship, the client's thoughts and feelings are summarized or simplified.[1] For example, the client may say, "When my doctor referred me to occupational therapy, I thought you would be the person who would help me get the use of my arm back. I've been coming to therapy for weeks now, and I still don't have full functioning in my arm. What am I supposed to do? Will I ever be able to use my hand again?" Clarification may sound something like, "When you came to occupational therapy, you expected to immediately get the function back in your arm. Now you realize that the return of arm and hand function is going to take longer than expected and is more than a matter of someone just fixing it?" Clarification is used when the OT practitioner wants to help the client look closer at the thoughts and feelings experienced. All of these active listening skills can be acquired with practice. The practitioner starts by using restatement, reflection, and clarification in his or her interactions with the client's family and friends. If the OT practitioner forgets to use the three processes, he or she can rehearse the conversations as if the active listening processes had been used. Recording statements made by family and friends, as well as the appropriate responses, are also helpful.

GROUP LEADERSHIP SKILLS

The final skill to consider is group leadership. Since group treatment is one technique of the profession, the OT student must expect to study group dynamics—how groups interact and function.

In the 1960s and 1970s, groups became a popular phenomenon. There were therapy groups, training groups, sensitivity groups, and encounter groups. This widespread interest led to critical examination of the group process. People have always gathered in groups, but the idea of analyzing the different elements of groups and using them as a treatment or learning approach is a contemporary discovery. As people interact in groups around shared concerns, patterns of behavior emerge. The awareness and understanding of these patterns allow the OT practitioner to guide and direct the interactions in positive, goal-oriented directions.

Most OT groups are task oriented and involve structure, activity, and goals. Common group activities include cooking, arts and crafts, exercise, activities of daily living, and reality orientation groups. The goals of the group and the techniques used depend, in large part, on the setting (inpatient or outpatient) in which the group meets. Other variables to consider include the size and composition of the group, the frame of reference, and the duration and frequency of the group meetings.[5]

Some people are natural group leaders, yet group leadership is a skill that can be developed. Group leadership involves incorporating the principles of the therapeutic use of self, as well as developing an awareness of group dynamics. As defined in *Merriam-Webster's Collegiate Dictionary*®, edition 10, group dynamics is "the interacting forces within a small human group; the sociological study of these forces."[6] Group leadership skills can be acquired only through involvement and practice, but awareness of the basic structures and processes provides the starting point for understanding the experience.

Studying group processes requires becoming a group participant and examining all aspects of the process. The "doing" and "understanding" are different. The study calls for examination of the skills needed by both leaders and group members. Leaders need to know how to exhibit leadership, convey knowledge about groups to group members, carry out organizational tasks, structure sessions, and guide members' performance. As group members, participants must be aware of task assignments (the specific responsibilities of the individuals), the importance of active listening, and the various roles that members assume as they interact in different ways.

The group leader needs to effectively take charge of the group. When a group lacks confidence in the leader's ability to lead, confusion often results. If an individual sounds and looks as if he or she is in charge, confidence will be communicated to group members, and they will support the activity. Assuming a leadership role is not becoming a dictator but appearing confident and clearly structuring the process so people know what is expected of them. As group interaction progresses, leadership can and does shift within the group—as part of the dynamics—but the OT practitioner is ultimately responsible for the form and structure. A group's success is highly dependent on early and clear leadership.

Box 15-1 provides guidelines for exercising leadership in the earliest stages of group formation and task identification. These are points of which to be aware before entering a formal course on group dynamics, and they will be useful in any situation of leadership. (See Activities, #5, for ways to practice the skill.)

APPLICATION OF THERAPEUTIC USE OF SELF TO OCCUPATIONAL THERAPY

To illustrate how the therapeutic use of self is applied in OT, several examples are presented. Consider an OT practitioner in a public school setting who has a personality that can be described as moderately cheerful and easygoing. Although this approach serves many children, successful interaction with the following two clients requires a style change. Client #1 is an overly indulged, whining child who acts out her feelings; client #2 is a child who is fearful, shy, and compliant.

As the OT practitioner works with client #1—if he is truly conscious of the use-of-self as a therapeutic tool and of the importance of building a therapeutic relationship—he quickly realizes that his usual easygoing, cheerful manner may be detrimental to therapy, especially since the child sees him as a "pushover" for her manipulative behavior. He elects to employ a stern, almost detached, no-nonsense approach. His plan for client #1 involves clearly defined expectations with rewards and consequences spelled out.

The first time the child "tests" him with a tantrum, he calmly allows the behavior to run its course and then unemotionally repeats his expectations of her. By using this approach, the OT practitioner convinces the child that he means what he says and is not going to be influenced by her manipulations. Once this relationship is established, he gradually relaxes and resumes his usual approach yet remains prepared to return to the no-nonsense approach if needed.

As this OT practitioner works with client #2, he again considers the child's personality and assesses her needs. He concludes that the client does not require

Box 15-1

TAKING CHARGE OF A GROUP

1. **PLAN AND PRACTICE OR REHEARSE THE ACTIVITY TO KNOW WHAT IS NEEDED.**

2. **ANTICIPATE! THINK HOW PEOPLE <u>MIGHT</u> INTERPRET THE INSTRUCTIONS.**

3. **CARRY A WRITTEN LIST OF ALL THE POINTS TO REMEMBER.**

4. **STAND TO ADDRESS THE GROUP.**

5. **GET EVERYONE'S ATTENTION BEFORE TALKING (EXPECT IT AND IT WILL HAPPEN).**

6. **REGULATE VOICE APPROPRIATELY (LOUD AND CLEAR, AS NEEDED).**

7. **TELL IN SEQUENCE. KEEP WORDS TO A MINIMUM AND DEMONSTRATE "FIRST," "NEXT," ETC.**

8. **TELL THE GROUP WHAT TO DO WHEN THE TASK IS COMPLETE.**

9. **INDICATE THE END OF INSTRUCTIONS AND THE BEGINNING OF THE ACTIVITY.**

the no-nonsense approach; she needs to have fun and exercise choice making. The OT practitioner approaches therapy with a "have-fun-and-be-silly" playtime attitude. Each time there is a media change, he presents her with several alternatives and expects her to choose. He allows her to share in planning when appropriate and listens to her concerns.

These two examples illustrate how a practitioner effectively works one-on-one, builds therapeutic relationships, and uses interaction as a tool to promote better function. Whether a practitioner works one-on-one or in a group, with children or adults, the same principles apply. The effective OT practitioner builds the relationship on the uniqueness of the client, applying the therapeutic use of self according to client needs.

Additional examples are examined that involve a second OT practitioner working with adults. This practitioner is intent, serious, competent, makes good technical treatment choices, and usually her approach is matter-of-fact and informative. Client #1 is 40 years of age and talks constantly, but has little content to his monologues. He agrees to his therapy plans, but never quite finishes the activities; he appears to be lazy and unmotivated. Client #2 is a young adult who is sullen and angry. He was in an automobile accident that has left him in a wheelchair. In therapy he either refuses to cooperate or deliberately sabotages treatment plans.

Adult client #1 has had several OT practitioners and has developed a reputation for being difficult. The practitioner has studied the client ahead of time to determine the best therapeutic relationship. She realizes that her normal approach—direct, informative, and matter-of-fact—may not be effective; as a result she decides on another approach. She schedules 1-hour, one-on-one sessions in an individual treatment room, rather than the usual $^1/_2$-hour time blocks. During this hour she also schedules other clients to overlap each end of the hour, leaving him as her "only" client for approximately 10 minutes, 20 minutes into the hour.

The OT practitioner meets with him, speaks in a friendly manner, and explains that she is aware that he works slowly and has allowed more time for treatment—but she must schedule others at the same time. She writes a checklist for his activities and informs him that she will regularly look in on him. The practitioner explains that although his schedule allows 1 hour, he can leave when the planned activities are completed. Since he is alone in the small treatment room, there is no one with whom he can talk.

As the treatment plan is implemented, the OT practitioner regularly checks the client. After 20 minutes she remains with him only when he has completed most of the activities, in which case she uses the remaining 10 minutes (of the usual $^1/_2$-hour session) to pleasantly talk about nontherapeutic things.

The OT practitioner's approach to client #2 is entirely different. When he comes for treatment, the practitioner schedules no other clients. She designs a step-by-step plan, explains it in detail (identifying its purpose and goals) but exerts no pressure on him to accept the plan or engage in the activities. She says she will spend time with him each day, regardless of whether he engages in therapy. She reads articles about his condition and sometimes shares the material with him. She encourages him to talk about what he is experiencing inside and is careful NOT to say she understands how he feels. Instead, the OT practitioner asks the client to describe what it is like to have his life changed so drastically, using active listening techniques to restate, reflect, and clarify what he says. She also asks him what he would like to accomplish in therapy and agrees to revise the plan to include his goals for treatment.

In each case the OT practitioner considers the needs of the client. Client #1 sabotages his own program by passive resistance—he agrees to work but wastes therapy time with no evidence of inner conflicts, only an unwillingness to accept responsibility for his program. Through effective planning and scheduling, the OT practitioner removes the opportunity for the client to waste therapy time. She extends the treatment time to facilitate the expectation that he will complete the activities and rewards his efforts by chatting in the manner he enjoys when he does so.

Client #2 is actively resistant to therapy and has not sufficiently dealt with the denial and anger of becoming paralyzed at a young age. In response the OT practitioner gives the client her full attention—making no demands. She explains the treatment plan and makes it clear that she is ready to work when the client is ready. She also encourages him to share his therapy goals so they can be included in the plan. In sharing reading materials on his condition, she signals a willingness to discuss any aspect of the trauma the client desires. The client believes he has lost control of his life; therefore the OT practitioner does not take more of his sense of control by forcing him into therapy for which he is not ready. She accepts his hostility and anger by simply being there. She is aware that often a person needs the patience of another who is willing to wait and listen.

SUMMARY

Important in therapy is the interaction between the client and OT practitioner—the therapeutic relationship. The practitioner is perepared to engage in high quality interaction skills by developing self-awareness. This awareness enables the OT practitioner to adapt her or his manner of relating to result in the greatest benefit to the client; this technique is called the therapeutic use of self. To the OT practitioner the use of the self is as important in the therapy process as technical skills and knowledge. In addition to self-awareness, several other skills are needed by the OT practitioner to sustain an effective therapeutic relationship. These skills include understanding verbal and nonverbal communication, developing empathy and trust, active listening, and leading a group treatment session. The clients in OT come from different backgrounds and have different needs. The OT practitioner must learn how to adapt his or her approach to each individual.

OT is an individual and personal form of treatment that focuses on the whole person. The OT practitioner's use of self creates a therapeutic relationship—an atmosphere supportive of improving the client's overall functioning.

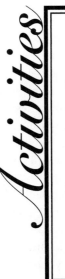

1. Make a list of desirable qualities for use in therapeutic relationships. Seek out a written description for each quality. Write a one- or two-sentence description for each, and make a self-rating scale.
2. Working with a partner, agree to monitor each other's communication (verbal and nonverbal) in a specific situation (i.e., class discussion, visit to a clinic, at luncheon table). Each person is to keep a "personal reaction log" on the events and a "report log" of the other's behavior. At the end of the monitored time, share the logs and compare the personal reactions against the reported behavior.
3. If a videotape library is available, watch videotapes of people with impairments, disabilities, or problem behaviors. Write a description of the therapeutic relationship you would develop in each case, should that person become your client. Include a rationale for your choice of therapeutic relationship.

Activities—cont'd

4. Select a partner. Each person is to write four to five verbal messages
that a client may say to an OT practitioner. Switch your messages
with those of your partner. On a separate piece of paper each person is
to write an appropriate active listening response to each message.
When finished, ask your partner to read his or her messages one at a
time as you give your response. Share feedback to the responses with
each other (i.e., How did it feel getting the response from your partner? Did the response demonstrate active listening?).

5. Practice taking charge of a group. The object is to "own" the activity
and demonstrate leadership. This can be accomplished in small groups
of six to ten in the following manner:

(a) On slips of paper equal in number to the people, write simple
activities (e.g., write a word on the board; form a line and walk
around the desk, etc.).

(b) Each member should draw one slip and not let the others know
the content.

(c) Given planning time, each member then leads the group in the
identified activity.

(d) After the activity, provide written feedback about leadership qualities displayed.

REFERENCES

1. Davis CM: *Patient practitioner interaction: an experiential manual for developing the art of health care*,
Thorofare, NJ, 1994, Slack.

2. Early MB: *Mental health concepts and techniques for the occupational therapy assistant*, ed 2, New York,
1993, Raven Press.

3. Goleman D: *Emotional intelligence*, New York, 1995, Bantam Books.

4. Kübler-Ross E: *On death and dying*, New York, 1969, Macmillan.

5. Schwartzberg SL: Therapeutic use of self. In Hopkins HL, Smith HD, editors: *Willard &
Spackman's occupational therapy*, ed 8, Philadelphia, 1993, JB Lippincott.

6. Mish F, editor: *Merriam-Webster's collegiate dictionary®*, ed 10, Springfield, Mass, 1994, Merriam-
Webster.

7. Tufano R: Therapeutic communication. In Sladyk K, editor: *OT student primer: a guide to college
success*, Thorofare, NJ, 1997, Slack.

Occupational therapy provides me with the unique opportunity to observe and to share my knowledge and my experiences in order to affect the well-being of another person. The potential to observe makes life interesting. It provides an opportunity to stand aside, note, and experience reality within its context, be it beautiful or painful. Observation further provides an opportunity to stand still and acknowledge. It provides the occupational therapist with an opportunity to apply activity analysis—the main method of occupational therapy—to detect function or dysfunction of task performance, as well as the performance components; but task performance is the focus of the human being. Observation thus allows the occupational therapist to view the human through activities or tasks, these tasks being crucial forces responsible for shaping the human being. In other words, an occupational therapist is an observer with a powerful tool, "activity analysis." Through observation the therapist can assess performance, set goals, treat the individual with the set goals in mind, and critically evaluate its impact, all by applying different forms of clinical reasoning.

The human being evolves around task performance. The human is shaped by what he or she performs, and life is meaningless without the ability and the motivation to perform at whatever small capacity. The smallest gains can be as rewarding and worthwhile for those involved as are the bigger accomplishments or achievements for others.

Occupational therapy has further allowed me to share my knowledge regarding occupational performance that could, in some instances, affect the quality of life of those involved. It has provided me with an opportunity to challenge limitations at different levels of performance, in a very exciting way, as some of these limitations have been at a level that I would have thought would be impossible to influence. Limitations have the potential to develop maturity in life, and many limitations not only bring about frustrations and negative aspects but the inner beauty of the person involved and unknown potentials that may flourish and thereby enhance maturity.

Task performance is, therefore, the force that molds the human being into an occupational being. It is a privilege to be an occupational therapist and to be involved with that powerful driving force. ■

Guorún Árnadóttir, MA, BOT
Private Practitioner
Reykjavík, Iceland

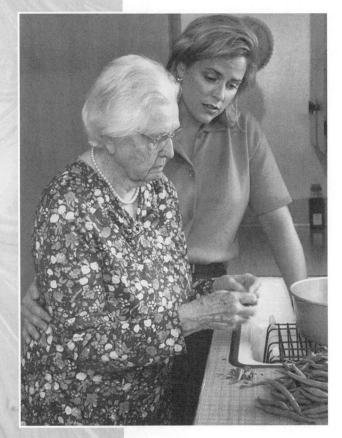

16

Treatment Modalities Used in Occupational Therapy

Objectives

After reading this chapter, the reader will be able to:

❖ Identify the principal tools of occupational therapy (OT) practice, and describe the primary therapeutic purposes for each

❖ Explain the purpose of activity analysis, and describe its application to purposeful activity

❖ Understand the role of the OT practitioner in splinting and in assistive technology

Key terms

Modality

Medium

Methods

Purposeful activity

Activity analysis

Grading

Adaptation

Assistive devices

Enabling activities

Adjunctive activities

Therapeutic exercise

Physical agent modalities

Splint

OT practitioners use a variety of modalities as tools of the trade. Through the selection and use of these modalities, OT practitioners aim to reach the goals identified in the treatment plan for each client. Selecting the modality to use and the time to use it becomes a skill through experience and practice. For the student entering the field, it may be confusing to understand how each modality fits into OT. It is important that the OT student learn the modalities of the profession and understand how they are used in practice.

What is meant by the term modality? A **modality** includes both media and methods.[7] Reed[8] defines **medium,** or media, as "the means by which the therapeutic effects are transmitted." For example, the medium used to treat a child in OT may be a scooter board. The steps, sequences, and approaches used to activate the therapeutic effect of a medium are the **methods.**[8] The OT practitioner may ask the child to use the scooter board in different ways to activate a therapeutic response. One method may be to ask the child to ride the board on his stomach down an

Chapter 16 photo: Lohman H, Padilla R, Byers-Connon S: *Occupational therapy with elders: strategies for the COTA,* St Louis, 1998, Mosby.

incline. In treatment, it is necessary that the OT practitioner consider the whole modality, that is, both the medium and the method used.

Since the beginning of the profession, purposeful activity (or occupation) has been used as an OT treatment modality. With the advent of the medical model, however, OT practitioners began using other modalities to enhance their treatment. These treatment modalities have included the use of exercise and activity modalities, the emergence of which has started a controversy regarding what constitutes legitimate tools of the profession. In her 1989 article, *Guidelines for Using Both Activity and Exercise,* Dutton maintains that, "The controversy over the role of occupational therapists has persisted because activity and exercise have been seen as mutually exclusive, philosophically opposed treatment approaches. Activity and exercise are really at complementary ends of the same continuum."[5]

A continuum of OT treatment that helps conceptualize the use of the various OT treatment modalities, including both activity and exercise, is described by Pedretti.[6] This continuum is based on the occupational performance model in which the ultimate goal for the client is to become as independent as possible in performance areas and resume occupational roles. There are four stages in this treatment continuum (Figure 16-1). They are (1) adjunctive methods, (2) enabling activities, (3) purposeful activity, and (4) occupational performance and occupational roles. The client does not necessarily proceed through this continuum one stage at a time. Stages may overlap or occur simultaneously.

In this chapter this continuum is used as a framework for helping the student to organize his or her thoughts around OT treatment modalities.

PURPOSEFUL ACTIVITY

Purposeful activity is the foundation upon which OT was built; to this day, it remains the central focus of OT treatment. In the American Occupational Therapy Association's (AOTA's) position paper, **purposeful activity** is defined as "goal-directed behaviors or tasks that comprise occupations."[2] This document states, "An activity is purposeful if the individual is an active, voluntary participant and if the activity is directed toward a goal that the individual considers meaningful."[2]

Purposeful activity should have an *inherent* goal. In other words, aside from the therapeutic goal(s) for which the activity is being used, the activity in and of itself has a goal or end product. For example, the inherent goal of a leather lacing kit is to make a leather coin holder (or whatever item the kit contains). The inherent goal of cooking is to prepare something to eat. The goals that are intrinsic to the activity make it purposeful. The OT practitioner will also have therapeutic reasons for asking the client to participate in a selected activity. For example, the practitioner may use the leather lacing activity for the therapeutic purpose of

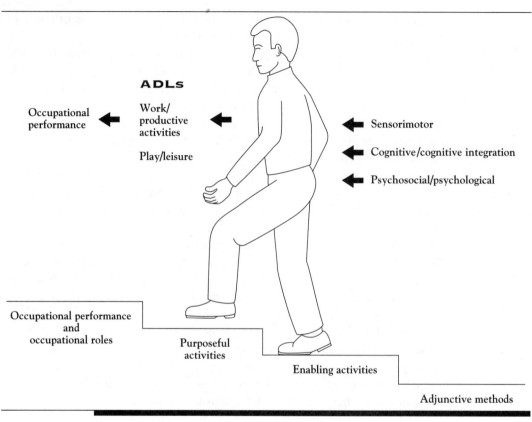

FIGURE 16-1. STAGES IN TREATMENT CONTINUUM. (ILLUSTRATION COURTESY OF KARIN BOYCE.)

improving the individual's fine motor or sequencing skills. The therapeutic goals of the cooking activity may be to increase safety awareness, improve self-esteem, or demonstrate problem-solving skills.

For purposeful activity to be an effective therapy tool, the OT practitioner needs to ensure that the activity has significance to the client. Further, purposeful activity requires client involvement and is geared toward either prevention, maintenance, or improvement of function. It reflects client involvement in life task situations, relates to the interests of the client, and is adaptable and gradable. Purposeful activity is considered beneficial by the OT practitioner through his or her judgment and knowledge of human development, pathology, interpersonal relationships, and the needs of the client being served.[9] To understand purposeful activity and how an activity is selected and implemented to reach occupational performance for a client, the OT practitioner must first understand and be able to analyze activities.

ACTIVITY ANALYSIS

Activity analysis is the process whereby the OT practitioner breaks down the steps of an activity and examines each of the components. Through the process of activity analysis, the practitioner determines the multiple demands required to perform a given activity successfully. This analysis is important because it provides information that allows the OT practitioner to determine the therapeutic value of a particular activity. With experience in analyzing activities, the OT practitioner is able to break down an activity quickly and easily and identify the possibilities.

There are many different ways to complete an activity analysis, yet beyond the differences there is a unifying theme. The type or focus of activity analysis relates to the frame of reference being used. The object of analysis is to identify possible demands that the activity may make on the one who engages in it. The OT practitioner must choose the category of demands to analyze. If the practitioner is using a biomechanical frame of reference, these aspects of the activity are emphasized. Therefore in this situation the activity analysis focuses on the range of motion, type of muscle contraction, and strength required to complete the activity.[7]

The approach to activity analysis used for the purposes of this text is based on the occupational performance model described in Chapter 9. The performance components (sensorimotor, cognitive, and psychological or psychosocial) are used to organize the thinking process for analysis. This approach forces the practitioner to look at the activity in relationship to how it affects the whole person, not just one component.

The practitioner must first determine the context of the activity and identify what is needed to perform it, including the space, equipment, materials, time, and cost required. Next, the practitioner breaks down the activity into a series of steps and then analyzes each step for the human skills and abilities normally needed to perform the activity. Most take for granted the number of steps an individual goes through and the complex components that are involved in simple activities that are performed everyday. An example illustrates the point:

Circumstance and steps involved: A woman is sitting in a chair and needs to respond to a caller who comes to the door. First, the woman hears the knock at the door. She identifies the specific door from which the sound is coming and determines where the door is located. The woman stands and walks to the door. She reaches out with her arm, while opening her hand, and grasps the door knob. She turns the knob and pulls the door open. She sees the caller and says, "Hello."

Activity analysis: Sensorimotor skills enable the woman to hear the sound of the knock, to distinguish the door from which the sound is coming, to see the door and a clear path to it, to rise out of the chair, to have the equilibrium and postural control to navigate across the room, and to exercise range of motion and strength to turn the door knob and pull the door open. Cognitive skills enable the woman to recognize the sound of the knock as a signal that indicates the caller's arrival at the door, to sequence the steps necessary to greet the caller, and to distinguish the desirability of the caller. Psychosocial or psychological skills enable the woman to manage the potential feelings (e.g., responsibility, anxiety, excitement) and the social aspects of how to acceptably answer the door, extend a greeting, and entertain the caller.

The final element of the activity analysis involves consideration of the client's age, occupational roles, culture, gender, interests, and preferences that may influence the meaningfulness of the activity.[2] Certain activities, for example, balancing a checkbook, may be more appropriate for a particular age group. Balancing a checkbook is an appropriate and possibly a meaningful activity for an adult, whereas a first grader is not expected to consider balancing a checkbook a purposeful activity. Gender and culture may also be considered when analyzing an activity. For many male clients and in some cultures, cooking is seen as an activity only women perform.

The OT practitioner must be fully aware of what is required to match an activity with the person's needs and abilities and to anticipate any potential problem that he or she may encounter.

APPLICATION OF ACTIVITY ANALYSIS TO PURPOSEFUL ACTIVITY

OT practitioners select activities for different reasons and for different therapeutic purposes. Purposeful activity is used to assist the client in mastering a new skill, restoring a deficit, compensating for a functional disability, maintaining health, or preventing dysfunction.[2] Prescribing purposeful activity does not rest solely on the analysis of the activity; it requires the integration of the client's needs and abilities (determined through evaluation) with the demands of the activity (determined through activity analysis).

Activity analysis focuses on the task that is to be performed, and it identifies the requirements of such. On the other hand, the focus of the evaluation is on the functioning level of the client, and it involves identification of the person's deficits for which compensation must be found and the assets upon which strength can be drawn. In the delivery of treatment, evaluation receives more attention, whereas activity analysis tends to be a "background awareness." To draw on an earlier analogy, activity analysis is a letter in the "OT alphabet," and it is basic to effective treatment planning.

Having analyzed the activity and evaluated the client, the practitioner determines whether the client can perform the particular activity. If the client cannot, the practitioner grades or adapts the activity to enable the individual to experience a measure of success, rather than endure a performance failure.

Grading involves changing the process, environment, tools, or materials of the activity to increase or decrease the performance demands of the client.[2] Grading an activity is used when the therapeutic goal is to improve or restore function and when the practitioner wants to challenge the client to a certain level. For example, if the practitioner feels the client is not maximally challenged while sanding a piece of wood for a project, the sand paper can be changed to provide greater resistance or the wood can be positioned on an incline. This is referred to as *grading up*. *Grading down* is used when the client is experiencing difficulty performing the activity. Perhaps on a particular day, the client is feeling tired as a result of having slept poorly the night before. He does not feel capable of completing his shaving routine while standing. The practitioner may decrease the requirements of the activity by allowing him to sit while shaving or by requiring him to shave only one side of his face while the practitioner shaves the other.

When the goal of an activity is to have the client perform it at the highest possible level of function, **adaptation** of the activity or the environment may need to be made. "Adaptation is the process that changes an aspect of the activity or the environment to enable successful performance and accomplish a therapeutic goal."[2] Adaptation may involve using assistive technologies or modifying the environment.

Assistive devices range from *low tech* to *high tech*. Typically, devices that are considered low tech do not have electronic components. Low-tech devices, such as those designed for self-feeding shown in Figure 16-2, have been a part of OT for many years. High-tech devices, however, were introduced to OT more recently and include those with electronic components. Examples of high-tech devices are augmentative communication equipment, environmental control systems, and power wheelchairs. Figure 16-3 shows an example of an augmentative communication device.

The use of devices to aid function has a long history in OT and is an integral part of the profession. In the early years, practitioners frequently fabricated or adapted devices on their own to meet some unique need of the client. Today, however, since there are companies that have a wide variety of devices available for purchase or rent, custom fabrication of devices is rarely necessary. Today, most OT practitioners have a general knowledge of assistive technology. In particular, they are involved in the implementation of low-tech devices that are used as part of an overall treatment plan. Other OT practitioners develop an expertise in this area through advanced training. These practitioners specialize in assistive technology and are involved with the implementation of devices that are high tech and more complex.

OT practitioners must also be alert to the need for modifications to a person's environment that could facilitate function. The primary environments (e.g., home, work, and school) in which an individual functions should be evaluated for accessibility. The OT practitioner evaluates the accessibility of the environment, makes recommendations for modifications, and follows up to ensure that the recommend-

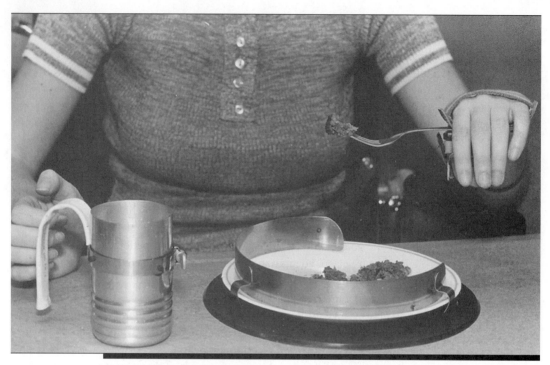

FIGURE 16-2. SELF-FEEDING USING SEVERAL LOW-TECH ASSISTIVE DEVICES TO COMPENSATE FOR ABSENT GRASP: UNIVERSAL CUFF, PLATE GUARD, NONSKID MAT, AND CLIP-TYPE CUP HOLDER. (FROM PEDRETTI LW: OCCUPATIONAL THERAPY: PRACTICE SKILLS FOR PHYSICAL DYSFUNCTION, ED 4, ST LOUIS, 1996, MOSBY.)

ed modifications have been properly made and are effectively used by the client. Examples of environmental modifications include the installation of ramps into buildings, installation of hand grip bars for bathroom safety, and arrangement of furniture in the home or at work.

A few simple examples illustrate the difference between grading and adapting. Suppose a client has a spinal cord injury and has lost the ability to grasp objects. The OT practitioner realizes that this deficit cannot be overcome; however, the goal is mealtime independence. Activity analysis has made the practitioner aware of the demands of self-feeding. After analyzing the activity, the OT practitioner realizes that the ability to perform hand grasp is normally needed to hold the utensil. Consequently, if the client is to be independent in self-feeding, a way must be found around his inability to grasp by adapting the activity. To do this, the practitioner begins with a utensil-holding appliance cuff (called a universal cuff), which slips on the hand, thus eliminating the need to grasp the fork or spoon (see Figure 16-2). With this device the OT practitioner and client can work together to train in the new method for performing self-feeding.

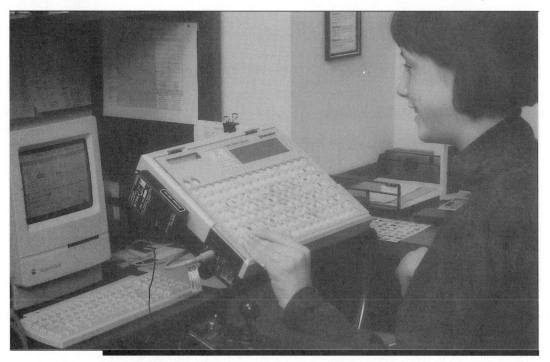

FIGURE 16-3. THIS INDIVIDUAL USES HER AUGMENTATIVE COMMUNICATION DEVICE TO ACCESS THE COMPUTER. (COURTESY OF PRENTKE ROMICH COMPANY, WOOSTER, OHIO.)

In another situation a practitioner is working with a woman who has a mental illness. She is withdrawn and avoids social contact. Available group activities are analyzed to determine which may be best for the client. Clinical judgment tells the practitioner not to begin with a cooking group (a highly social activity); instead, the practitioner seeks a craft activity that is simple, undemanding, and can be performed in an area of the room where she can be among others but need not interact with them. As the woman improves and becomes more comfortable with social interaction, the activity is graded up to make it more challenging. The OT practitioner begins by asking the client to work independently on a craft activity at the same table as other clients. The goal is that eventually the client will be able to participate in a group that is preparing a meal. The practitioner uses activity analysis to determine the demands of the activity, recalling the client's strengths and weaknesses. To meet the goal, the OT practitioner grades the activity by selecting one with low social demands, gradually increasing the level of social contact until the client is able to relate to others without being threatened.

Every OT practitioner must be able to assess the demands of an activity at many levels, to integrate the information with knowledge of the client's needs and abilities in order to select appropriate activities, and to grade and adapt activities as needed. The profession is still engaged in the work of defining OT's use of purposeful activity and its approach to the analysis of activity. Everyone entering the field should develop an appreciation for how important this work is.

ENABLING ACTIVITIES

Another type of modality used in OT treatment is enabling activities. **Enabling activities** are those that simulate a purposeful activity. The key difference between enabling and purposeful activities is that enabling activities do not have an inherent goal and therefore are not considered purposeful.[7]

Examples of enabling activities are the use of clothing fastener boards that simulate dressing tasks such as buttoning a button or zipping a zipper, or the use of manipulation boards (Figure 16-4, *left*) that simulate different types of hand grips for tasks such as opening a door lock, turning on a water faucet, or switching on a light. The inclined sanding board (Figure 16-4, *right*) is an enabling activity, which has a long history in OT and is used to exercise muscles of the arm through simulated sanding of wood; however, there is no actual end product. There is a variety of table-top media used to train cognitive and perceptual skills that are also considered enabling activities.

The use of enabling activities as a part of treatment should be carefully considered. Enabling activities are valuable in retraining motor, perceptual, and cognitive skills, but they should only be a part of a comprehensive treatment plan that also includes purposeful and adjunctive activities.[7]

ADJUNCTIVE ACTIVITIES

Adjunctive activities are those that are used to prepare the client for purposeful activity; they are therapeutic exercise and physical agent modalities (including orthotics and sensory stimulation) and splinting.[7] The purpose of adjunctive activities is to prepare the client for occupational performance.

THERAPEUTIC EXERCISE

Therapeutic exercise is a modality that has been used more recently in OT as the profession has evolved. *Taber's Cyclopedic Medical Dictionary* describes therapeutic exercise as the "scientific supervision of exercise for the purpose of preventing muscular atrophy, restoring joint and muscle function, and improving efficiency of cardiovascular and pulmonary function."[10]

The general goals of therapeutic exercise are to (1) increase muscle strength, (2) maintain or increase joint range of motion and flexibility, (3) improve muscle endurance, (4) improve physical conditioning and cardiovascular fitness, and (5)

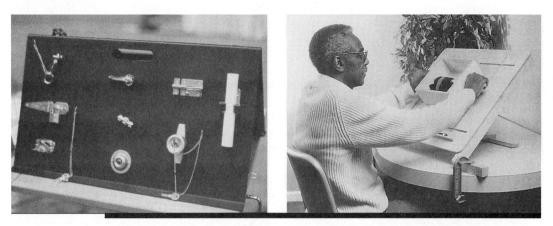

FIGURE 16-4. (LEFT) MANIPULATION BOARD SIMULATES THE DIFFERENT
HAND GRASPS USED IN EVERYDAY ACTIVITIES. (RIGHT) INCLINE SANDING BOARD
SIMULATES SANDING WOOD ON AN INCLINED PLANE AND IS USED TO EXERCISE
ELBOW AND SHOULDER MUSCULATURE. (PHOTOGRAPH AT RIGHT COURTESY OF
S & S WORLDWIDE, ADAPTABILITY, 1995.)

improve coordination.[7] The OT practitioner selects an appropriate therapeutic
exercise from available options on the basis of client needs, his or her treatment
goals, client's capabilities, and any precautions related to the client's condition.[7]
Although a description of each therapeutic exercise is beyond the scope of this
entry-level text, Table 16-1 provides a summary of the types of therapeutic exercise
used for each of the general goals.

The advantage of therapeutic exercise is that the practitioner can target specific muscle groups and motor movements by asking the client to perform particular
exercises. The amount of resistance and number of repetitions can also be controlled. The disadvantage of using therapeutic exercise is that it does not involve
the whole person, whereas purposeful activity provides a holistic approach to treatment in that it requires the individual to use many different performance components (e.g., gross and fine motor, visual, emotional). Therapeutic exercise should
not be used exclusively but to prepare a client for purposeful activity and occupational performance.

PHYSICAL AGENT MODALITIES

Physical agent modalities are also considered adjunctive activities. **Physical
agent modalities** (PAMs) are used to bring about a response in soft tissue and are
most commonly used by OT practitioners for treating hand and arm injuries and
disorders. PAMs use light, sound, water, electricity, and temperature. For example, modalities that involve heat transfer to an injured area (i.e., warm paraffin
baths, hot packs, whirlpools, or ultrasound) and modalities that involve cold

TABLE 16-1	SUMMARY OF TYPES OF THERAPEUTIC EXERCISE	
General Goal	**Type of Exercise**	**Description of Exercise**
Increase muscle strength	Active assisted	Client moves body part as much as he or she can and is assisted to complete movement by practitioner or therapeutic equipment
	Active range of motion	Client actively moves body part through complete range of motion without assistance or resistance
	Resistive	Client moves body part through available range of motion against resistance; resistance may be applied manually, by special therapeutic equipment, or through the use of weights; the amount of resistance increases as the person's strength increases
Maintain or increase joint range of motion and flexibility	Passive range of motion	Client is not able to move the body part, so movement is provided by an outside force such as a practitioner or a therapeutic device (e.g., continuous passive motion device); no muscle contraction takes place
	Active range of motion	See above
Improve muscle endurance	Low load, high repetition program	Practitioner determines client's maximum capacity for a strengthening program, then reduces the maximum resistance load and increases the number of repetitions
Improve physical conditioning and cardiovascular fitness	Sustained rhythmic, aerobic	Examples include jogging, bicycle riding, swimming, and walking
Improve coordination	Coordination training	Repetitious activities and exercises that require smooth, controlled movement patterns (e.g., placing pegs in holes, stacking blocks, picking up marbles)

transfer (i.e., cold packs and ice) are examples of PAMs. Electrical modalities include media such as transcutaneous electrical nerve conduction units (TENs), functional electrical stimulation (FES), and neuromuscular electrical stimulation devices (NMES).

The use of PAMs in OT is very controversial.[5,7,11] After debate and discussion, AOTA developed a position statement on the use of PAMs that states, "Physical agent modalities may be used by OT practitioners when used as an adjunct to or in preparation for purposeful activity to enhance occupational performance."[1] Another important detail outlined in this document is that PAMs are not to be used by entry-level practitioners; in fact, the practitioner needs to complete specialized postprofessional training before using PAMs. With proper application, the use of PAMs in OT allows the practitioner to provide a comprehensive treatment program for the client.[7]

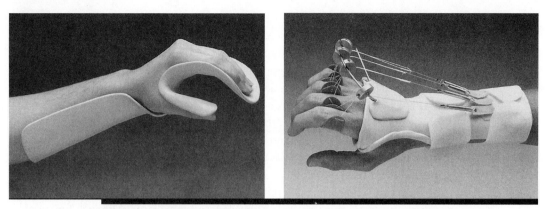

FIGURE 16-5. (LEFT) STATIC SPLINT: RESTING PAN SPLINT. (RIGHT) DYNAMIC SPLINT: FOREARM-BASED FOUR-DIGIT OUTRIGGER WITH DYNAMIC EXTENSION ASSIST SUPPLIED BY SPRINGS. (PHOTOGRAPHS FROM PEDRETTI LW: OCCUPATIONAL THERAPY: PRACTICE SKILLS FOR PHYSICAL DYSFUNCTION, ED 4, ST LOUIS, 1996, MOSBY.)

SPLINTING

Mosby's Medical, Nursing, and Allied Health Dictionary defines a **splint** as "an orthopedic device for immobilization, restraint, or support of any part of the body."[3] A splint may be rigid or flexible. Three primary purposes of a splint are to (1) restrict movement, (2) immobilize, or (3) mobilize a body part.[4] The OT practitioner is expected to recognize when there is a need for a splint, select a design that is correct for the problem, fit or fabricate it, and educate the client in its proper use and care.

There are two main classifications of splints—static splints and dynamic splints. The *static splint* has no moving components; as the name implies, it remains in a fixed position. Static splints are used to protect or rest a joint, diminish pain, or prevent shortening of the muscle.[4] Figure 16-5, *left*, shows an example of one type of static splint called a resting pan splint. The *dynamic splint* has one or more flexible components that move. The purpose of the dynamic splint is to increase passive motion, enhance active motion, or replace lost motion.[4] The movable components (elastic, rubber band, or spring) are attached to a static base. Figure 16-5, *right*, shows an example of a dynamic splint.

Both static and dynamic splints can be purchased either ready-made or custom fabricated by the OT practitioner. Custom-made splints are easily fabricated using low-temperature plastics, which become flexible and moldable when heated in hot water or with a heat gun. Several manufacturers offer various types of low-temperature plastics, each having different properties. Often the client leaves a therapy session with the needed splint the same day it is prescribed.

The Registered Occupational Therapist (OTR) is responsible for evaluating the client and recommending the type of splint. Either the OTR or the Certified

Occupational Therapy Assistant (COTA) may fabricate the splint. The OT practitioner must consider how the splint fits, both initially and throughout its use. Whether a commercial splint is used or one is custom fabricated, it is the responsibility of the OT practitioner to see that the attachments that hold it in place are comfortably located and that the device keeps the body part aligned in the correct position. The client should be educated about the wearing of the splint—how to correctly put it on and take it off, the amount of time the split should be worn, and how to keep the affected area and the splint clean. At each therapy session, the practitioner looks for pressure areas and signs of distress such as redness, swelling, or reported discomfort.

Splinting requires an in-depth knowledge of body structure, motion analysis, and disability precautions, as well as knowledge of the client. Although functional considerations are the primary concern, the practitioner must also keep in mind cosmetic and psychological factors. Client cooperation and support are essential, for the best-designed splint will not help the client who refuses to wear it.

SUMMARY

In the field of OT, there is a wide range of therapeutic modalities that is used to achieve the goals of the client. These modalities can be conceptualized along a four-stage treatment continuum. Stage 1 of this continuum pertains to the use of adjunctive modalities. Adjunctive modalities are used to prepare the client for purposeful activity and include therapeutic exercise modalities, physical agent modalities, and splints.

Stage 2 of the treatment continuum uses enabling activities, which simulate purposeful activities. They include dressing practice boards, moving cones from one side of the table to the other, and work-hardening tasks such as putting piping together.

Stage 3 of the treatment continuum uses purposeful activity. For an activity to be considered purposeful, it must have an inherent goal (in addition to the therapeutic goal) and be meaningful to the client. Activity analysis requires a skill that is learned through practice and is second nature to the experienced OT practitioner. Part of activity analysis and implementation is knowing how to grade activities and when and how to provide adaptations and assistive technology.

Stage 4 of the continuum is occupational performance and includes the performance of activities of daily living, work and school tasks, and play or leisure tasks by the client to the maximum possible level of independence. This is the ultimate goal of OT intervention.

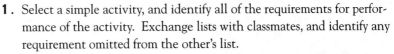

Activities

1. Select a simple activity, and identify all of the requirements for performance of the activity. Exchange lists with classmates, and identify any requirement omitted from the other's list.

2. For each performance component of the *Uniform Terminology for OT Checklist*, edition 3 (see Appendix D), identify an activity that can be therapeutically used for the individual who has a deficit in that area.

3. Find and read an article on splinting (with picture or design) from *American Journal of Occupational Therapy* or another professional source. Report on the article to your class or to a small group of students from your class.

4. Gather available resources on assistive devices. This can be done two ways: (a) In your community, research companies that provide assistive devices and study the types of equipment and services they provide. (b) Select one particular category of assistive devices (e.g., feeding equipment, augmentative communication devices, power wheelchairs), and search the Internet for companies that produce or sell these devices. Summarize the information that you find in a report.

5. Research and write a paper on the history of purposeful activity in OT.

REFERENCES

1. American Occupational Therapy Association: Position paper: physical agent modalities, *Amer J Occup Ther* 46(12):1090, 1992.

2. American Occupational Therapy Association: Position paper: purposeful activity, *Amer J Occup Ther* 47(12):1081, 1993.

3. Anderson KN, editor: *Mosby's medical, nursing, and allied health dictionary*, ed 4, St Louis, 1994, Mosby.

4. Belkin J, English CB: Hand splinting: principles, practice, and decision making. In Pedretti LW, editor: *Occupational therapy: practice skills for physical dysfunction*, ed 4, St Louis, 1996, Mosby.

5. Dutton R: Guidelines for using both activity and exercise, *Amer J Occup Ther* 43:573, 1989.

6. Pedretti LW: Occupational performance: a model for practice in physical dysfunction. In Pedretti LW, editor: *Occupational therapy: practice skills for physical dysfunction*, ed 4, St Louis, 1996, Mosby.

7. Pedretti LW, Wade IE: Therapeutic modalities. In Pedretti LW, editor: *Occupational therapy: practice skills for physical dysfunction*, ed 4, St Louis, 1996, Mosby.

8. Reed KL: Tools of practice: heritage or baggage, *Amer J Occup Ther* 40:597, 1986.

9. Simon CJ: Use of activity and activity analysis. In Hopkins HL, Smith HD, editors: *Willard & Spackman's occupational therapy*, ed 8, Philadelphia, 1993, JB Lippincott.

10. Thomas CL, editor: *Tabers' cyclopedic medical dictionary*, ed 18, Philadelphia, 1997, FA Davis.

11. West WL, Wiemer RB: Should the representative assembly have voted as it did, when it did, on occupational therapists' use of physical agent modalities? *Amer J Occup Ther* 45:1143, 1991.

The most effective COTA is someone who has developed a personal view of humanity and has acquired mastery in occupational therapy knowledge and skills. This level of practitioner understands when engaging others in the occupational therapy process, he or she is also participating in the occupational therapy process itself. ▄

Roberta Murphy, BPS, COTA, ROH
Faculty, Allied Health Division
Sacramento City College
Sacramento, California

I found out about occupational therapy when I was 23 years of age, and it immediately appealed to me. I learned that occupational therapy helps people perform activities that make life worth living—cooking a good dinner, eating food, playing a game with friends, or completing a project. What could be more important? I was right; occupational therapy is about the power of engagement in occupations. It is one of the best-kept secrets of our American health care system. Over the years I have found working directly with clients tremendously rewarding—and challenging—but it is also extremely gratifying to plan programs, educate student therapists, and conduct research. I have been an occupational therapy practitioner for 23 years; at this stage in my career I find that I help shape the future of the profession by contributing to our knowledge base through research, a particularly rewarding and fun part of being a practitioner. I keep coming back to the insight I had when I was 12 years of age—occupations have a powerful influence on who we are as individuals and who we will become as we grow older. What could be more fascinating than exploring how occupation works? What could be more exciting than working with a group of people who share the commitment to understand occupation and how it can be used to help people lead healthy, fulfilling lives? ▄

L. Diane Parham, PhD, OTR, FAOTA
Associate Professor
Occupational Therapy Department
University of Southern California
Los Angeles, California

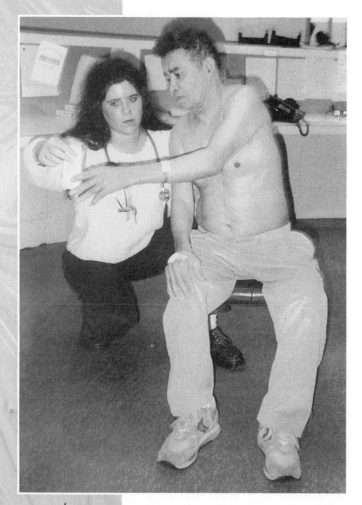

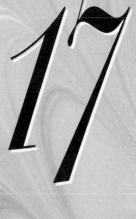

Clinical Reasoning

Objectives

After reading this chapter, the reader will be able to:

✤ Explain the nature of clinical reasoning
✤ Understand the three elements of clinical reasoning
✤ Describe the thought processes and strategies of clinical reasoning that are used by occupational therapy (OT) practitioners
✤ Compare the clinical reasoning skills of the novice with those of the expert
✤ Identify ways the OT practitioner can develop clinical reasoning skills

Key terms

Clinical reasoning
Scientific element
Ethical element
Artistic element
Procedural reasoning
Interactive reasoning
Conditional reasoning
Narrative reasoning
Pragmatic reasoning
Novice practitioner
Expert practitioner

At this point in the text, one may ask, "How does all of this get put together?" Why is it that a therapist working in a pediatric setting selects the sensory integration evaluation tool over other choices to evaluate her young child client? How does the therapist working with a severely disabled young adult know that he has the potential to drive a powered wheelchair? How does an OT practitioner working in an outpatient hand clinic know which splint to recommend for his client with arthritis? As the student of OT progresses in school and moves closer to beginning his or her first fieldwork, questions such as these may arise. How does one ever put all of the pieces together and perform as an OT practitioner?

These types of clinical questions involve clinical reasoning. **Clinical reasoning** is a process that involves complex cognitive and affective skills, that is, it involves both thinking and feeling. Clinical reasoning is used throughout the OT process—from screening to discharge. All OT practitioners must use clinical reasoning. It is used in the treatment choices when the practitioner weighs the possibilities and options, then chooses a course of action. Joan Rogers states that the goal of clinical reasoning is for the practitioner to "select the right therapeutic action for the

Chapter 17 photo: Gillen G, Burkhardt A: *Stroke rehabilitation: a function-based approach*, St Louis, 1998, Mosby.

patient."[6] The therapeutic course of action is designed to improve the occupational performance of the client and is individualized according to his or her interests.

Many, if not most, OT practitioners are unable to explain how they reach certain treatment decisions. A typical response from a practitioner when asked how he or she decided on a particular course of action is, "I don't know. I just know that it is right." Only recently have members of the OT profession begun to direct their attention toward studying clinical reasoning in hopes of learning more about the processes OT practitioners use to arrive at the decisions they make.

Joan Rogers' 1983 Eleanor Clarke Slagle lecture in which she discussed the art and science of clinical reasoning clinical reasoning.[6] In 1986 a 2-year research project jointly funded by the American Occupational Therapy Association (AOTA) and the American Foundation of Occupational Therapy (AOTF) was initiated. The study, known as the *Clinical Reasoning Study*, examined the clinical reasoning processes and strategies used by OT practitioners. An examination of the ways in which practitioners perform clinical reasoning enabled the practice of OT to be better understood. Information and strategies gleaned from these studies on clinical reasoning can be imparted to students to assist them in developing effective methods for solving the problems of future clients.

ELEMENTS OF CLINICAL REASONING

Clinical reasoning is a complex, multifaceted process. Rogers characterizes three elements of clinical reasoning: the scientific, the ethical, and the artistic.[6] There is no particular order in which these elements are applied by the OT practitioner. The **scientific element** addresses the question, "What are the possible things that can be done for this client?" The answer to this question is found in the assessment and the evaluation procedures used to determine strengths and weaknesses of the client, the writing of a plan to guide and direct the change process, and the selection of therapeutic modalities that result in successful occupational performance outcomes. The scientific element demands careful and accurate assessments, analysis, and recording.

The **ethical element** poses the question, "What should be done for this client?" The answer must take into account the client's perspective and his or her goals for treatment. Each individual has different views on what is health, what is important in life, and how things are accomplished. When the OT practitioner comes from the client's place of understanding, a treatment plan that preserves the client's values can be developed.[6] It is the OT practitioner's responsibility to supply information to the client so that he or she can participate in making decisions regarding treatment goals and methods. The OT practitioner considers all the scientific information, but ultimately, the decision of what should be done is an ethical one based on the individual's particular needs, goals, culture, environment, and lifestyle.[6]

The **artistic element** of clinical reasoning is evident in the skill used by the OT practitioner when he or she guides the treatment process and selects the "right action" in the face of uncertainties that are inherent in the clinical process.[6] The therapeutic process involves integrating and blending many separate components —the deficiencies to be addressed, the client's interests and wishes, the medium or activity to be used, and the interpersonal climate that is to support the therapy process. The therapeutic relationship and the way in which the OT practitioner interacts with the client play a major role in the artistic element. The therapeutic process is indeed an art, for there is no preexisting formula for success. The artistic element of clinical reasoning does not have a set of rules or procedures to follow. To the student and entry-level practitioner, the artistic element may seem the most difficult to grasp and pursue.

THOUGHT PROCESS DURING CLINICAL REASONING

This text has described clinical reasoning as a cognitive thought process through which the practitioner goes. One may ask, "What exactly does this thought process involve?" In the therapy process, many diverse bits of information are gathered together (evaluation), many outside factors that may affect the process are considered (e.g., life space, prognosis, and desires), the demands of activities are analyzed (activity analysis), time investment choices are made (plan), and a progressive approach in terms of identifiable goals is organized (treatment). The clinical reasoning used throughout the therapy process requires the analysis of data, the use of specific knowledge bases, and the synthesis of awareness. The OT practitioner must actively think and process information, not just remember something once learned. The process demands the use of critical thinking—the ability to think independently.

Rogers and Holm[7] describe an information processing view of cognition that is used during the OT assessment to form an OT diagnosis. During the different steps in the approach, the OT practitioner's mind works with specific processing capabilities to gather, organize, analyze, and synthesize information.[6,7]

In the first step, the OT practitioner forms a *preassessment image* of the client, an outline that will be used for further assessment of the client. To form this image the OT practitioner gathers initial information. Two important factors that the practitioner will consider are the diagnosis and age of the client. These two factors allow the practitioner to see particular things about the situation. The OT practitioner asks himself or herself, "What am I going to consider in regard to this client?" "What do I know about this condition (in general and how it affects this person)?" Another important factor to consider is the client's life roles and functional status before he or she was referred to OT. All of this information about the client is linked to the practitioner's frame of reference to construct the preassessment image.

Using the preassessment image, the OT practitioner begins the *cue acquisition* step. This second step involves gathering the data regarding the client's functional status and occupational roles. Although the practitioner may not choose to use all data, the data used are called *cues*.

After cue acquisition, the practitioner proceeds to the third step, *hypothesis generation*. With this step, the practitioner organizes the data that have been gathered and makes tentative assumptions, which will serve as the basis for therapeutic action. For example, in evaluating a female client's ability to feed herself, the OT practitioner notices that the client is having difficulty and does not eat all of the food on her plate (cues). The practitioner's hypothesis in this situation is that the difficulty is the result of a left-sided neglect caused by the client's stroke. There can be one or more hypotheses; the practitioner's hypothesis can also conclude that the client's dysfunction is due to the fact that she must use her nondominant hand to feed herself.

The process continues with step four, *cue interpretation*. Further cues are gathered as the practitioner continues the search for data. Each cue is compared with the hypothesis being considered to determine if there is relevancy. The practitioner interprets whether the cue confirms the hypothesis, does not confirm the hypothesis, or does not contribute in either way to the hypothesis.[6]

Eventually the OT practitioner completes the initial collection phase and begins the fifth step, an examination of the data that has been collected. Rogers and Holm[7] refer to this as the *hypothesis evaluation* step. The practitioner weighs the evidence for and against each of the diagnostic hypotheses. The hypothesis with the most supporting evidence is selected and forms the basis for treatment intervention.

The outcome of this process is an OT diagnosis that describes the occupational performance deficits of the client. The diagnosis also provides information on the likely cause of the deficit, the signs and symptoms that led the practitioner to the diagnosis, and the pathologic condition that caused the deficit.[7] Through this thought process the OT practitioner has gone from sensing that there is a problem to defining the problem.

The clinical reasoning thought processes are also used to determine what treatment options are available. The OT practitioner asks, "What treatment approaches will be most effective in this situation, and how long can they be expected to achieve the desired results?" Each time an OT practitioner treats a client, he or she searches long-term memory to retrieve scientific knowledge and practical experience that relate to the situation of the current client.[6] The practitioner may change the approach used if its similarity to the current situation is minimal or if the outcome was not totally successful. The practitioner may compare a number of treatment situations to determine the most suitable approach for the current client.

The actual therapy also represents many levels of analysis and synthesis. The results of the treatment are closely monitored and evaluated by the practitioner to determine if the modalities that were selected achieved the intended goal(s). The practitioner continues to process in his or her mind knowledge about the disorder, a holistic view of the client, his or her skill and ability as the practitioner, and the modalities to be used to facilitate change and enhance the client's occupational performance. It is important that the OT practitioner collaborate with the client throughout the process in order to validate the practitioner's findings and confirm that therapy is proceeding on a track that is meaningful to the client.

CLINICAL REASONING STRATEGIES

It was often believed that OT practitioners used a single strategy for clinical reasoning. However, research conducted by Cheryl Mattingly and Maureen Fleming discovered this was not the case. In the article, *The Therapist with the Three-Track Mind,* Fleming describes three distinct strategies, or three tracks, that are used by OT practitioners for clinical reasoning.[2] These three tracks are the procedural, the interactive, and the conditional track. Practitioners shift easily and frequently among the three tracks, depending on what they are addressing in therapy with a specific client.

Procedural reasoning is a strategy used by the OT practitioner when he or she focuses on the client's disease or disability and determines what will be the most appropriate modalities to use to improve the functional performance. Central tasks for the OT practitioner during procedural reasoning are problem identification, goal setting, and treatment planning.[2] The problem-solving skills discussed in Chapter 12 are used during procedural reasoning. This track is similar to the scientific element of clinical reasoning.

Interactive reasoning is a strategy used by the OT practitioner when he or she wants to understand the client as a person. This type of reasoning takes place during face-to-face interactions between the practitioner and the client.[2] OT practitioners use interactive reasoning strategies to (1) understand the disability from the client's point of view, (2) engage the client in treatment, (3) individualize the treatment setting by matching treatment goals and procedures to the particular client and his or her life experiences and disability, (4) impart a sense of trust and acceptance to the client, (5) relieve tension by using humor, (6) develop a common language of actions and meanings, and (7) determine whether the treatment is going well.[2]

The third type of strategy used by OT practitioners is **conditional reasoning.** Conditional reasoning has several aspects.[2] During conditional reasoning, the practitioner first considers the client's condition as a whole, including the disease or disability and what it means to the person—the physical context and the social context. Next, the OT practitioner conceives of how the client's condition may change. A change in the client's present condition is dependent on his or her active involvement in treatment. This imagined condition is dependent on the practitioner's ability to motivate the client to participate in treatment, as well as to share the same vision for improvement of his or her condition.[2] With these images in mind, the practitioner implements treatment and mentally checks along the way to compare the client with what he or she was before the disability, how he or she is progressing in treatment, and where he or she wants to be in the future.[2]

Another clinical reasoning strategy described in the literature is called **narrative reasoning.** Mattingly describes two different ways in which OT practitioners use narrative reasoning—storytelling and story creation.[3] In storytelling, OT practitioners tell stories about clients to each other. Storytelling helps the practitioners reason how particular clients may be experiencing their disabilities and how treatments might proceed. Storytelling may take place informally over lunch or more formally in a case study presentation at a staff meeting.

OT practitioners also create stories. The practitioner envisions how the future may be for the client so that he or she may guide the treatment process. This technique is similar to conditional reasoning. In another aspect of story creation, OT practitioners create experiences for clients to make the activities meaningful. As an example, an OT practitioner is treating a stroke patient who is gaining improved movement in his affected arm and hand. The practitioner has asked him to make a tile mosaic trivet. The practitioner must create a vision for the client that explains why he needs to work hard to complete this project. Part of storytelling is explaining to the client how this activity relates to other meaningful activities and how completing the project can help him overcome his disability. In summarizing the use of narrative reasoning, Mattingly states, "Narratives make sense of reality by linking the outward world of actions and events to the inner world of human intention and motivation."[3]

Pragmatic reasoning is another strategy that has been suggested by Schell and Cervero as contributing to the clinical reasoning process. Pragmatic reasoning takes into consideration factors in the context of the practice setting and in the personal context of the OT practitioner that may inhibit or facilitate treatment. Factors related to the context of the practice setting include reimbursement and the availability of equipment and space.[8] An example of how reimbursement may be a factor in clinical reasoning is the client who has a need for OT services but does not have the insurance coverage or ability to pay for services. An example of how equipment and space may be a factor in clinical reasoning is the practitioner who wants a client to participate in a particular activity; however, the facility in which he or she works does not have the space or equipment necessary to perform the activity. These factors, which relate to the availability of resources, will influence the clinical reasoning process.

Factors related to the personal context of the OT practitioner include the repertoire of therapeutic and negotiation skills, personal motivation, and willingness to read the practice culture.[8] Decisions made regarding the treatment of a client are likely to be a reflection of what the practitioner knows how to do and that which he or she is willing to do.

DEVELOPMENT OF CLINICAL REASONING SKILLS

Clinical reasoning is not a skill that can be taught; it is developed over time with practical experience. Slater and Cohn describe variations in clinical reasoning at five different stages of career development. These stages are on a continuum beginning with the novice practitioner, followed by the advanced beginner practitioner, the competent practitioner, the proficient practitioner, and the expert practitioner.[9] Differences have been noted when comparing the clinical reasoning skills of the novice practitioner versus the expert practitioner.

The focus of the **novice practitioner** (stage 1) is on the learning of the procedural skills (e.g., assessment, diagnostic, and treatment planning procedures) necessary to practice.[2,9] The novice practitioner feels most comfortable with performing the techniques and procedures learned in school and refining these skills. Novice practitioners do not feel comfortable using interactive reasoning strategies. At stage 2, the *advanced beginner* is learning to recognize additional cues and beginning to see the client as an individual.[9] However, the advanced beginner still does not see the whole picture.

Slater and Cohn describe the *competent practitioner* (stage 3) as being able to see more facts and to determine the importance of these facts and observations.[9] The practitioner at stage 3 has a broader understanding of the client's problems and is more likely to individualize treatment. However, flexibility and creativity are still lacking. The *proficient practitioner* (stage 4) is able to view situations as a whole instead of as isolated parts.[9] The practical experience of the proficient practitioner allows him or her to develop a direction and vision of where the client should be going. If the initial plans do not work, the proficient therapist is easily able to modify them.

Expert practitioners (stage 5) recognize and understand rules of practice; however, for this group of practitioners the rules shift to the background.[9] The expert practitioner is described as using intuition to know what to do next. "This intuitive judgment is based on correct identification of relevant cues at a particular time in the patient's therapy, and a variety of medical, physical and psychosocial factors are considered."[9] Expert practitioners use both procedural and interactive skills without difficulty.[2] Conditional reasoning is also carried out more easily by the expert practitioner, who can rely on past clinical situations to help process imagined outcomes for the client.

Rogers relates some of the differences in clinical reasoning to the way in which novice and expert practitioners remember information and solve problems.[6] Novices record information in individual cues; experts use chunking to sort and record information. Chunking is a strategy that is used to remember several units of information. For example, it is easier to remember a phone number if it is divided into chunks instead of trying to remember individual numbers (e.g., 501-555-9487 instead of 5015559487). Expert practitioners use the technique of chunking to categorize information about clients according to how it applies to practice.[6]

Without the experience of the expert, how can the student or novice practitioner enhance his or her clinical reasoning skills? The clinical reasoning process cannot be taught in customary ways, such as reading about it in a textbook, but it can be learned.[1,4] Learning clinical reasoning skills can be facilitated through coaching and role modeling.[1,5,9] It is important that the student begins to become aware of the processes and strategies used in clinical reasoning, which will facilitate the development of clinical reasoning skills. The novice practitioner can read personal experiences of individuals with disabilities to learn to develop narrative reasoning skills.[5] The student can use case studies presented throughout his or her course work to analyze the clinical reasoning strategies that are used or to practice developing the skills on his or her own. The novice practitioner can observe other practitioners in action or in a simulated treatment session, consciously aware of the clinical reasoning processes and strategies that are being used; he or she should ask whether the approach seems appropriate and whether he or she would do things the same way. How might the strategies used be improved? Finally, the novice practitioner can use his or her fieldwork opportunities to learn the clinical reasoning processes used by the different OT practitioners. Before beginning fieldwork, he or she should set some personal goals related to the development of clinical reasoning skills that he or she would like to achieve. During fieldwork placement, the practitioner should identify strategies that he or she sees as successful and model them in his or her treatment. Finally, the novice practitioner should ask his or her supervisor for feedback on the development of his or her clinical reasoning skills.

Understandably, a student normally wants to know everything immediately and wants it to fit together perfectly. Unfortunately, because of the nature of the therapeutic process, it does not happen that way. The student should gather all the knowledge that he or she can while in school, being patient and allowing skills to develop. Perhaps sooner than expected, clinical reasoning skills will be developed, and the therapeutic process will come naturally.

SUMMARY

The value of the OT process rests on the clinical reasoning of its practitioners. Good clinical judgment is perhaps the single, most important quality an OT practitioner can have. Using good clinical reasoning enables the practitioner to make the choices that improve client independence and reduce the need for therapy. Even the most experienced practitioner can make errors in judgment. When risks are taken and new ideas are tried, failure may be the outcome. Remember, however, it is the ongoing quality of reasoning that is significant. The OT practitioner must use clinical reasoning in evaluation, goal setting, media selection, and personal interactions, since OT does not have "formula" answers for solving problems.

The elements of science, ethics, and art are combined in the therapy process. It is in this realm of clinical reasoning that the uniqueness of the profession is found. OT practitioners use a variety of clinical reasoning strategies throughout the therapy process. These strategies include procedural, interactive, conditional, narrative, and pragmatic reasonings.

There is a difference between the clinical reasoning of novice and expert practitioners. Practical experience allows expert practitioners to use a wider range of clinical reasoning strategies, whereas novice practitioners rely primarily on procedural reasoning strategies. As a student, however, it is not necessary to wait for clinical reasoning skills to be perfected. He or she must begin to develop skills by becoming aware of the different strategies used in simulated and actual clinical situations. Eventually, clinical reasoning skills will come effortlessly with little conscious thought given to how the decisions are made.

Activities

1. When an instructor gives you an assignment or learning experience, determine which type of clinical reasoning the assignment is meant to promote.
2. View a videotape of a case study of a client in a therapy session. Analyze the clinical reasoning strategies used by the practitioner. Were the strategies effective? What would you have done differently?
3. Write a short story about someone you know who has a disability. Report how this individual's past and present may reflect on his or her possible future.[5]
4. Read a literary work about an individual who has experienced a disabling condition. Using the narrative reasoning strategy, analyze the person's experiences. In your own words, describe the person's story. Your instructor can provide suggestions for books to read.
5. Set some personal goals that will help you develop clinical reasoning skills in your fieldwork placements. Think of ways you can monitor your progress in attaining these goals (e.g., asking a supervisor for feedback). Role play with a fellow student how you might ask your supervisor for feedback.

REFERENCES

1. Benamy BC: *Developing clinical reasoning skills: strategies for the occupational therapist,* San Antonio, 1996, Therapy Skill Builders.

2. Fleming MH: The therapist with the three-track mind, *Amer J Occup Ther* 45:1007, 1991.

3. Mattingly C: The narrative nature of clinical reasoning, *Amer J Occup Ther* 45:998, 1991.

4. Mattingly C: What is clinical reasoning? *Amer J Occup Ther* 45:979, 1991.

5. Neistadt ME: Teaching strategies for the development of clinical reasoning, *Amer J Occup Ther* 50:676, 1996.

6. Rogers JC: Clinical reasoning: the ethics, science and art, *Amer J Occup Ther* 37:601, 1983.

7. Rogers JC, Holm MB: Occupational therapy diagnostic reasoning: a component of clinical reasoning, *Amer J Occup Ther* 45:1045, 1991.

8. Schell BA, Cervero RM: Clinical reasoning in occupational therapy: an integrative review, *Amer J Occup Ther* 47:605, 1993.

9. Slater DY, Cohn ES: Staff development through analysis of practice, *Amer J Occup Ther* 45:1038, 1991.

EPILOGUE

In the preceding chapters, we have examined occupational therapy—its historical roots, requirements of education, focus of treatment, variety of applications, and skills required to become a practitioner. Throughout this exploration, the theme of the holistic approach has been both emphasized and demonstrated.

Human life is both an external and internal experience; yet, our health care system has focused on the external aspect and devoted little attention to the internal. We should not, however, find fault; there have been many external threats that have demanded attention, including disease, trauma, developmental anomalies, and degenerative disorders. Many technical advances have saved lives and have improved the quality of life.

We are suggesting that the internal experience has been neglected. Consequently, there is a need in rehabilitation to give attention to the inner traumas that result from disability and dysfunction. Although not every client needs such a therapeutic focus, many do. As our world and society become more technically and objectively oriented, there is an increased danger of neglecting the delicate, inner subjective reality—which is where our humanity resides. We suggest that the field of occupational therapy increase awareness of the *importance* of the subtle inner reality. The profession functions from a mind-set that is different from technical specialties. An occupational therapy practitioner is the facilitator of a client's struggle toward independence—of how little or how much a person is capable. The practitioner is not the repository of some "cure"; rather, he or she is the link for helping clients find their own abilities or capabilities.

Quality changes—not measurable, quantitative changes—mend the spirit. The spirit either prevents or enables a person to fight the limitations that threaten. This raises the question of the appropriateness of "spirit mending." The term is an acknowledgment that the person has an inner being that is a source of energy and courage. Each of us is a unique person with an identity that is more than the sum of its parts. If a *person* is to be truly rehabilitated, more than physical function is at stake. The following questions are implied in various parts of the text and are specifically raised here for the readers' consideration:

Is there a place in our objectively oriented and technological world for spirit mending?

When a person is stricken by a disorder or trauma, or if she or he has been impaired since birth or infancy, it is not only the physical body that suffers but also the psyche and spirit.

Is there a time and place in our human services delivery system that addresses the inner person in the face of trauma and disability?

Since its earliest beginnings, occupational therapy has been concerned with both the physical and nonphysical aspects of a person. Historically, the roots of occupational therapy can be traced to a nineteenth century movement, "Moral Treatment," which claimed a concern for more than physical function.

Is occupational therapy a proper discipline for a measure of spirit mending?

All students must study psychology, as well as physical function and technical skills. This educational emphasis confirms the assertion that occupational therapy is the proper discipline for a measure of spirit mending. The concern for the whole person is an expected perspective of any individual treatment plan.

*Can we afford **not** to include the subjective, the feeling or nonmaterial dimension of our clients in service delivery and remain true to the purpose we profess?*

The holistic perspective is the foundation of occupational therapy. With economic measures exerting great force on restructuring the field, occupational therapy must deal with the question of where to place priorities in service delivery.

Will we continue to regard the subjective aspects of rehabilitation as valid focuses for treatment planning?

There are practical considerations, such as who will pay for nonmeasurable services; perhaps it is our responsibility to convince others—by data research—that professional attention to this area leads to greater overall improved and, in the long run, results in cost-effective delivery of services.

We will chart our future with the choices we make now. Can we draw upon our rich heritage? When a person is viewed as a "living machine" made up of separate parts, it may be appropriate that each discipline identify and focus only on the part it is most suited to serve. If, instead, a person is viewed as a living organism, one becomes aware that the whole is **more** than the sum of its parts. It has been a conviction of our profession since its beginning that a healthy person is body, mind, and spirit—in total integration. Dysfunction in any part affects the entire being, that is, if a person loses the ability to walk, it is not only the legs that are the focus, the total being is profoundly affected!

To articulate the unique contribution that occupational therapy makes to rehabilitation, we have chosen "spirit mending," since the term captures an essential, though nebulous, dimension of human needs that occupational therapy strives to meet. Whatever the term, those entering the field should consider and debate the issue—for it can be easily lost in accountability demands that continue to escalate. A profession's strength and respect grows by setting its own parameters.

We unequivocally state our position. Nothing—no technical expertise or health-promoting activity—is **more** important than regard for the total humanness of the persons we serve. This priority, in no way, devalues the importance of technical expertise, which is of prime importance. Both are needed if we truly are to help gain greater dignity and independence for those whose spirits have been assaulted by life.

APPENDIXES

Appendix A

OCCUPATIONAL THERAPY ROLES

This document is a guide to major roles common in the profession of occupational therapy. It is intended to assist the practitioner in identifying career options and developing career paths. "Practitioner" refers to anyone who is certified by the American Occupational Therapy Certification Board (AOTCB) as an occupational therapist (OTR) or an occupational therapy assistant (COTA). Practitioners work in a variety of systems including health care, educational, academic, governmental, social, corporate, and industrial settings. This document can be a resource for planning career ladders, developing job descriptions, and suggesting educational content for formal and continuing education programs.

This document is to be used and distributed as a whole. Use of individual pages or sections will distort the intent and purpose for which it was intended.

Roles listed in this document are those frequently held by certified practitioners and are not all inclusive. The nature of the experience as an occupational therapy practitioner prepares individuals for other specialized roles (e.g., activity director, case manager, rehabilitation coordinator, dean). Roles described in this document are valued equally. Although different roles may vary in their scope and in the experience required to perform them, each role fulfills specific function within the profession and contributes to the profession's growth, development, and strength.

An individual's employment setting, method of service delivery, performance competence, and career goals are all interdependent and result in an individualized composite of roles during actual job performance. In this document, roles are not exclusive because jobs performed by practitioners may include aspects of more than one role. For example, an occupational therapist may have a job that includes practitioner and fieldwork educator roles. Another individual may function as a faculty member, researcher, and consultant.

Career progression involves advancement within roles, as well as transition to different roles. When transitioning occurs, practitioners need to have demonstrated performance potential and appropriate educational preparation for the new role. Individuals entering into a new role typically require closer supervision and will begin at a relatively lower level of expertise than in their other roles. Preparation for new roles often involves self-reflection, continuing or advanced education, and acquisition of experience and skills required for the new role. The development of a mentoring relationship assists in understanding the context in which role performance will occur. For example, an individual who is an advanced-level administrator in a practice setting may move into an entry-level faculty role in an academic setting. Preparation for this transition may include acquiring appropriate academic degrees; understanding the educational environment; and demonstrating potential for teaching, scholarly activity, and professional service.

ROLE DESCRIPTIONS

Each role in this document consists of the following components: major function, scope of a role, performance areas, qualifications, and supervision. These components are described as follows:

Major function: Describes the primary purpose(s) of the role.

Scope of role: Delineates the range of responsibility and complexity that typically occurs within the role.

Key performance areas: Specifies common activities and expectations associated with role function. Performance that occurs within each area is built upon the unique philosophy and perspective of occupational therapy. Practitioners are expected to take personal responsibility for functioning within the ethical code and standards of the profession. Specific knowledge, skills, and attitudes fundamental for performance are beyond the scope of this document.

Individuals develop varying degrees of expertise in role performance. Levels of expertise are those skills that are fundamental to the entry level (noted by ●), those skills that are intermediate (noted by ●●), or those skills that require a high degree of proficiency (noted by ●●●). These three levels describe the professional development process for each role and are described in Figure 1. Progression within a role through the three levels of professional development is based on accumulation of higher level skills through experience, education, guided self-development, and professional socialization. Progression is not simply the amount of time in a role. Each person progresses along this continuum at an individualized pace. Some individuals may remain at one level for the duration of

ROLE	MAJOR FOCI	SUPERVISION
Entry	• Development of skills • Socialization in the expectations related to the organization, peer, and profession. *Acceptance of responsibilities and accountability for role-relevant professional activities is expected.*	Close
Intermediate	• Increased independence • Mastery of basic role functions • Ability to respond to situations based on previous experience • Participation in the education of personnel *Specialization is frequently initiated, along with increased responsibility for collaboration with other disciplines and related organizations. Participation in role-relevant professional activities is increased.*	Routine or general
Advanced	• Refinement of specialized skills • Understanding of complex issues affecting role functions *Contribution to the knowledge base and growth of the profession results in being considered an expert, resource person, or consultant within a role. This expertise is recognized by others inside and outside of the profession through leadership, mentoring, research, education, and volunteerism.*	Minimal

FIGURE 1. LEVELS OF ROLE PERFORMANCE.

their career and not everyone progresses to the advanced level. An individual may function in more than one role simultaneously. When this occurs, it is possible to function at different levels within each role. For example, a new faculty member may be at an entry level in teaching, though at an advanced level in clinical practice. All roles described in this document build on the performance expectations of the Practitioner-OTR and Practitioner-COTA, as this is the entry point into the profession. Consequently, the entry-level performance areas are considered to be an inherent part of all other roles described in this document.

Supervision: Describes the typical oversight required or recommended for individuals at the various levels of role performance. The amount of supervision required is closely linked to both the role and the level of exper-

TYPE	DESCRIPTION
Close	Daily, direct contact at the site of work
Routine	Direct contact at least every 2 weeks at the site of work, with interim supervision through other methods such as telephone or written communication
General	Monthly direct contact with supervision available as needed by other methods
Minimal	Contact only on an as-needed basis; maybe less than monthly

FIGURE 2. TYPES OF FORMAL SUPERVISION.

tise in a role. The supervision recommended is intended to be a collaborative relationship that serves to promote quality service and the professional development of the individuals involved. All COTAs will require more than a minimal level of supervision by an OTR when providing services. Formal supervision occurs along a continuum including close, routine, general, and minimal. Refer to Figure 2 for descriptions of these levels.

In addition to formal supervision, individuals may provide or receive functional supervision. Functional supervision implies the provision of information and feedback to coworkers. Individuals who provide functional supervision have specialized knowledge as a result of their own experience and expertise. Based on this specialized knowledge or skill, the individual supervises peers relative to this expertise in a particular function. For example, a fieldwork educator may provide functional supervision to coworkers who are supervising students, although he or she is not responsible for evaluating the overall performance of the other therapists.

Qualifications: Lists the critical credentials, education, and work experience necessary as a prerequisite to adequate role performance. Qualifications are listed in a range to reflect changing expectations associated with higher levels of role functioning. As all roles are within the profession, professional certification as a practitioner is a consistent requirement. Additionally, all practitioners are expected to meet state and federal regulatory mandates, adhere to relevant Association policies, and participate in continuing professional development.

PRACTITIONER—OTR

Major function: Provide quality occupational therapy services, including assessment, intervention, program planning and implementation, discharge planning-related documentation, and communication. Service provision may include direct, monitored, and consultative approaches.

Scope of role: OTR practitioners advance along a continuum form entry to advanced level based on experience, education, and practice skills. The OTR has the ultimate responsibility for service provision (AOTA, 1990, p. 1093).

Key performance areas (● entry-level skills, ●● intermediate skills, ●●● high-proficiency skills):

● Responds to requests for service and initiates referrals when appropriate.

● Screens individuals to determine the need for intervention.

● Evaluates individuals to obtain and interpret data necessary for planning intervention and for intervention.

● Interprets evaluation findings to appropriate individuals.

● Develops and coordinates intervention plans, including goals and methods to achieve stated goals.

● Implements the intervention plan directly or in collaboration with others.

● Adapts environment, tools, materials, and activities according to the needs of the individual and his or her social cultural context.

● Monitors the individual's response to intervention and modifies plan as needed.

● Communicates and collaborates with other team members, individuals, family members, or caregivers.

● Follows policies and procedures required in the setting.

● Develops appropriate home and community programming to support performance in natural environment.

● Terminates services when maximum benefit is received and formulates discontinuation and follow-up plans.

- Documents services as required.
- Maintains records required by practice setting, third-party payers, and regulatory agencies.
- Performs continuous quality improvement activities and program evaluation using predetermined criteria.
- Provides inservice education to team members and the community.
- Maintains treatment area, equipment, and supply inventory.
- Identifies and pursues own professional growth and development.
- Schedules and prioritizes own workload.
- Participates in professional and community activities.
- Monitors own performance and identifies supervisory needs.
- Functions according to the AOTA *Code of Ethics* (AOTA, 1988) and *Standards of Practice* (AOTA, 1992) of the profession.
- •• Supervises/teaches occupational therapy practitioners, students, and other staff performing supportive services and/or other aspects of service provision.
- •• Assists other practitioners in the development of professional skills.
- •• Participates in committees and activities of larger systems in the development of service operations, policies, and procedures.
- •• Participates in the fieldwork education process.
- •• Critically examines own practice and integrates new knowledge.
- ••• Performs advanced, specialized evaluations or interventions.
- ••• Develops protocols and procedures for intervention programs based on current occupational therapy theory and practice.
- ••• Provides expert consultation to practitioners and outside groups about area of expertise.

Qualifications:
❑ Certified by the American Occu-

pational Therapy Certification Board (AOTCB) as an OTR.

❑ Meets state regulatory requirements.

❑ Progressive levels of expertise will require one or more of the following: work experience, self-study, continuing education, special certification, or postprofessional education.

Supervision: Practice supervision must be performed by an experienced OTR. Administrative supervision is determined by individual settings and may or may not be performed by an OTR.

❑ *Entry-level practitioners-OTRs* in a particular practice area will require close supervision for service delivery aspects and routine supervision for administrative aspects (AOTA, 1981).

❑ *Intermediate practitioners-OTRs* require routine to general supervision from advanced practitioners.

❑ *Advanced practitioners-OTRs* require minimal supervision within area of expertise and general supervision for administrative aspects.

PRACTITIONER—COTA

Major function: Provides quality occupational therapy services to assigned individuals under the supervision of an OTR.

Scope of role: COTA practitioners advance along a continuum from entry to advanced level, based on experience, education, and practice skills. Development along this continuum is dependent on the development of service competency. The OTR has ultimate overall responsibility for service provision (AOTA, 1990, p. 1093).

Key performance areas (• entry-level skills, •• intermediate skills, ••• high-proficiency skills):
- Responds to request for services in accordance with service agency's policies and procedures.

- Assists with data collection and evaluation under the supervision of an OTR.
- Develops treatment goals under the supervision of an OTR.
- Implements and coordinates intervention plan under the supervision of an OTR.
- Provides direct service that follows a documented routine and accepted procedure under the supervision of an OTR.
- Adapts intervention environment, tools, materials, and activities according to the needs of the individual and his or her sociocultural context under the supervision of an OTR.
- Communicates and interacts with other team members and the individual's family or caregivers in collaboration with an OTR.
- Monitors own performance and identifies supervisory needs.
- Follows policies and procedures required in a setting.
- Performs continuous quality improvement activities or program evaluation in collaboration with an OTR.
- Maintains treatment area, equipment, and supply inventory as required.
- Identifies and pursues own professional growth and development.
- Maintains records and documentation required by work settings under the supervision of an OTR.
- Participates in professional and community activities.
- Functions according to the AOTA *Code of Ethics* (AOTA, 1988) and *Standards of Practice* (AOTA, 1992) of the profession.
- ●● Schedules and prioritizes own workload.
- ●● Supervises volunteers, COTAs, OTA students, and personnel other than OT practitioners under the direction of an OTR.
- ●● Participates in development of policies and procedures in collaboration with an OTR.
- ●● Participates in the fieldwork education process under the direction of an OTR.
- ●● Selects, adapts, and implements intervention under the supervision of an OTR.
- ●● Administers standardized tests under the supervision of an OTR after service competency has been established.
- ●● Modifies treatment approaches to reflect changing needs under the supervision of an OTR.
- ●● Formulates discontinuation and follow-up plans under the supervision of an OTR.
- ●● Participates in organizational activities and committees.
- ●●● Serves as a resource person to the agency in areas of specific expertise.
- ●●● Educates others in the area of established service competency under the supervision of an OTR.
- ●●● Contributes to program planning and development in collaboration with an OTR.

Qualifications:

❑ Certified by the American Occupational Therapy Certification Board (AOTCB) as a COTA.

❑ Meets state regulatory requirements.

❑ Progressive levels of expertise will require one or more of the following: work experience, self-study, continuing education, and formal education including advanced degrees.

Supervision: COTAs at all levels require at least general supervision by an OTR. The level of supervision is related to the ability of the COTA to safely and effectively provide those interventions delegated by an OTR. Typically, entry-level COTAs and COTAs new to a particular practice environment will require close supervision, intermediate-level practitioners routine supervision, and advanced-level practitioners general supervision. COTAs will require closer supervision for interventions that are more complex or evaluative in nature and for areas in which service competencies have not been developed. Service competency is the ability to use the identified intervention in a safe and effective manner.

EDUCATOR (CONSUMER, PEER)

Major function: Develops and provides educational offerings or training related to occupational therapy to consumer, peer, and community individuals or groups.

Scope of roles: Practitioners advance along a continuum of providing informal education to individuals and small groups in the course of service provision, to developing and providing comprehensive educational programs targeted to consumers and peers. At entry level of role, education typically occurs with peers and consumers within the individual's own service system (e.g., patient education, department, or school district inservice). At higher levels of expertise, provision of educational offerings may involve individuals or groups from multiple systems (e.g., provision of injury-prevention programs to industry, caregiver education programs to community, and continuing education seminars).

Key performance areas (● entry-level skills, ●● intermediate skills, ●●● high-proficiency skills):

● Implements strategies to assist individual learner to identify own learning needs.

● Develops or collaborates with individual learner in developing learning objectives.

● Implements educational methods designed to support learner's objectives.

● Responds to feedback about the teaching-learning process, and modifies own educational strategies to support learning.

● Supports the evaluation of educational effectiveness.

● Monitors own performance and identifies own development needs.

● Functions according to the AOTA *Code of Ethics* (AOTA, 1988) and *Standards of Practice* (AOTA, 1992) of the profession.

●● Selects or designs strategies to identify individual learner needs.

●● Develops program plans and materials for formal program offerings (e.g., conference presentations, workshops, seminars).

●● Uses a variety of teaching-learning methods appropriate to the learning objectives and learner needs.

●●● Evaluates strategies to identify learning needs of individuals and groups.

●●● Develops program plans and educational methods for extended or multiple program offerings.

●●● Designs evaluation strategies to assess impact of educational programs.

Qualifications:

❑ Certified by the American Occupational Therapy Certification Board (AOTCB) as an OTR or a COTA.

❑ Progressive levels of expertise will require combinations of the following: self-study continuing education, experience, and post–entry-level formal education.

❑ Appropriate level of practice or service expertise is necessary as it relates to provision of these education services.

Supervision: Supervision depends on the nature of the project and the skills of the educator. COTAs at all levels usually will require OTR supervision for educational activities that occur related to occupational therapy consumers.

FIELDWORK EDUCATOR (practice setting)

Major function: Manages Level I or II fieldwork in a practice setting. Provides occupational therapy or occupational therapy assistant students with opportunities to practice and carry out practitioner competencies.

Scope of role: The fieldwork educator role may range from supervision of an individual student to full responsibility for an entire fieldwork program.

Key performance areas (● entry-level skills, ●● intermediate skills, ●●● high-proficiency skills):

● Establishes, mediates, and supports relationships between practice-based and academic personnel.

● Initiates and maintains communication and correspondence between the practice and academic settings.

● Schedules students in collaboration with the academic fieldwork coordinator.

● Provides orientation for student to fieldwork site including policies, procedures, and student responsibilities.

● Facilitates student learning activities to achieve desired student competence.

● Facilitates student's clinical reasoning and reflective practice.

● Evaluates student performance throughout fieldwork.

● Provides the student with both formative and cumulative feedback and supervision.

● Ensures student's integration of professional standards and ethics into practice.

● Ensures students' compliance with agencies' standards, goals, and objectives.

● Attends meetings, programs, or continuing education related to fieldwork education.

● Develops learning objectives for fieldwork in collaboration with academic institution(s) and consistent with current student fieldwork evaluation(s).

● Functions according to the AOTA *Code of Ethics* (AOTA, 1988) and *Standards of Practice* (AOTA, 1992) of the profession.

●● Provides functional supervision to OTRs and COTAs specific to their roles as student fieldwork supervisors.

●● Facilitates assignment of students to appropriate practitioners for supervision.

●● Counsels or arbitrates students' concerns.

●● Oversees the administrative aspects of the fieldwork program, including formal agreement with academic programs.

●● Conducts ongoing fieldwork program evaluations and monitors changes in program.

●● Organizes or participates in appropriate fieldwork education support groups (e.g., local fieldwork councils, Commission on Education).

●● Coordinates continuing education and inservice opportunities to develop staff fieldwork education skills.

●●● Participates at leadership level in appropriate fieldwork groups.

●●● Facilitates the development of clinical fieldwork programs and related student supervision skills.

●●● Contributes to student learning by modeling leadership in professional organizations and facilitating student involvement.

Qualifications:

❏ Certified by the American Occupational Therapy Certification Board (AOTCB) as an OTR or a COTA.

❏ Meets appropriate state regulatory requirements.

❏ Continuing education regarding fieldwork education and supervision.

❏ Entry-level OTRs and COTAs may supervise Level I fieldwork students.

❏ OTRs with 1 year of practice-based experience may supervise OT and OTA Level II fieldwork students.

❏ COTAs with 1 year of practice-based experience may supervise OTA Level II fieldwork students.

❏ Three years of experience are recommended for individuals overseeing programs involving multiple student supervisors and multiple students.

Supervision: Supervision provided by an administrator or specifically designated individual. Level of supervision varies with skills of educator, complexity of setting, and nature of student's learning needs.

SUPERVISOR

Major function(s): Manages the overall daily operation of occupational therapy services in a defined practice area(s).

Scope of role: The supervisor is involved in managing other occupational therapy practitioners, personnel, and volunteers in a defined practice setting or program.

Key performance areas (● entry-level skills, ●● intermediate skills, ●●● high-proficiency skills):

● Assists in selection, orientation, and training of staff, students, and volunteers.

● Promotes professional growth through staff development.

● Coordinates scheduling of work assignments.

● Evaluates, monitors, and provides feedback regarding job performance of assigned staff.

● Assists in establishment, implementation, and evaluation of agency goals and objectives.

● Monitors and facilitates staff compliance with established standards and guidelines.

● Provides for acquisition, care, and maintenance of physical facilities, supplies, and equipment.

● Oversees implementation of continuous quality improvement activities.

● Represents personnel, fiscal, professional, and program needs to occupational therapy administrator.

● Functions according to the AOTA *Code of Ethics* (AOTA, 1988) and *Standards of Practice* (AOTA, 1992) of the profession.

●● Develops, implements, and monitors department policies and procedures in collaboration with occupational therapy administrator.

●● Coordinates specific activities for department or service unit.

●● Facilitates collaboration among occupational therapy and non–occupational therapy personnel and administrators.

●●● Serves as liaison to specialty program coordinators and administrators.

Qualifications:

❑ Certified by AOTCB as an OTR or COTA.

❑ Meets appropriate state regulatory requirements.

❑ Two to 3 years of practice experience in service area prior to supervising others is recommended.

❑ One year of experience is recommended prior to supervising a COTA. Experienced COTAs may supervise other COTAs administratively, as long as service protocols and documentation are supervised by an OTR.

❑ Continuing or postprofessional education relevant to supervisory function.

Supervision: Routine to minimal supervision provided by the occupational therapy administrator. Supervision ranges from routine to minimal, depending on the experience and expertise of the supervisor. Consultation from more advanced practitioners should be available as needed.

ADMINISTRATOR (PRACTICE SETTING)

Major function: Manages department, program, services, or agency providing occupational therapy services.

Scope of role: This role encompasses those individuals who organize and manage occupational therapy service units.

Key performance areas (● entry-level skills, ●● intermediate skills, ●●● high-proficiency skills):

● Plans, develops, and monitors occupational therapy services to ensure quality service.

● Achieves service unit goals and objectives through allocation of resources.

● Recruits and hires employees.

● Conducts performance evaluation and staff development activities.

● Establishes policies and standard operating procedures.

● Formulates and manages budget.

● Maintains effective information management systems.

● Assures safe work environments, procedures, and methods.

● Develops and monitors reimbursement processes to support services.

● Monitors the acquisition and maintenance of supplies, equipment, and facilities.

● Develops and supervises a continuous quality improvement program.

● Ensures compliance with accreditation, certification, and government standards.

● Advocates for appropriate use of occupational therapy services.

● Oversees fieldwork education process.

● Functions according to the AOTA *Code of Ethics* (AOTA, 1988) and *Standards of Practice* (AOTA, 1992) of the profession.

●● Establishes a long-range plan for staff recruitment, development, and retention.

●● Collaborates with other administrators within the organization to develop and manage organizational systems.

●● Collaborates with others outside of the organization regarding pertinent administrative management issues.

●● Participates at a leadership level in professional, community organizations.

●●● Participates in organizational strategic planning and establishes strategic plan for assigned areas.

●●● Develops and implements marketing strategies for assigned areas.

●●● Facilitates development of systems supporting clinical research.

●●● Assumes leadership role within the organization and in interorganizational projects.

Qualifications:

❑ Certified by AOTCB as an OTR.

❑ Meets appropriate state regulatory requirements.

❑ Graduate degree or continuing education relevant to management.

❑ Recommended experience varies with size and scope of department; a minimum of 3 years experience is preferred for small programs and 5 or more years for larger programs.

Supervision: General supervision by administrative personnel within the organization is required. Individuals with fewer than 3 years experience should have access to an occupational therapy management consultant. Consultation from more advanced practitioners should be available as needed.

Consultant

Major function: Provides occupational therapy consultation to individuals, groups, or organizations.

Scope of role: Consultative services may take place within the case, colleague, or systems model. Consultation may relate to practice, education, administration, or research.

Key performance areas (● entry-level skills, ●● intermediate skills, ●●● high-proficiency skills):

● Communicates scope of professional expertise.

• Assists consumers in identifying problems to be addressed in the consultative process.

• Collaborates with consumers in developing appropriate consultation outcomes.

• Develops recommendations that are relevant within the cultural context of the consumers' environment.

• Assists consumers in developing and implementing interventions, or identifying alternate resources necessary to obtain consumer objectives.

• Complies with applicable local, state, and federal laws and regulations.

• Functions according to the AOTA *Code of Ethics* (AOTA, 1988) and *Standards of Practice* (AOTA, 1992) of the profession.

•• Assesses quality of own consultative efforts, and identifies own continuing professional development needs.

••• Participates at a leadership level in professional, community organizations.

Qualifications:

❑ Certified by AOTCB as an OTR or COTA.

❑ Meets appropriate state regulatory requirements.

❑ Intermediate or advanced practice level.

❑ Recommend minimum of 6 months experience for case consultation, 1 year for colleague consultation, and 3 to 5 years for systems consultation.

Supervision: Practitioners are expected to function as consultants within the scope of practice appropriate to their level of competence. The OTR functioning as a consultant is responsible for obtaining supervision when needed to meet regulatory and professional standards. The COTA functioning as a consultant is expected to seek the appropriate level of OTR supervision to meet regulatory and professional standards.

FIELDWORK COORDINATOR (ACADEMIC SETTING)

Major function: Manages student fieldwork program within the academic setting.

Scope of role: The fieldwork coordinator role may be decentralized among the faculty or may be managed entirely by one individual. This encompasses all fieldwork experiences required by a curriculum.

Key performance areas (• entry-level skills, •• intermediate skills, ••• high-proficiency skills):

• Identifies and secures sites for fieldwork education.

• Reviews the quality and appropriateness of fieldwork sites in collaboration with other academic faculty.

• Develops fieldwork objectives in collaboration with the fieldwork sites.

• Initiates and maintains communication and correspondence between the academic and fieldwork sites.

• Communicates with fieldwork educators regarding the curriculum model, course content, and fieldwork expectations.

• Oversees the administrative aspects of the fieldwork program including agreements with fieldwork sites.

• Assigns students to fieldwork settings.

• Orients students to responsibilities and protocol for fieldwork.

• Maintains communication with fieldwork educators and students during fieldwork.

• Monitors the facilitation of clinical reasoning and reflective practice in Level II fieldwork settings.

• Counsels and arbitrates with students and fieldwork educators on matters of concern.

• Collaborates with the fieldwork educator in assigning the final appraisal (grading) of the student.

• Supports research.

• Functions according to the AOTA *Code of Ethics* (AOTA, 1988) and *Standards of Practice* (AOTA, 1992) of the profession.

• Participates in appropriate fieldwork educational support groups (e.g., local fieldwork councils, Commission on Education).

•• Provides educational opportunities to prepare and enhance fieldwork educators' knowledge and skills.

•• Coordinates continuing education pertaining to fieldwork education processes for clinical fieldwork educators.

•• Participates actively in professional, volunteer organizations.

•• Supervises support personnel carrying out administrative aspects of fieldwork.

••• Participates at leadership level in appropriate fieldwork group.

••• Facilitates the development of fieldwork programs and related student supervision skills.

Qualifications:

❑ Certified by AOTCB as an OTR or COTA.

❑ Three years of practice experience and experience in supervising and advising fieldwork students are recommended.

Supervision: General supervision by academic administrator who is usually the program director. Close to routine supervision for new faculty.

FACULTY

Major function: Provides formal academic education for occupational therapy or occupational therapy assistant students.

Scope of role: This role varies among institutions and the subsequent balance expected between teaching, service, and scholarly activities. Progression within this role typically advances from lecturer and instructor to the professional ranks, including assistant, associate,

full, and emeritus professorships. Included in the faculty role may be adjunct, clinical, or academic appointments.

Key performance areas (• entry-level skills, •• intermediate skills, ••• high-proficiency skills):

• Develops educational course objectives and sequences the content to promote optimal learning.

• Designs and structures effective educational experiences, including methods, media, content areas, and types of student interactions.

• Facilitates students' learning through lectures, discussions, practical and laboratory exercises, or practice-related experiences.

• Evaluates and addresses student learning needs within their social and cultural environmental context.

• Reviews educational media and published resources and selects class readings or supplemental materials.

• Plans and prepares course materials to include course syllabi, lectures, case studies, teaching/learning handouts, and questions for group discussion.

• Prepares evaluation materials and measures student attainment of stated course objectives.

• Develops and maintains proficiency in teaching areas through investigation, formal education, continuing education, or practice.

• Participates in curriculum development.

• Participates in teaching evaluation and uses outcome data to modify teaching.

• Advises students and student groups.

• Serves on department, school, college, or university committees.

• Assists with designated departmental administrative tasks such as student admissions, recruitment, and course scheduling.

• Maintains students' records according to regulations and procedures.

• Functions according to the AOTA *Code*

of Ethics (AOTA, 1988) and *Standards of Practice* (AOTA, 1992) of the profession.

● Engages in service to the university or community.

●● Prepares innovative curriculum or instructional methods.

●● Evaluates and incorporates emerging research findings and technology into teaching and research.

●● Participates in research and scholarly activities

●● Collaborates in the preparation of academic reports and accreditation self-studies.

●● Participates actively in professional organizations.

●●● Provides expert consultation to practitioners, educators, and outside groups about area of expertise.

●●● Chairs or leads groups or organizations outside the department.

●●● Mentors students through scholarly investigation process to develop student skills in research.

●●● Mentors other faculty in the development of their teaching, research, and practice skills.

Qualifications:

❏ Certified by AOTCB as an OTR or COTA.

❏ For OTR, in professional programs, a doctoral degree is preferred (a master's degree is recommended).

❏ In technical programs, a master's degree is preferred (a bachelor's degree is recommended).

❏ Intermediate to advanced skills in primary area of teaching.

❏ Skills as a classroom instructor and understanding of the educational system.

Supervision: General supervision by academic program director and other appropriate academic administrators. Close to routine supervision by academic program directors for new, adjunct, and part-time faculty.

PROGRAM DIRECTOR (ACADEMIC SETTING)

Major function: Manages the occupational therapy educational program.

Scope of role: The program director's role varies depending on the level of the program (e.g., technical, professional, or postprofessional level) and the demands of the academic setting (e.g., technical school, community college, college, university, or health sciences center). The academic program director facilitates the education of competent graduates through faculty development and supervision and effective program management. Dependent on their academic environment, program directors may oversee both academic and practice-related activities, externally funded projects, and continuing education programs.

Key performance areas (● entry-level skills, ●● intermediate skills, ●●● high-proficiency skills):

● Oversees student recruitment, selection, evaluation, advisement, retention, and professional development.

● Oversees institutional and professional accreditation activities and reports.

● Manages faculty recruitment, development, evaluation, and retention.

● Assigns and monitors faculty and staff responsibilities.

● Ensures the quality of the program.

● Formulates and implements a fiscal plan.

● Represents the program to university administrators and negotiates for the needs of the program.

● Fosters an academic climate that facilitates faculty, student, and staff learning and professional growth.

● Promotes effective instructional techniques for faculty.

● Oversees student and faculty rights and responsibilities.

● Produces narrative and data-based reports for internal and external communication.

● Facilitates library acquisitions of resources for teaching and research.

● Fosters beneficial relationships among faculty and practitioners.

● Functions according to the AOTA *Code of Ethics* (AOTA, 1988) and *Standards of Practice* (AOTA, 1992) of the profession.

●● Develops and implements long-range or strategic plans.

●● Produces scholarly work.

●● Facilitates the development of useful information management systems.

●● Participates at the leadership level in professional and community organizations.

●●● Leads in the acquisition of externally funded projects.

●●● Designs and implements marketing for program enhancement.

●●● Promotes central theme within the occupational therapy programs that contributes to the knowledge base of the profession.

Qualifications:

Technical-Level Program Director:

❑ An OTR with a bachelor's degree (a master's degree is preferred) who is certified by AOTCB.

❑ Recommend 3 years of professional practice with experience supervising COTAs.

❑ Recommend 3 years experience as a faculty member.

❑ Experience or continuing education in academic management.

Professional-Level Program Director:

❑ An OTR with a master's degree (a doctoral degree is preferred) who is certified by AOTCB.

❑ Recommend 5 years experience in practice.

❑ Recommend 5 years experience as a faculty member.

❑ Experience or continuing education in academic management.

Post–Professional-Level Program Director:

❑ An OTR with a doctoral degree who is certified by AOTCB.

❑ Recommend 5 years experience in practice.

❑ Recommend 5 years experience as a faculty member.

❑ Experience or continuing education in academic management.

❑ Intermediate to advanced competence as a researcher/scholar.

Supervision: General to minimal supervision from designated administrative officer. Individuals with fewer than 3 years experience should have access to occupational therapy education and accreditation consultants.

RESEARCHER/SCHOLAR

Major function: Performs scholarly work of the profession including examining, developing, refining, and evaluating the profession's body of knowledge, theoretical base, and philosophical foundations.

Scope of role: The role of the researcher ranges from the individual who critically examines and interprets empirical studies to independent investigator. The scholar is an individual who has in-depth knowledge and who engages in examination, development, or refinement of the profession's body of knowledge.

Key performance areas (● entry-level skills, ●● intermediate skills, ●●● high-proficiency skills):

● Promotes and engages in research/scholarly activities.

● Reads, interprets, and applies scholarly information relative to occupational therapy.

● Collects research data.

● Assumes responsibility for the ethical

concerns in research and complies with institutional bioethics committee protocols.

● Functions according to the AOTA *Code of Ethics* (AOTA, 1988) and *Standards of Practice* (AOTA, 1992) of the profession.

●● Directs the completion of studies, including data analysis, interpretation, and dissemination of results.

●● Collaborates with others to facilitate studies of concern to the profession.

●● Monitors resources which facilitate research and scholarly activities.

●●● Probes methods of science, theoretical information, or research designs to answer questions important to the profession.

●●● Conceptualizes the body of knowledge in the profession to develop new theories, frames of reference, or models of practice.

●●● Mentors novice researchers.

●●● Participates at the leadership level in professional, volunteer organizations.

Qualifications:

❏ Certified by AOTCB as an OTR or a COTA.

❏ Progressive levels of expertise will require combinations of the following: self-study, continuing education, experience, and formal education for independent research or scholarly activities.

❏ COTAs can contribute to the research process. COTAs need additional academic qualifications to be a principal investigator.

Supervision: Supervision ranges from close to minimal, depending on the nature of the project and the skills of the researcher/scholar.

ENTREPRENEUR

Major function: Entrepreneurs are partially or fully self-employed individuals who provide occupational therapy services.

Scope of role: Entrepreneurs may function in a variety of roles, including independent contractor and private practice owner or operator. The form of organization may be sole proprietorship, partnership, corporation, group practice, or joint venture.

Key performance areas (● entry-level skills, ●● intermediate skills, ●●● high-proficiency skills):

● Delivers quality occupational therapy services within scope of endeavor.

● Develops and implements business plans designed to ensure viability using financial and legal consultation.

● Establishes a business organization appropriate to nature and scope of activities.

● Negotiates contractual relationships that take into account the setting, services, and reimbursement.

● Uses legal, financial, and practice consultation as needed to support business operations.

● Establishes and collects fees for service, complying with reimbursement requirements.

● Manages business support services.

● Complies with local, state, and federal laws and regulations related to business and practice.

● Complies with standards and guidelines of accrediting or regulating organizations.

● Develops and maintains personnel policies and records.

● Develops and implements marketing strategies, as appropriate.

● Evaluates consumer satisfaction and business operations.

● Develops and implements risk management plan that includes business property, liability, and employee or employer benefits.

● Functions according to the AOTA *Code of Ethics* (AOTA, 1988) and *Standards of Practice* (AOTA, 1992) of the profession, as well as business ethics.

●● Participates in, supervises, or oversees fieldwork program.

●● Participates at a leadership level in professional, community organizations.

Qualifications:

❑ Certified by AOTCB as an OTR or COTA.

❑ Meets appropriate state regulatory requirements.

❑ A minimum of 3 years of practice experience.

Supervision: In cases in which a COTA provides direct service, it is the COTA's responsibility to obtain the appropriate level of supervision from an OTR. Expert consultation or mentorship is obtained as needed to support the business, legal, financial, regulatory, and practice aspects of role performance.

REFERENCES

American Occupational Therapy Association: Guide to supervision of occupational therapy personnel, *Amer J Occup Ther*, 35:815, 1981.

American Occupational Therapy Association: Occupational therapy code of ethics, *Amer J Occup Ther*, 42:795, 1988.

American Occupational Therapy Association: Entry-level delineation for registered occupational therapists (OTRs) and certified occupational therapy assistants (COTAs), *Amer J Occup Ther*,44:1091, 1990.

American Occupational Therapy Association: Standards of practice, *Amer J Occup Ther*, 46:1082, 1992.

RELATED BACKGROUND MATERIALS

American Occupational Therapy Association: Essentials and guidelines for an accredited educational program for the occupational therapist, *Amer J Occup Ther*, 45:1077, 1991.

American Occupational Therapy Association: Essentials and guidelines for an accredited educational program for the occupational therapist, *Amer J Occup Ther*, 45:1085, 1991.

American Occupational Therapy Association: Guide to supervision of occupational therapy personnel (in press). In Reference manual of official documents of the American Occupational Therapy Association, Inc, Rockville, Md, 1988. (Original work published *Amer J Occup Ther*, 35:815, 1981.)

Beeler JL, Young, PA, Dull, SM: Professional development framework: pathway to the future, *J Nurs Staff Develop* 6:296, 1990.

Mitchell, MM: Professional development: clinician to academician, *Amer J Occup Ther*, 39:368, 1985.

BACKGROUND

The need for a broader description of career options for occupational therapy was identified as part of the Entry-Level Study Report (AOTA, 1987) presented to the Representative Assembly (RA). The RA charged the Executive Board to study the recommendation of the Entry-Level Report and develop an action plan. The Executive Board formed a Directions for the Future (DFF) Coordinating Committee and charged that committee to develop an overall action plan. Part of the action plan was the implementation of a DFF Symposium to examine the future needs of practice and education.

Following the symposium, the DFF Coordinating Committee directed the Commission on Education (COE) and Commission on Practice (COP) to form a combined task force of members to develop a document describing a hierarchy of occupational therapy roles. The chairpersons of both commissions selected representatives from a wide variety of arenas in both practice and education. The task force included individuals directly involved in both professional and technical levels of education and practice. Special Interest Section Steering Committee (SISSC) representation was added to the task force to further broaden the scope of the task force. Reference to current professional literature provided a foundation for committee work. The most important references are listed at the end of this section.

Throughout the entire document development process, the document was reviewed by the members of the full COE, COP, COTA Task Force, and SISSC, as well as program directors for professional and technical curricula, thus ensuring both OTR and COTA perspectives.

One preliminary review of this document was followed by two formal reviews of drafts. The commission chairpersons recommended that the task force report be sent to the Intercommission Council (ICC) to further ensure that all facets of the Association were represented in the document development process.

As a result of the task force and review processes, an integrated education and practice taxonomy was recommended by the task force rather than a hierarchy. The taxonomy was preferred because it would provide practical information for a variety of uses within the profession. Since this taxonomy is a classification of categories of professional roles, it was decided to entitle the document *Occupational Therapy Roles*.

An ad hoc task force representing the Commission on Education Steering Committee (COESC), the Commission on Practice (COP), and the Special Interest Sections Steering Committee (SISSC) met in 1991 to 1992 and developed this draft entitled, *Occupational Therapy Roles*. This document is expected to replace and expand on the *Guide to Classification of Occupational Therapy Personnel* (AOTA, 1987).

REFERENCES

American Occupational Therapy Association: Guide to classification of occupational therapy personnel, *Amer J Occup Ther*, 39:803, 1987.

This document was prepared by the Occupational Therapy Roles Task Force:
  Patricia A. Crist, PhD, OTR, FAOTA—Chairperson
  Julie A. Halom, OTR;
  Jim Hinojosa, PhD, OTR, FAOTA;
  Scott McPhee, DrPH, OTR/L, FAOTA;
  Marlys M. Mitchell, PhD, OTR/L, FAOTA;
  Barbara A. Boyt Schell, MS, OTR/L, FAOTA;
  Mary Jane Youngstrom, MS, OTR;
  Carolyn Harsh, ScD, OTR/L—Staff Liaison;
  Sarah D. Hertfelder, Med, MOT, OTR—Staff
    Liaison for the Intercommission Council;
  Catherine Nielson, MPH, OTR/L—Chairperson.
Approved by the Representative Assembly (6/93)

  This document replaces the following documents rescinded by the Representative Assembly in June of 1993:

American Occupational Therapy Association (in press): Guide to classification of occupational therapy personnel. In Reference manual of official documents of The American Occupational Therapy Association, Inc., Rockville, Md. (Original work published 1985, *Amer J Occup Ther*, 39:803, 1987.

American Occupational Therapy Association: Supervision guidelines for certified occupational therapy assistants, *Amer J Occup Ther*, 44:1089, 1990.

The source of Appendix A is: *American Journal of Occupational Therapy*, 47:1087-1099. Also available with Companion Guide from AOTA Products Dept., 301-652-2682 (800-SAY AOTA, members).

(From the American Occupational Therapy Association, Inc., Bethesda, Md.)

Appendix B

OCCUPATIONAL THERAPY CODE OF ETHICS: THE AMERICAN OCCUPATIONAL THERAPY ASSOCIATION

The American Occupational Therapy Association's Code of Ethics is a public statement of the values and principles used in promoting and maintaining high standards of behavior in occupational therapy. The American Occupational Therapy Association and its members are committed to furthering people's ability to function within their total environment. To this end, occupational therapy personnel provide services for individuals in any stage of health and illness, to institutions, to other professionals and colleagues, to students, and to the general public.

The *Occupational Therapy Code of Ethics* is a set of principles that applies to occupational therapy personnel at all levels. The roles of practitioner (registered occupational therapist and certified occupational therapy assistant), educator, fieldwork educator, supervisor, administrator, consultant, fieldwork coordinator, faculty program director, researcher/scholar, entrepreneur, student, support staff, and occupational therapy aide are assumed.

Any action that is in violation of the spirit and purpose of this Code shall be considered unethical. To ensure compliance with the Code, enforcement procedures are established and maintained by the Commission on Standards and Ethics. Acceptance of membership in the American Occupational Therapy Association commits members to adherence to the Code of Ethics and its enforcement procedures.

Principle 1. Occupational therapy personnel shall demonstrate a concern for the well-being of the recipients of their services. (beneficence)

A. Occupational therapy personnel shall provide services in an equitable manner for all individuals.

B. Occupational therapy personnel shall maintain relationships that do not exploit the recipient of services sexually, physically, emotionally, financially, socially, or in any other manner. Occupational therapy personnel shall avoid these relationships or activities that interfere with professional judgment and objectivity.

C. Occupational therapy personnel shall take all reasonable precautions to avoid harm to the recipient of services or to his or her property.

D. Occupational therapy personnel shall strive to ensure that fees are fair, reasonable, and commensurate with the service performed and are set with due regard for the service recipient's ability to pay.

Principle 2. Occupational therapy personnel shall respect the rights of the recipients of their services (e.g., autonomy, privacy, confidentiality).

A. Occupational therapy personnel shall collaborate with service recipients or their surrogate(s) in determining goals and priorities throughout the intervention process.

B. Occupational therapy personnel shall fully inform the service recipients of the nature, risks, and potential outcomes of any interventions.

C. Occupational therapy personnel shall obtain informed consent from subjects involved in research activities indicating they have been fully advised of the potential risks and outcomes.

D. Occupational therapy personnel shall respect the individual's right to refuse professional services or involvement in research or educational activities.

E. Occupational therapy personnel shall protect the confidential nature of information gained from educational, practice, research, and investigational activities.

Principle 3. Occupational therapy personnel shall achieve and continually maintain high standards of competence (e.g., duties)

A. Occupational therapy practitioners shall hold the appropriate national and state credentials for providing services.

B. Occupational therapy personnel shall use procedures that conform to the Standards of Practice of the American Occupational Therapy Association.

C. Occupational therapy personnel shall take responsibility for maintaining competence by participating in professional development and educational activities.

D. Occupational therapy personnel shall perform their duties on the basis of accurate and current information.

E. Occupational therapy practitioners shall protect service recipients by ensuring that duties assumed by or assigned to other occupational therapy personnel are commensurate with their qualifications and experience.

F. Occupational therapy practitioners shall provide appropriate supervision to individuals for whom the practitioners have supervisory responsibility.

G. Occupational therapists shall refer recipients to other service providers or consult with other service providers when additional knowledge and expertise are required.

Principle 4. Occupational therapy personnel shall comply with laws and Association policies guiding the profession of occupational therapy (e.g., justice).

A. Occupational therapy personnel shall understand and abide by applicable Association policies: local, state, and federal laws; and institutional rules.

B. Occupational therapy personnel shall inform employers, employees, and colleagues about those laws and Association policies that apply to the profession of occupational therapy.

C. Occupational therapy practitioners shall require those they supervise in occupational therapy related activities to adhere to the Code of Ethics.

D. Occupational therapy personnel shall accurately record and report all information related to professional activities.

Principle 5. Occupational therapy personnel shall provide accurate information about occupational therapy services (e.g., veracity).

A. Occupational therapy personnel shall accurately represent their qualifications, education, experience, training, and competence.

B. Occupational therapy personnel shall disclose any affiliations that may pose a conflict of interest.

C. Occupational therapy personnel shall refrain from using or participating in the use of any form of communication that contains false, fraudulent, deceptive, or unfair statements or claims.

Principle 6. Occupational therapy personnel shall treat colleagues and other professionals with fairness, discretion, and integrity (e.g., fidelity, veracity)

A. Occupational therapy personnel shall safeguard confidential information about colleagues and staff.

B. Occupational therapy personnel shall accurately represent the qualifications, views, contributions, and findings of colleagues.

C. Occupational therapy personnel shall report any breaches of the Code of Ethics to the appropriate authority.

Author: Commission on Standards and Ethics (SEC)
Ruth Hansen, PhD, OTR, FAOTA, Chairperson
Approved by the Representative Assembly: 4/77
Revised: 1979, 1988, 1994
Adopted by the Representative Assembly: 7/94.
Note: This document replaces the 1988 Occupational Therapy Code of Ethics, which was rescinded by the 1994 Representative Assembly.
(From the American Occupational Therapy Association, Inc., Bethesda, Md.)

Appendix C

STANDARDS OF PRACTICE FOR OCCUPATIONAL THERAPY

PREFACE

These standards are intended as recommended guidelines to assist occupational therapy practitioners in the provision of occupational therapy services. These standards serve as a minimum standard for occupational therapy practice and are applicable to all individual populations and the programs in which these individuals are served.

These standards apply to those registered occupational therapists and certified occupational therapy assistants who are in compliance with regulation where it exists. The term occupational therapy practitioner refers to the registered occupational therapist and to the certified occupational therapy assistant, both of whom are in compliance with regulation where it exists.

The minimum educational requirements for the registered occupational therapist are described in the current Essentials and Guidelines of an Accredited Educational Program for the Occupational Therapist (American Occupational Therapy Association [AOTA], 1991a). The minimum educational requirements for the certified occupational therapy assistant are described in the current Essentials and Guidelines of an Accredited Educational Program for the Occupational Therapy Assistant (AOTA, 1991b).

STANDARD I: PROFESSIONAL STANDING

1. An occupational therapy practitioner shall maintain a current license, registration, or certification as required by law.

2. An occupational therapy practitioner shall practice and manage occupational therapy programs in accordance with applicable federal and state laws and regulations.

3. An occupational therapy practitioner shall be familiar with and abide by AOTA's (1988) Occupational Therapy Code of Ethics.

4. An occupational therapy practitioner shall maintain and update professional knowledge, skills, and abilities through appropriate continuing education or inservice training or higher education. The nature and minimum amount of continuing education must be consistent with state law and regulation.

5. A certified occupational therapy assistant must receive supervision from a registered occupational therapist as defined by the current Supervision Guidelines for Certified Occupational Therapy Assistants (AOTA, 1990) and by official AOTA documents. The nature and amount of supervision must

be provided in accordance with state law and regulation.

6. An occupational therapy practitioner shall provide direct and indirect services in accordance with AOTA's standards and policies. The nature and scope of occupational therapy services provided must be in accordance with state law and regulation.

7. An occupational therapy practitioner shall maintain current knowledge of the legislative, political, social, and cultural issues that affect the profession.

STANDARD II: REFERRAL

1. A registered occupational therapist shall accept referrals in accordance with AOTA's Statement of Occupational Therapy Referral (AOTA, 1989) and in compliance with appropriate laws.

2. A registered occupational therapist may accept referrals for assessment or assessment with intervention in occupational performance areas or occupational performance components when individuals have or appear to have dysfunctions or potential for dysfunctions.

3. A registered occupational therapist, responding to requests for service, may accept cases within the parameters of the law.

4. A registered occupational therapist shall assume responsibility for determining the appropriateness of the scope, frequency, and duration of services within the parameters of the law.

5. A registered occupational therapist shall refer individuals to other appropriate resources when the therapist determines that the knowledge and expertise of other professionals is indicated.

6. A registered occupational therapist shall educate current and potential referral sources about the process of initiating occupational therapy referrals.

STANDARD III: SCREENING

1. A registered occupational therapist, in accordance with state and federal guidelines, shall conduct screening to determine whether intervention or further assessment is necessary and to identify dysfunctions in occupational performance areas.

2. A registered occupational therapist shall screen independently or as a member of an interdisciplinary team. A certified occupational therapy assistant may contribute to the screening process under the supervision of a registered occupational therapist.

3. A registered occupational therapist shall select screening methods that are appropriate to the individual's age and developmental level; gender; education; cultural background; and socioeconomic, medical, and functional status. Screening methods may include, but are not limited to, interviews, structured observations, informal testing, and record reviews.

4. A registered occupational therapist shall communicate screening results and recommendations to appropriate individuals.

STANDARD IV: ASSESSMENT

1. A registered occupational therapist shall assess an individual's occupational performance components and occupational performance areas. A registered occupational therapist conducts assessments individually or as part of a team of professionals, as appropriate to the practice settings and the purposes of the assessments. A certified occupational therapy assistant may contribute to the assessment process under the supervision of a registered occupational therapist.

2. An occupational therapy practitioner shall educate the individual, or the individual's family or legal guardian, as appropriate,

about the purposes and procedures of the occupational therapy assessment.

3. A registered occupational therapist shall select assessments to determine the individual's functional abilities and problems as related to occupational performance areas; occupational performance components; physical, social, and cultural environments; performance safety; and prevention of dysfunction.

4. Occupational therapy assessment methods shall be appropriate to the individual's age and developmental level; gender; education; socioeconomic, cultural, and ethnic background; medical status; and functional abilities. The assessment methods may include some combination of skilled observation, interview, record review, or the use of standardized or criterion-referenced tests. A certified occupational therapy assistant may contribute to the assessment process under the supervision of a registered occupational therapist.

5. An occupational therapy practitioner shall follow accepted protocols when standardized tests are used. Standardized tests are tests whose scores are based on accompanying normative data that may reflect age ranges, gender, ethnic groups, geographic regions, and socioeconomic status. If standardized tests are not available or appropriate, the results shall be expressed in descriptive reports, and standardized scales shall not be used.

6. A registered occupational therapist shall analyze and summarize collected evaluation data to indicate the individual's current functional status.

7. A registered occupational therapist shall document assessment results in the individual's records, noting the specific evaluation methods and tools used.

8. A registered occupational therapist shall complete and document results of occupational therapy assessments within the time frame established by practice settings, government agencies, accreditation programs, and third-party payers.

9. An occupational therapy practitioner shall communicate assessment results, within the boundaries of client confidentiality, to the appropriate persons.

10. A registered occupational therapist shall refer the individual to the appropriate services or request additional consultations if the results of the assessments indicate areas that require intervention by other professionals.

STANDARD V: INTERVENTION PLAN

1. A registered occupational therapist shall develop and document an intervention plan based on analysis of the occupational therapy assessment data and the individual's expected outcome after the intervention. A certified occupational therapy assistant may contribute to the intervention plan under the supervision of a registered occupational therapist.

2. The occupational therapy intervention plan shall be stated in goals that are clear, measurable, behavioral, functional, and appropriate to the individual's needs, personal goals, and expected outcome after intervention.

3. The occupational therapy intervention plan shall reflect the philosophical base of occupational therapy (AOTA, 1979) and be consistent with its established principles and concepts of theory and practice. The intervention planning processes shall include
   a. Formulating a list of strengths and weaknesses.
   b. Estimating rehabilitation potential.
   c. Identifying measurable short-term and long-term goals.

　　d. Collaborating with the individual, family members, other caregivers, professionals, and community resources.

　　e. Selecting the media, methods, environment, and personnel needed to accomplish the intervention goals.

　　f. Determining the frequency and duration of occupational therapy services.

　　g. Identifying a plan for reevaluation.

　　h. Discharge planning.

4. A registered occupational therapist shall prepare and document the intervention plan within the time frames and according to the standards established by the employing practice settings, government agencies, accreditation programs, and third-party payers. The certified occupational therapy assistant may contribute to the formation of the intervention plan under the supervision of the registered occupational therapist.

STANDARD VI: INTERVENTION

1. An occupational therapy practitioner shall implement a program according to the developed intervention plan. The plan shall be appropriate to the individual's age and developmental level, gender, education, cultural and ethnic background, health status, functional ability, interests and personal goals, and service provision setting. The certified occupational therapy assistant shall implement the intervention under the supervision of a registered occupational therapist.

2. An occupational therapy practitioner shall implement the intervention plan through the use of specified purposeful activities or therapeutic methods to enhance occupational performance and achieve stated goals.

3. An occupational therapy practitioner shall be knowledgeable about relevant research in the practitioner's areas of practice. A registered occupational therapist shall interpret research findings as appropriate for application to the intervention process.

4. An occupational therapy practitioner shall educate the individual, the individual's family or legal guardian, noncertified occupational therapy personnel, and nonoccupational therapy staff, as appropriate, in activities that support the established intervention plan. An occupational therapy practitioner shall communicate the risk and benefit of the intervention.

5. An occupational therapy practitioner shall maintain current information on community resources relevant to the practice area of the practitioner.

6. A registered occupational therapist shall periodically reassess and document the individual's levels of functioning and changes in levels of functioning in the occupational performance areas and occupational performance components. A certified occupational therapy assistant may contribute to the reassessment process under the supervision of a registered occupational therapist.

7. A registered occupational therapist shall formulate and implement program modifications consistent with changes in the individual's response to the intervention. A certified occupational therapy assistant may contribute to program modifications under the supervision of a registered occupational therapist.

8. An occupational therapy practitioner shall document the occupational therapy services provided, including the frequency and duration of the services within the time frames and according to the standards established by the employing facility, government agencies, accreditation programs, and third-party payers.

STANDARD VII: DISCONTINUATION

1. A registered occupational therapist shall discontinue service when the individual has achieved predetermined goals or has achieved maximum benefit from occupational therapy services.

2. A registered occupational therapist, with input from a certified occupational therapy assistant where applicable, shall prepare and implement a discharge plan that is consistent with occupational therapy goals, individual goals, interdisciplinary team goals, family goals, and expected outcomes. The discharge plan shall address appropriate community resources for referral for psychosocial, cultural, and socioeconomic barriers and limitations that may need modification.

3. A registered occupational therapist shall document the changes between the initial and current states of functional ability and deficit in occupational performance areas and occupational performance components. A certified occupational therapy assistant may contribute to the process under the supervision of a registered occupational therapist.

4. An occupational therapy practitioner shall allow sufficient time for the coordination and effective implementation of the discharge plan.

5. A registered occupational therapist shall document recommendations for follow-up or reevaluation when applicable.

STANDARD VIII: CONTINUOUS QUALITY IMPROVEMENT

1. An occupational therapy practitioner shall monitor and document the continuous quality improvement of practice, which may include outcomes of services, using predetermined practice criteria reflecting professional consensus, recent developments in research, and specific employing facility standards.

2. An occupational therapy practitioner shall monitor all aspects of individual occupational therapy services for effectiveness and timeliness. If actual care does not meet the prescribed standard, it must be justified by peer review or other appropriate means within the practice setting. Occupational therapy services shall be discontinued when no longer necessary.

3. A registered occupational therapist shall systematically assess the review process of patient care to determine the success or appropriateness of interventions. Certified occupational therapy assistants may contribute to the process in collaboration with the registered occupational therapist.

STANDARD IX: MANAGEMENT

1. A registered occupational therapist shall provide the management necessary for efficient organization and provision of occupational therapy services.

2. A certified occupational therapy assistant, under the supervision of a registered occupational therapist, may perform the following management functions:
   a. Education of members of other related professions and physicians about occupational therapy.
   b. Participation in (1) orientation, supervision, training, and evaluation of the performance of volunteers and other noncertified occupational therapy personnel, and (2) developing plans to remediate areas of skill deficit in the performance of job duties by volunteers and other noncertified occupational therapy personnel.

c. Design and periodic review of all aspects of the occupational therapy program to determine its effectiveness, efficiency, and future directions.

d. Systematic review of the quality of service provided, using criteria established by professional consensus and current research, as well as established standards for state regulation; accreditation; American Occupational Therapy Certification Board (AOTCB) certification; and related laws, policies, guidelines, and regulations.

e. Incorporation of a fair and equitable system of admission, discharge, and charges for occupational therapy services.

f. Participation in cross-disciplinary activities to ensure that the total needs of the individual are met.

g. Provision of support (i.e., space, time, money as feasible) for clinical research or collaborative research when such projects have the approval of the appropriate governing bodies (e.g., institutional review board), and the results of which are deemed potentially beneficial to individuals of occupational therapy services now or in the future.

REFERENCES

American Occupational Therapy Association: The philosophical base of occupational therapy, *Amer J Occup Ther* 33:785, 1979.

American Occupational Therapy Association: Occupational therapy code of ethics, *Amer J Occup Ther* 42:795-796, 1988.

American Occupational Therapy Association: Statement of occupational therapy referral. In *Reference manual of the official documents of American Occupational Therapy Association, Inc. (AOTA) (p VIII.1)*, Rockville, Md, 1989. (Original work published 1969, revised 1980).

American Occupational Therapy Association: Supervision guidelines for certified occupational therapy assistants, *Amer J Occup Ther* 44:1089-1090, 1990.

American Occupational Therapy Association: *Essentials and guidelines of an accreditation educational program for the occupational therapist*, Rockville, Md, 1991a, AOTA.

American Occupational Therapy Association: *Essentials and guidelines of an accreditation educational program for the occupational therapy assistant*, Rockville, Md, 1991b, AOTA.

Prepared by the Commission of Practice (Jim Hinojosa, PhD, OTR, FAOTA, Chair).

Approved by the Representative Assembly March 1992.

This document replaces the 1983 Standards of Practice for Occupational Therapy (*Amer J Occup Ther* 37:802-804), which was rescinded.

(From the American Occupational Therapy Association, Inc., Bethesda, Md.)

Appendix D

UNIFORM TERMINOLOGY FOR OCCUPATIONAL THERAPY*

This is an official document of The American Occupational Therapy Association. This document is intended to provide a generic outline of the domain of concern of occupational therapy and is designed to create common terminology for the profession and to capture the essence of occupational therapy succinctly for others.

It is recognized that the phenomena that constitute the profession's domain of concern can be categorized, and labeled, in a number of different ways. This document is not meant to limit those in the field, formulating theories or frames of reference, who may wish to combine or refine particular constructs. It is also not meant to limit those who would like to conceptualize the profession's domain of concern in a different manner.

INTRODUCTION

The first edition of Uniform Terminology was approved and published in 1979 (AOTA, 1979). In 1989, the *Uniform Terminology for Occupational Therapy*— second edition (AOTA, 1989) was approved and published. The second document presented an organized structure for understanding the areas of practice for the profession of occupational therapy. The document outlined two domains. **Performance areas** (activities of daily living [ADL], work and productive activities, and play or leisure) include activities that the occupational therapy practitioner[1] emphasizes when determining functional abilities. **Performance components** (sensorimotor, cognitive, psychosocial, and psychological aspects) are the elements of performance that occupational therapists assess and, when needed,

in which they intervene for improved performance.

This third edition has been further expanded to reflect current practice and to incorporate contextual aspects of performance. *Performance Areas, Performance Components,* and *Performance Contexts* are the parameters of occupational therapy's domain of concern. *Performance areas* are broad categories of human activity that are typically part of daily life. They are activities of daily living, work and productive activities, and play or leisure activities. *Performance components* are fundamental human abilities that—to varying degrees and in differing combinations—are required for successful engagement in performance areas.

These components are sensorimotor, cognitive, psychosocial, and psychological. *Performance contexts* are situations or factors that influence an individual's engagement in desired and/or required performance areas. Performance contexts consist of *temporal* aspects (chronological age, developmental age, place in the life cycle, and health status); and *environmental* aspects (physical, social, and cultural considerations). There is an interactive relationship among performance areas, performance components, and performance contexts. Function in performance areas is the ultimate concern of occupational therapy, with performance components considered as they relate to participation in performance areas. Performance areas and performance components are always viewed within performance contexts. Performance contexts are taken into consideration when determining function and dysfunction relative to performance areas and performance components, and in plan-

---

*Third edition

[1]"Occupational therapy practitioner" refers to both registered occupational therapists and certified occupational therapy assistants.

ning intervention. For example, the occupational therapist does not evaluate strength (a performance component) in isolation. Strength is considered as it affects necessary or desired tasks (performance areas). If the individual is interested in homemaking, the occupational therapy practitioner would consider the interaction of strength with homemaking tasks. Strengthening could be addressed through kitchen activities, such as cooking and putting groceries away. In some cases, the practitioner would employ an adaptive approach and recommend that the family switch from heavy stoneware to lighter-weight dishes, or use lighter weight pots on the stove to enable the individual to make dinner safely without becoming fatigued or compromising safety.

Occupational therapy assessment involves examining performance areas, performance components, and performance contexts. Intervention may be directed toward elements of performance areas (e.g., dressing, vocational exploration), performance components (e.g., endurance, problem solving),or the environmental aspects of performance contexts. In the latter case, the physical and/or social environment may be altered or augmented to improve and/or maintain function. After identifying the performance areas the individual wishes or needs to address, the occupational therapist assesses the features of the environments in which the tasks will be performed. If an individual's job requires cooking in a restaurant as opposed to leisure cooking at home, the occupational therapy practitioner faces several challenges to enable the individual's success in different environments. Therefore, the third critical aspect of performance is the performance context, the features of the environment that affect the person's ability to engage in functional activities.

This document categorizes specific activities in each of the performance areas (ADL, work and productive activities, play or leisure). This categorization is based on what is considered "typical," and is not meant to imply that a particular individual characterizes personal activities in the same manner as someone else. Occupational therapy practitioners embrace individual differences, and so would document the unique pattern of the individual being served, rather than forcing the "typical" pattern on him or her and family. For example, because of experience or culture, a particular individual might think of home management as an ADL task rather than "work and productive activities" (current listing). Socialization might be considered part of a play or leisure activity instead of its current listing as part of "activities of daily living," because of life experience or cultural heritage.

EXAMPLES OF USE IN PRACTICE

Uniform Terminology—third edition, defines occupational therapy's domain of concern, which includes performance areas, performance components, and performance contexts. While this document may be used by occupational therapy practitioners in a number of different areas (e.g., practice, documentation, charge systems, education, program development, marketing, research, disability classifications, and regulations), it focuses on the use of uniform terminology in practice. This document is not intended to define specific occupational therapy programs or specific occupational therapy interventions. Examples of how performance areas, performance components, and performance contexts translate into practice are provided below.

- An individual who is injured on the job may have the potential to return to work and productive activities, which is a performance area. In order to achieve the outcome of returning to work and productive activities, the individual may need to address specific performance components, such as strength, endurance, soft-tissue integrity, time management, and the physical features of performance contexts, like structures and objects in his or her environment. The occupational therapy practitioner, in collaboration with the individual and other members of the vocational team, uses planned interventions to achieve the desired outcome. These interventions may include activities such as an exercise program, body mechanics instruction, and job site modifications, all of which may be provided in a work-hardening program.

- An elderly individual recovering from a cerebral vascular accident may wish to live in a community setting, which combines the performance areas of ADL with work and productive activities. In order to achieve the outcome of community living, the individual may need to address specific performance components, such as muscle tone, gross motor coordination, postural control, and self-management. It is also necessary to consider the sociocultural and physical features of performance contexts, such as support available from other persons, and adaptations of structures and objects within the environment. The occupational therapy practitioner, in cooperation with the team, utilizes planned interventions to achieve the desired outcome. Interventions may include neuromuscular facilitation, practice of object manipulation, and instruction in the use of adaptive equipment and home safety equipment. The practitioner and individual also pursue the selection and training of a personal assistant to ensure the completion of ADL tasks. These interventions may be provided in a comprehensive inpatient rehabilitation unit.

- A child with learning disabilities is required to perform educational activities within a public school setting. Engaging in educational activities is considered the performance area of work and productive activities for this child. To achieve the educational outcome of efficient and effective completion of written classroom work, the child may need to address specific performance components. These include sensory processing, perceptual skills, postural control, motor skills, and the physical features of performance contexts, such as objects (e.g., desk, chair) in the environment. In cooperation with the team, occupational therapy interventions may include activities like adapting the student's seating in the classroom to improve postural control and stability, and practicing motor control and coordination. This program could be developed by an occupational therapist and supported by school district personnel.

- The parents of an infant with cerebral palsy may ask to facilitate the child's involvement in the performance areas of activities of daily living and play. Subsequent to assessment, the therapist identifies specific performance components, such as sensory awareness and neuromuscular control. The practitioner also addresses the physical and cultural features of performance contexts. In collaboration with the parents occupational therapy interventions may include activities such as seating and positioning for play, neuromuscular facilitation techniques to enable eating, facilitating parent skills in caring for and playing with their infant, and modifying the play space for accessibility. These interventions may be provided in a home-based occupational therapy program.

- An adult with schizophrenia may need and want to live independently in the community, which represents the performance areas of activities of daily living, work and productive activities, and leisure activities. The specific performance categories may be medication routine, functional mobility, home management, vocational exploration, play or leisure performance, and social interaction. In order to achieve the outcome of living independently, the individual may need to address specific performance components, such as topographical orientation; memory; categorization; problem solving; interests; social conduct; time management; and sociocultural features of performance contexts, such as social factors (e.g., influence of family and friends) and roles. The occupational therapy practitioner, in cooperation with the team, utilizes activities such as training in the use of public transportation, instruction in budgeting skills, selection and participation in social activities, instruction in social conduct, and participation in community reintegration activities. These interventions may be provided in a community-based mental health program.

• An individual with a history of substance abuse may need to reestablish family roles and responsibilities, which represent the performance areas of activities of daily living, work and productive activities, and leisure activities. In order to achieve the outcome of family participation, the individual may need to address performance components of roles; values; social conduct; self-expression; coping skills; self-control; and the sociocultural features of performance contexts, such as custom, behavior, rules, and rituals. The occupational therapy practitioner, in cooperation with the team, utilizes planned interventions to achieve the desired outcomes. Interventions may include roles and values exercises, instruction in stress management techniques, identification of family roles and activities, and support to develop family leisure routines. These interventions may be provided in an inpatient acute care unit.

PERSON-ACTIVITY-ENVIRONMENT FIT

Person-activity-environment fit refers to the match among the skills and abilities of the individual; the demand of the activity; and the characteristics of the physical, social, and cultural environments. It is the interaction among the performance areas, performance components, and performance contexts that is important and determines the success of the performance. When occupational therapy practitioners provide services, they attend to each individual's unique personal history. The personal history includes one's skills and abilities (performance components), the past performance or specific life tasks (performance areas), and experience within particular environments (performance contexts). In addition to personal history, anticipated life tasks and role demands influence performance.

When considering the person-activity-environment fit, variables such as novelty, importance, motivation, activity tolerance, and quality are salient. Situations range from those that are completely familiar, to those that are novel and have never been experienced. Both the novelty and familiarity within a situation contribute to the overall task performance. In each situation, there is an optimal level of novelty that engages the individual sufficiently and provides enough information to perform the task. When too little novelty is present, the individual may miss cues and opportunities to perform. When too much novelty is present, the individual may become confused and distracted, inhibiting effective task performance.

Humans determine that some stimuli and situations are more meaningful than others. Individuals perform tasks they deem important. It is critical to identify what the individual wants or needs to do when planning interventions.

The level of motivation an individual demonstrates to perform a particular task is deter-

I. PERFORMANCE AREAS	II. PERFORMANCE COMPONENTS	III. PERFORMANCE CONTEXTS

A. Activities of Daily Living
  1. Grooming
  2. Oral Hygiene
  3. Bathing/Showering
  4. Toilet Hygiene
  5. Personal Device Care
  6. Dressing
  7. Feeding and Eating
  8. Medication Routine
  9. Health Maintenance
  10. Socialization
  11. Functional Communication
  12. Functional Mobility
  13. Community Mobility
  14. Emergency Response
  15. Sexual Expression
B. Work and Productive Activities
  1. Home Management
    a. Clothing Care
    b. Cleaning
    c. Meal Preparation/Cleanup
    d. Shopping
    e. Money Management
    f. Household Maintenance
    g. Safety Procedures
  2. Care of Others
  3. Educational Activities
  4. Vocational Activities
    a. Vocational Exploration
    b. Job Acquisition
    c. Work or Job Performance
    d. Retirement Planning
    e. Volunteer Participation
C. Play or Leisure Activities
  1. Play or Leisure Exploration
  2. Play or Leisure Performance
	A. Sensorimotor Component
	  1. Sensory
	    a. Sensory Awareness
	    b. Sensory Processing
	      (1) Tactile
	      (2) Proprioceptive
	      (3) Vestibular
	      (4) Visual
	      (5) Auditory
	      (6) Gustatory
	      (7) Olfactory
	    c. Perceptual Processing
	      (1) Stereognosis
	      (2) Kinesthesia
	      (3) Pain Response
	      (4) Body Scheme
	      (5) Right-Left Discrimination
	      (6) Form Constancy
	      (7) Position in Space
	      (8) Visual-Closure
	      (9) Figure Ground
	      (10) Depth Perception
	      (11) Spatial Relations
	      (12) Topographical Orientation
	  2. Neuromusculoskeletal
	    a. Reflex
	    b. Range of Motion
	    c. Muscle Tone
	    d. Strength
	    e. Endurance
	    f. Postural Control
	    g. Postural Alignment
	    h. Soft Tissue Integrity
	  3. Motor
	    a. Gross Coordination
	    b. Crossing the Midline
	    c. Laterally
	    d. Bilateral Integration
	    e. Motor Control
	    f. Praxis
	    g. Fine Coordination/Dexterity
	    h. Visual-Motor Integration
	    i. Oral-Motor Control
	B. Cognitive Integration and Cognitive Components
	  1. Level of Arousal
	  2. Orientation
	  3. Recognition
	  4. Attention Span
	  5. Initiation of Activity
	  6. Termination of Activity
	  7. Memory
	  8. Sequencing
	  9. Categorization
	  10. Concept Formation
	  11. Spatial Operations
	  12. Problem Solving
	  13. Learning
	  14. Generalization
	C. Psychosocial Skills and Psychological Components
	  1. Psychological
	    a. Values
	    b. Interests
	    c. Self-Concept
	  2. Social
	    a. Role Performance
	    b. Social Conduct
	    c. Interpersonal Skills
	    d. Self-Expression
	  3. Self-Management
	    a. Coping Skills
	    b. Time Management
	    c. Self-Control
		A Temporal Aspects
		  1. Chronological
		  2. Developmental
		  3. Life Cycle
		  4. Disability Status
		B. Environment
		  1. Physical
		  2. Social
		  3. Cultural

mined by both internal and external factors. An individual's biobehavioral state (e.g., amount of rest, arousal, tension) contributes to the potential to be responsive. The features of the social and physical environments (e.g., persons in the room, noise level) provide information that is either adequate or inadequate to produce a motivated state.

Activity tolerance is the individual's ability to sustain a purposeful activity over time. Individuals must not only select, initiate, and terminate activities, but they must also attend to a task for the needed length of time to complete the task and accomplish their goals.

The quality of performance is measured by standards generated by both the individual and others in the social and cultural environments in which the performance occurs. Quality is a continuum of expectations set within particular activities and contexts.

"Occupational Therapy" is the use of purposeful activity or interventions to promote health and achieve functional outcomes. "Achieving functional outcomes" means to develop, improve, or restore the highest possible level of independence of any individual who is limited by a physical injury or illness, a dysfunctional condition, a cognitive impairment, a psychosocial dysfunction, a mental illness, a developmental or learning disability, or an adverse environmental condition. Assessment means the use of skilled observation or nonstandardized test and measurements to identify areas for occupational therapy services.

Occupational therapy services include, but are not limited to:

1. the assessment, treatment, and education of or consultation with the individual, family, or other persons; or
2. interventions directed toward developing, improving, or restoring daily living skills, work readiness or work performance, play

skills or leisure capacities, or enhancing educational performance skills; or
3. providing for the development, improvement, or restoration of sensorimotor, oral motor, perceptual or neuromuscular functioning; or emotional, motivational, cognitive, or psychosocial components of performance.

These services may require assessment of the need for and use of interventions such as the design, development, adaptation, application, or training in the use of assistive technology devices; the design, fabrication, or application of rehabilitative technology such as selected orthotic devices; training in the use of assistive technology, orthotic or prosthetic devices; the application of physical agent modalities as an adjunct to or in preparation for purposeful activity; the use of ergonomic principles; the adaptation of environments and processes to enhance functional performance; or the promotion of health and wellness (AOTA, 1993, p.1117).

I. **Performance Areas**

Throughout this document, activities have been described as if individuals performed the tasks themselves. Occupational therapy also recognizes that individuals arrange for tasks to be done through others. The profession views independence as the ability to self-determine activity performance, regardless of who actually performs the activity.

A. Activities of Daily Living—Self-maintenance tasks.

1. *Grooming*—Obtaining and using supplies; removing body hair (use of razors, tweezers, lotions, etc.); applying and removing cosmetics; washing, drying, combing, styling, and brushing hair; caring for nails (hands

and feet), caring for skin, ears, and eyes; and applying deodorant.

2. *Oral Hygiene*—Obtaining and using supplies; cleaning mouth; brushing and flossing teeth; or removing, cleaning, and reinserting dental orthotics and prosthetics.

3. *Bathing/Showering*—Obtaining and using supplies; soaping, rinsing, and drying body parts; maintaining bathing position; and transferring to and from bathing positions.

4. *Toilet Hygiene*—Obtaining and using supplies; clothing management; maintaining toilet position; transferring to and from toileting position; cleaning body; and caring for menstrual and continence needs (including catheters, colostomies, and suppository management).

5. *Personal Device Care*—Cleaning and maintaining personal care items, such as hearing aids, contact lenses, glasses, orthotics, prosthetics, adaptive equipment, and contraceptive and sexual devices.

6. *Dressing*—Selecting clothing and accessories appropriate to time of day, weather, and occasion; obtaining clothing from storage area; dressing and undressing in a sequential fashion; fastening and adjusting clothing and shoes; and applying and removing personal devices, prostheses, or orthoses.

7. *Feeding and Eating*—Setting up food; selecting and using appropriate utensils and tableware; bringing food or drink to mouth; cleaning face, hands, and clothing; sucking, masticating, coughing, and swallowing; and management of alternative methods of nourishment.

8. *Medication Routine*—Obtaining mediation, opening and closing containers, following prescribed schedules, taking correct quantities, reporting problems and adverse effects, and administering correct quantities using prescribed methods.

9. *Health Maintenance*—Developing and maintaining routines for illness prevention and wellness promotion, such as physical fitness, nutrition, and decreasing health risk behaviors.

10. *Socialization*—Accessing opportunities and interacting with other people in appropriate contextual and cultural ways to meet emotional and physical needs.

11. *Functional Communication*—Using equipment or systems to send and receive information, such as writing equipment, telephones, typewriters, computers, communication boards, call lights, emergency systems, Braille writers, telecommunication devices for the deaf, and augmentative communication systems.

12. *Functional Mobility*—Moving from one position or place to another, such as in-bed mobility, wheelchair mobility, transfers (wheelchair, bed, car, tub, toilet, tub/shower, chair, floor). Performing functional ambulation and transporting objects.

13. *Community Mobility*—Moving self in the community and using public

or private transportation, such as driving, or accessing buses, taxi cabs, or other public transportation systems.

14. *Emergency Response*—Recognizing sudden, unexpected hazardous situations, and initiating action to reduce the threat to health and safety.

15. *Sexual Expression*—Engaging in desired sexual and intimate activities.

B. Work and Productive Activities— Purposeful activities for self-development, social contribution, and livelihood.

1. *Home Management*—Obtaining and maintaining personal and household possessions and environment.

   a. Clothing Care—Obtaining and using supplies; sorting, laundering (hand, machine, and dry clean); folding; ironing; storing; and mending.

   b. Cleaning—Obtaining and using supplies; picking up; putting away; vacuuming; sweeping and mopping floors; dusting; polishing; scrubbing; washing windows; cleaning mirrors; making beds; and removing trash and recyclables.

   c. Meal Preparation and Cleanup—Planning nutritious meals; preparing and serving food; opening and closing containers, cabinets, and drawers; using kitchen utensils and appliances; cleaning up and storing food safely.

   d. Shopping—Preparing shopping lists (grocery and other); selecting and purchasing items; selecting method of payment; and completing money transactions.

   e. Money Management— Budgeting, paying bills, and using bank systems.

   f. Household Maintenance— Maintaining home, yard, garden, appliances, vehicles, and household items.

   g. Safety Procedures—Knowing and performing prevention and emergency procedures to maintain a safe environment and to prevent injuries.

2. *Care of Others*—Providing for children, spouse, parents, pets, and others, such as giving physical care, nurturing, communicating, and using age-appropriate activities.

3. *Educational Activities*— Participating and learning environment through school, community, or work-sponsored activities, such as exploring educational interests, attending to instruction, managing assignments, and contributing to group experiences.

4. *Vocational Activities*—Participating in work-related activities.

   a. Vocational Exploration— Determining aptitudes; developing interests and skills, and selecting appropriate vocational pursuits.

   b. Job Acquisition—Identifying and selecting work opportuni-

ties, and completing application and interview process.

   c. Work or Job Performance—
Performing job tasks in a timely
and effective manner; incorporating necessary work behaviors.

   d. Retirement Planning—
Determining aptitudes; developing interests and skills; and
selecting appropriate avoca-
tional pursuits.

   e. Volunteer Participation—
Performing unpaid activities
for the benefit of selected individuals, groups, or causes.

C. Play or Leisure Activities—
Intrinsically motivating activities for
amusement, relaxation, spontaneous
enjoyment, or self-expression.

   1. *Play or Leisure Exploration—*
Identifying interests, skills, opportunities, and appropriate play or
leisure activities.

   2. *Play or Leisure Performance—*
Planning and participating in play
or leisure activities. Maintaining a
balance of play or leisure activities
with work and productive activities, and activities of daily living.
Obtaining, utilizing, and maintaining equipment and supplies.

II. Performance Components

A. Sensorimotor Component—The ability to receive input, process information, and produce output.

   1. *Sensory*

     a. Sensory Awareness—
Receiving and differentiating
sensory stimuli.

     b. Sensory Processing—
Interpreting sensory stimuli.

     (1) Tactile—Interpreting
light touch, pressure, temperature, pain, and vibra-
tion through skin contact/
receptors.

     (2) Proprioceptive—
Interpreting stimuli origi-
nating in muscles, joints,
and other internal tissues
that give information about
the position of one body
part in relation to another.

     (3) Vestibular—Interpreting
stimuli from the inner ear
receptors regarding head
position and movement.

     (4) Visual—Interpreting stim-
uli through the eyes,
including peripheral vision
and acuity, and awareness
of color and pattern.

     (5) Auditory—Interpreting
and localizing sounds, and
discriminating back-
ground sounds.

     (6) Gustatory—Interpreting
tastes.

     (7) Olfactory—Interpreting
odors.

   c. Perceptual Processing—
Organizing sensory input into
meaningful patterns.

     (1) Stereognosis—Identifying
objects through proprio-
ception, cognition, and
the sense of touch.

     (2) Kinesthesia—Identifying
the excursion and direc-
tion of joint movement.

     (3) Pain Response—Inter-
preting noxious stimuli.

(4) Body Scheme—Acquiring an internal awareness of the body and the relationship of body parts to each other.

(5) Right-Left Discrimination—Differentiating one side from the other.

(6) Form Constancy—Recognizing forms and objects as the same in various environments, positions, and sizes.

(7) Position in Space—Determining the spatial relationship of figures and objects to self or other forms and objects.

(8) Visual Closure—Identifying forms or objects from incomplete presentations.

(9) Figure Ground—Differentiating between foreground and background forms and objects.

(10) Depth Perception—Determining the relative distance between objects, figures, or landmarks and the observer, and changes in planes of surfaces.

(11) Spatial Relations—Determining the position of objects relative to each other.

(12) Topographical Orientation—Determining the location of objects and settings and the route to the location.

2. *Neuromusculoskeletal*

a. Reflex—Eliciting an involuntary muscle response by sensory input.

b. Range of Motion—Moving body parts through an arc.

c. Muscle Tone—Demonstrating a degree of tension or resistance in a muscle at rest and in response to stretch.

d. Strength—Demonstrating a degree of muscle power when movement is resisted, as with objects of gravity.

e. Endurance—Sustaining cardiac, pulmonary, and musculoskeletal exertion over time.

f. Postural Control—Using righting and equilibrium adjustments to maintain balance during functional movements.

g. Postural Alignment—Maintaining biomechanical integrity among body parts.

h. Soft Tissue Integrity—Maintaining anatomical and physiological condition of interstitial tissue and skin.

3. *Motor*

a. Gross Coordination—Using large muscle groups for controlled, goal-directed movements.

b. Crossing the Midline—Moving limbs and eyes across the midsagittal plane of the body.

c. Laterality—Using a preferred unilateral body part for activities requiring a high level of skill.

d. Bilateral Integration—
Coordinating both body sides
during activity.

e. Motor Control—Using the
body in functional and versatile
movement patterns.

f. Praxis—Conceiving and planning a new motor act in response
to an environmental demand.

g. Fine Coordination/Dexterity—
Using small muscle groups for
controlled movements, particularly in object manipulation.

h. Visual-Motor Integration—
Coordinating the interaction of
information from the eyes with
body movement during activity.

i. Oral-Motor Control—
Coordinating oropharyngeal
musculature for controlled
movements.

B. Cognitive Integration and Cognitive
Components—The ability to use higher brain functions.

1. *Level of Arousal*—Demonstrating
alertness and responsiveness to
environmental stimuli.

2. *Orientation*—Identifying person,
place, time, and situation.

3. *Recognition*—Identifying familiar
faces, objects, and other previously
presented materials.

4. *Attention Span*—Focusing on a
task over time.

5. *Initiation of Activity*—Starting a
physical or mental activity.

6. *Termination of Activity*—Stopping
an activity at an appropriate time.

7. *Memory*—Recalling information
after brief or long periods of time.

8. *Sequencing*—Placing information,
concepts, and actions in order.

9. *Categorization*—Identifying similarities of and differences among pieces
of environmental information.

10. *Concept Formation*—Organizing a
variety of information to form
thoughts and ideas.

11. *Spatial Operations*—Mentally
manipulating the position of
objects in various relationships.

12. *Problem Solving*—Recognizing a
problem, defining a problem, identifying alternative plans, selecting
a plan, organizing steps in a plan,
implementing a plan, and evaluating the outcome.

13. *Learning*—Acquiring new concepts and behaviors.

14. *Generalization*—Applying previously learned concepts and behaviors to a variety of new situations.

C. Psychosocial Skills and Psychological
Components—The ability to interact
in society and to process emotions.

1. *Psychological*

a. Values—Identifying ideas or
beliefs that are important to self
and others.

b. Interests—Identifying mental
or physical activities that create
pleasure and maintain attention.

c. Self-Concept—Developing the
value of the physical, emotional, and sexual self.

2. *Social*

a. Role Performance—Identifying,
maintaining, and balancing
functions one assumes or

acquires in society (e.g., worker, student, parent, friend, religious participant).

   b. Social Conduct—Interacting by using manners, personal space, eye contact, gestures, active listening, and self-expression appropriate to one's environment.

   c. Interpersonal Skills—Using verbal and nonverbal communication to interact in a variety of settings.

   d. Self-Expression—Using a variety of styles and skills to express thoughts, feelings, and needs.

  3. *Self-Management*

   a. Coping Skills—Identifying and managing stress and related factors.

   b. Time Management—Planning and participating in a balance of self-care, work, leisure, and rest activities to promote satisfaction and health.

   c. Self-Control—Modifying one's own behavior in response to environmental needs, demands, constraints, personal aspirations, and feedback from others.

III. Performance Contexts

Assessment of function in performance areas is greatly influenced by the contexts in which the individual must perform. Occupational therapy practitioners consider performance contexts when determining feasibility and appropriateness of interventions. Occupational therapy practitioners may choose interventions based on an understanding of contexts, or may choose interventions directly aimed at altering the contexts to improve performance.

A. Temporal Aspects

  1. *Chronological*—Individual's age.

  2. *Developmental*—Stage or phase of maturation.

  3. Life cycle—Place in important life phases, such as career cycle, parenting cycle, or educational process.

  4. Disability status—Place in continuum of disability, such as acuteness of injury, chronicity of disability, or terminal nature of illness.

B. Environment

  1. *Physical*—Nonhuman aspects of contexts. Includes the accessibility to and performance within environments having natural terrain, plants, animals, buildings, furniture, objects, tools, or devices.

  2. *Social*—Availability and expectations of significant individuals, such as spouse, friends, and caregivers. Also includes larger social groups which are influential in establishing norms, role expectations, and social routines.

  3. *Cultural*—Customs, beliefs, activity patterns, behavior standards, and expectations accepted by the society of which the individual is a member. Includes political aspects, such as laws that affect access to resources and affirm personal rights. Also includes opportunities for education, employment, and economic support.

REFERENCES

American Occupational Therapy Association: *Occupational therapy product output reporting systems and uniform terminology for reporting occupational therapy services,* Rockville, Md, 1979, AOTA.

American Occupational Therapy Association: Uniform terminology for occupational therapy—second edition, *Amer J Occup Ther* 43:808-815, 1989.

American Occupational Therapy Association: Definition of occupational therapy practice for state regulation (Policy 5.3.1), *Amer J Occup Ther* 47:1117-1121, 1993.

Authors

The Terminology Task Force:

Winifred Dunn, PhD, OTR, FAOTA, Chairperson

Mary Foto, OTR, FAOTA

Jim Hinojosa, PhD, OTR, FAOTA, Chairperson

Barbara Schell, PhD, OTR/L, FAOTA

Linda Kohlman Thomson, MOT, OTR, FAOTA

Sarah D. Hertfelder, Med, MOT, OTR/L—Staff Liaison for The Commission on Practice

Adopted by the Representative Assembly 7/94

NOTE: This document replaces the following documents, all of which were rescinded by the 1994 Representative Assembly:

Occupational Therapy Product Output Reporting System (1979)

Uniform Terminology for Reporting Occupational Therapy Services—First Edition (1979)

Uniform Occupational Therapy Evaluation Checklist (1981)

Uniform Terminology for Occupational Therapy—Second Edition (1989)

Uniform Terminology: Application to Practice*

Introduction

This document was developed to help occupational therapists apply *Uniform Terminology, Third Edition,* to practice. The original grid format (Dunn, 1988) enabled occupational therapy practitioners to systematically identify deficit and strength areas of an individual and to select appropriate activities to address these areas in occupational therapy intervention (Dunn & McGourty, 1990). For the third edition, the profession is highlighting "Contexts" as another critical aspect of performance. A second grid provides therapy practitioners with a mechanism to consider the contextual features of performance in activities of daily living (ADL), work and productive activity, and play/leisure. "Performance Areas" and "Performance Components" (Figure A) focus on the individual. These features are imbedded in the "Performance Contexts" (Figure B).

On the original grid (Dunn, 1988), the horizontal axis contains the Performance Areas of Activities of Daily Living, Work and Productive Activities, and Play or Leisure Activities (see Figure A). These Performance Areas are the functional outcomes occupational therapy addresses. The vertical axis contains the Performance Components, including Sensorimotor components, Cognitive Components, and Psychosocial Components. The Performance Components are the skills and abilities that an individual uses to engage in the Performance Areas. During an occupational therapy assessment, the occupational therapy practitioner determines an individual's abilities and limitations in the Performance Components and how they affect the individual's functional outcomes in the Performance Areas.

(continued on page 284)

*Third edition

Performance Components	Activities of Daily Living	Grooming	Oral hygiene	Bathing/showering	Toilet hygiene	Personal device care	Dressing	Feeding and eating	Medication routine	Health maintenance	Socialization	Functional communication	Functional mobility	Community mobility	Emergency response	Sexual expression	Work and Productive Activities	Home management	Care of others	Educational activities	Vocational activities	Play or Leisure Activities	Play or leisure exploration	Play or leisure performance
A. Sensorimotor component																								
1. Sensory																								
a. Sensory awareness																								
b. Sensory processing																								
(1) Tactile																								
(2) Proprioceptive																								
(3) Vestibular																								
(4) Visual																								
(5) Auditory																								
(6) Gustatory																								
(7) Olfactory																								
c. Perceptual processing																								
(1) Stereognosis																								
(2) Kinesthesia																								
(3) Pain response																								
(4) Body Scheme																								
(5) Right-left discrimination																								
(6) Form constancy																								
(7) Position in space																								
(8) Visual—closure																								
(9) Figure ground																								
(10) Depth perception																								
(11) Spatial relations																								
(12) Topographical orientation																								
2. Neuromusculoskeletal																								
a. Reflex																								
b. Range of motion																								
c. Muscle tone																								
d. Strength																								
e. Endurance																								
f. Postural control																								
g. Postural alignment																								
h. Soft-tissue integrity																								
3. Motor																								
a. Gross coordination																								
b. Crossing the midline																								
c. Laterality																								

FIGURE A. UNIFORM TERMINOLOGY GRID (PERFORMANCE AREAS AND PERFORMANCE COMPONENTS).

Performance Components—cont'd	**Activities of Daily Living**	Grooming	Oral hygiene	Bathing/showering	Toilet hygiene	Personal device care	Dressing	Feeding and eating	Medication routine	Health maintenance	Socialization	Functional communication	Functional mobility	Community mobility	Emergency response	Sexual expression	**Work and Productive Activities**	Home management	Care of others	Educational activities	Vocational activities	**Play or Leisure Activities**	Play or leisure exploration	Play or leisure performance
d. Bilateral integration																							
e. Motor control																							
f. Praxis																							
g. Fine coordination/dexterity																							
h. Visual-motor integration																							
i. Oral-motor control																							
B. Cognitive integration and cognitive components																							
1. Level of arousal																							
2. Orientation																							
3. Recognition																							
4. Attention span																							
5. Initiation of activity																							
6. Termination of activity																							
7. Memory																							
8. Sequencing																							
9. Categorization																							
10. Concept formation																							
11. Spatial operations																							
12. Problem solving																							
13. Learning																							
14. Generalization																							
C. Psychosocial skills and psychological components																							
1. Psychological																							
a. Values																							
b. Interests																							
c. Self-concept																							
2. Social																							
a. Role performance																							
b. Social conduct																							
c. Interpersonal skills																							
d. Self-expression																							
3. Self-management																							
a. Coping skills																							
b. Time management																							
c. Self-control																							

FIGURE A. CONT'D.

Special Note: The first application document (Dunn & McGourty, 1989) describes how to use the original *Uniform Terminology* grid with a variety of individuals. It is quite useful to introduce these concepts. However, the third edition of *Uniform Terminology* contains some changes in the Performance Areas and Performance Components lists. Be sure to check for the terminology currently approved in the third edition before applying this information in current practice environments.

With the addition of Performance Contexts into *Uniform Terminology*, occupational therapy practitioners must consider how to interface what the individual wants to do (i.e., performance area) with the contextual features that may support or block performance. Figure B illustrates the interaction of Performance Areas and Performance Contexts as a model for therapists' planning.

The grid in Figure B can be used to analyze the contexts of performance for a particular individual. For example, when working with a toddler with a developmental disability who needs to learn to eat, the occupational therapy practitioner would consider all the Performance Contexts features as they might impact on this toddler's ability to master eating. Unlike the grid in Figure A, in which the occupational therapy practitioner selects *both* Performance Areas (i.e., what the individual wants or needs to do) and the Performance Component (i.e., a person's strengths and needs), in this grid (Figure B) the occupational therapy practitioner only selects the Performance Area. After the Performance Area is identified through collaboration with the individual and significant others, the occupational therapy practitioner considers ALL Performance Contexts features as they might impact on performance of the selected task.

INTERVENTION PLANNING

Intervention planning occurs both within the general domain of concern of occupational thera-

FIGURE B. UNIFORM TERMINOLOGY GRID (PERFORMANCE AREAS AND PERFORMANCE COMPONENTS).

py (i.e., uniform terminology) and by considering the profession's theoretical frames of reference that offer insights about how to approach the problem. In Figure A, the occupational therapy practitioner considers the Performance Areas that are of interest to the individual and the individual's strengths and concerns within the Performance Components. The intervention strategies would emerge from the cells on the grid that are placed at the intersection of the Performance Areas and the targeted Performance Components (strength and/or concern). For example, if a child needed to improve sensory processing and fine coordination for oral hygiene and grooming, an occupational therapy practitioner might select a sensory integrative frame of reference to create intervention strategies, such as adding textures to handles and teaching the child sand and bean digging games. Dunn and McGourty (1989) discuss this in more detail.

When using Figure B, the occupational therapy practitioner considers the Performance Contexts features in relation to the desired Performance Area. The occupational therapy practitioner would analyze the individual's temporal, physical, social, and cultural contexts to determine the relevance of particular interventions. For example, if the child mentioned above was a member of a family in which having messy hands from sand play was unacceptable, the occupational therapy practitioner would consider alternate strategies that are more compatible with their lifestyle. For example, perhaps the family would be more interested in developing puppet play. This would still provide the child with opportunities to experience the textures of various puppets and the hand movements required to manipulate the puppets in play context, without adding the messiness of sand. When occupational therapy practitioners consider contexts, interventions become more relevant and applicable to individual's lives.

CASE EXAMPLE 1

Sophie is a 75-year-old lady, who was widowed 3 years ago, is recovering from a cerebral vascular accident and has been transferred from an acute care unit to an inpatient medical rehabilitation unit. Prior to her admission, she was living in a small house in an isolated location and has no family living nearby. She was driving independently and frequently ran errands for her friends. She is adamant in her goal to return to her home after discharge. All of her friends are quite elderly and are not able to provide many resources for support.

Sophie and the team collaborated to identify her goals. Sophie decided that she wanted to be able to meet her daily needs with little or no assistance. Almost all of the Performance Areas are critical in order to achieve the outcome of community living in her own home. Being able to cook all of her meal, bathe independently, and have alternative transportation available is necessary. Because of their significant impact on the patient's function in the Performance Areas, some of the Performance Components that may need to be addressed are figure ground, muscle tone, postural control, fine coordination, memory, and self-management.

In the selection of occupational therapy interventions, it is critical to analyze the elements of Performance Contexts for the individual. The physical and social elements of her home environment do not support returning home without modifications to her home and additional social supports being established. Railings must be added to the front steps, provision of and instruction in the use of a tub seat, and instruction in the use of specialized transportation may need to occur. If this same individual had been living in an apartment in a retirement community prior to her CVA, the contexts of her performance would support a return home with fewer environmental modifications being needed. Being independent in cooking might not be necessary due to meals being provided, and the bathroom might already be accessible and safe. If the individual had friends and family available, the social support network might already be established to assist with shopping and transportation needs. The occupational therapy interventions would be different due to the contexts in which the individual will be performing. Interventions must be selected with the impact of the Performance Contexts as an essential element.

CASE EXAMPLE 2

Malcolm is a 9-year-old boy who has a learning disability which causes him to have a variety of problems in the school. His teachers complain that he is difficult to manage in the classroom. Some of the Performance Components that may need to be addressed are his self control such as interrupting, difficulty sitting during instruction, and difficulty with peer relations. Other children avoid him on the playground, because he doesn't follow rules, doesn't play fair, and tends to anger quickly when confronted. The performance component impairment with concept formation is reflected in his sloppy and disorganized classroom assignments.

The critical elements of the Performance Contexts are the temporal aspect of age-appropriateness of his behavior and the social environmental aspect of his immature socialization. The significant cultural and temporal aspects of his family are that they place a high premium on athletic prowess.

The occupational therapy practitioner intervenes in several ways to address his behavior in the school environment. The occupational therapy practitioner focuses on structuring the classroom environment and facilitating consistent behavioral expectations for Malcolm by educational personnel. She also consults with the teachers to develop ways to structure activi-

ties which will support his ability to relate to other children in a positive way.

In contrast, another child with similar learning disabilities, but who is 12 years old in the 7th grade might have different concerns. Elements of the Performance Contexts are the temporal aspect of the age-appropriateness of his behavior; and the social environmental context of school where "bullying" behavior is unacceptable and in which completing assignments is expected. In addressing the cultural Performance Contexts the occupational therapy practitioner recognizes from meeting with parents that they have only average expectations for academic performance but value athletic accomplishments.

Since teachers at his school consider completion of home assignments to be part of average performance, the occupational therapy practitioner works with the child and parents on time management and reinforcement strategies to meet this expectation. After consultation with the coach, she works with the father to create activities to improve his athletic abilities. When occupational therapy practitioners consider family values as part of the contexts of performance, different intervention priorities may emerge.

AUTHORS

The Terminology Task Force:
Winnie Dunn, PhD, OTR, FAOTA—Chairperson
Mary Foto, OTR, FAOTA
Jim Hinojosa, PhD, OTR, FAOTA, Chairperson
Barbara A. Boyt Schell, PhD, OTR, FAOTA
Linda Kohlman Thomson, MOT, OTR, OT(C), FAOTA
Sarah D. Hertfelder, Med, MOT, OTR—Staff Liaison
    for The Commission on Practice—1994

Note: This document replaces the 1989 Application of
    Uniform Terminology to Practice that accompanied the
    *Uniform Terminology for Occupational Therapy—Second
    Edition*. (From the American Occupational Therapy
    Association, Inc., Bethesda, Md.)

INDEX

A

Abduction, as basic medical term, *195, 196*
Abuses, addressed in Code of Ethics, 76
Acceptance, stage of loss, 201
Accreditation
    definition of, 84-85
    of educational programs, 85-86
    of health care agencies, 85
Accreditation Council for Occupational
        Therapy Education (ACOTE)
    duties of, 86
    regulating education, 47
"Active being," defining humans in occu-
        pational therapy terms, 38
Active listening, developing skills in, 207-
        208
Activities; *see also* occupations; purposeful
        activities
    adjunctive, 224-228
    arts and crafts, 21
    basis in occupational therapy philoso-
        phy, 37
    definition of, 5
    dimensions of, 39
    enabling, 224, *225*
    gathering information concerning, 140,
        141
    group, 208-209
    versus occupations, 39
    play and leisure, *113,* 114-115
    terminology, 269-280
    types used in treatment, 8-9
    work and productive, *113,* 114
Activities of daily living (ADLs); *see also*
        Appendix D
    definition and types of, *113,* 114
    self-care tasks, 274-276
    in treatment continuum, *218*
Activity accommodation approach, to solu-
        tion development, 164, *165*
Activity analysis
    clinical reasoning in, 234
    description and steps in, 219-220
    frames of reference in, 219
    purposeful activities in, 220-224
Activity batteries, using for observation,
        144-147
Activity configurations, description of, 140
Activity Directors, occupational therapists
        as, 69
Acute care
    description of, 59
    within hospitals, 64-65
Adaptation
    basis in occupational therapy philoso-
        phy, 37
    definition of, 40

Adaptation—continued
    to reach goals, 221
Addictions, and supervised living, 67
Adduction, as basic medical term, *195, 196*
Adjunctive activities, definition of, 224-228
Adolescents, chemical dependency in, *12*
Advanced levels,
    classifying, 51, 52t
    function and supervision of, *246*
Aesthetics, philosophical questions of, 37
Alcoholism, and supervised living, 67
Altruism, in occupational therapy philoso-
        phy, 41
Alzheimer's disease, day treatment for
        clients with, 67
American Journal of Occupational Therapy
        (AJOT), 99-100
American Occupational Therapy
        Association (AOTA)
    accreditation of educational programs,
        85-86
    adapting to change, 30-31
    annual conference of, 100-101
    certification and registration guidelines,
        86-89
    classifying experience levels, 51, 52t
    dedication to quality, 98-99
    defining occupational therapy, 4-5
    defining personnel terminology, 46,
        244-258
    demographic statistics from, 54
    formal ethical code, 75-79
    imposing disciplinary sanctions, 90
    issuing Standards of Practice, 77
    lobbying efforts by, 31
    membership in, 97
    membership statistics of, 31
    mission of, 97
    occupational therapy career roles, 244-
        258
    photographic essay by, 9, *10-15*
    on physical agent modalities, 226
    promoting professional development,
        99-101
    public relations efforts by, 185
    Slagle's role in developing, 23
    sponsoring continuing education, 100-
        101
    structure of, 98
    summary of historical highlights, *25*
    uniform terminology, 269-280
American Occupational Therapy
        Foundation (AOTF), conducting
        research, 99
American Society of Hand Therapists, 88
American Student Committee of the Occu-
        pational Therapy Association, 98

Americans with Disabilities Act (ADA),
        25, 30
Anatomic position, as basic medical term,
        195, 196
Anger, stage of loss, 201
Anterior, as basic medical term, *195, 196*
Anthropology, as an educational founda-
        tion, 8
Antibiotics, changing focus of occupational
        therapy, *25,* 29
Antipsychotics, discovery of, 28
Appointments, scheduling, 181-182
Arms, injuries of, 225-226
Árnadóttir, Guorún, on observation and
        human potential, 214
Artistic elements, of clinical reasoning, 234
Arts and crafts
    early twentieth century work in, 21-23
    in groups, 208
    Herbert Hall, on uses in treatment, 21
    workshops in mental health centers, 67
Assessment
    activity battery method, *145*
    defining in the occupational therapy
        process, 127-128
    documenting, 149
    standards of practice, 264-265
    steps in the process, 137-150
    of treatment plan results, 168
Assistive devices, in occupational therapy,
        221-223
Assistive technology approach, to solution
        development, 164, *165*
Augmentative communication devices, 221,
        223
Autonomy, defining within ethical code, 76-
        77
Axiology components, of philosophy, 37

B

Bargaining, stage of loss, 201
Barton, George Edward, on value of occupa-
        tion, 21-22
Bathing/showering, AOTA definition of, 275
Batteries; *see* activity batteries
Behavioral sciences, as an educational foun-
        dation, 8
Beneficence, principle of, 75
Bertolotti, Diane, on the rewards of the pro-
        fession, 34
Bing, Robert, linking present and future, 18
Biochemical imbalances, within psychologi-
        cal and sociological spheres, 63
Biological (medical) spheres
    clinics providing care, 65
    occupational therapist's role within, *62,*
        64-66

Biological (medical) spheres—continued
   within occupational therapy practice,
      62-63
   role of home health agencies in, 65-66
Biology, as an educational foundation, 8
Boarding homes, 66
Brainstorming, in problem solving, 159, 160
Burkhardt, Ann, on rewards of occupation-
   al therapy, 120
Byers-Connon, Sue, on occupational thera-
   py as a "way of life," 44

C

Cardiopulmonary resuscitation (CPR), staff
   awareness of, 178
Case-Smith, Jane, on occupational therapy
   assessment, 134
Caudal, as basic medical term, *195, 196*
Centers for Disease Control (CDC), 179
Cephalo, as basic medical term, *195, 196*
Cerebral palsy
   photograph showing patient with, *11*
   special schools for impaired individuals,
      66
   United, 59
Certification
   definition of, 86
   entry-level, 86-87
   specialty, 88
   state requirements for, 88-89
Certified Occupational Therapy Assistants
   (COTAs)
   certification and registration guidelines,
      86-88
   distinctions of practitioner levels, 5
   educational requirements, *49*
   employment trends for, 69-70
   experience and performance levels of,
      51, 52t
   fieldwork required by, 47
   introduction of, 30
   major functions of, 50t, 248-250
   membership in AOTA, 97
   paths to becoming, 48-49
   role within occupational therapy
      process, 123-132
   statistics on degrees earned, 54
Checklists
   interests, 140, *141*
   for learning terminology, 194
Chemical dependency units, photo of, *12*
Children
   day treatment for, 66-67
   groups for, 202
   learning concepts, 109
   legislation protecting disabled, *25, 29*-30
   photograph showing splints, *10*
   play activities, 115
   special hospitals for, 65
Civil War, 19
Clarification, as a communication tool,
   207-208
Clinical reasoning
   definition and importance of, 232-233

Clinical reasoning—continued
   diagnoses with, 235
   ethics and, 233
   hypotheses evaluation, 235
   Joan Rogers on, 233
   preassessment images, 234-235
   thought process during, 234-236
Clinical training, importance of, 8
Clinics, addressing medical problems, 65
Close supervision, description of, 52-53
Code of Ethics, American Occupational
      Therapy Association, 261-263
   definition of, 74-75
   dilemmas concerning, 79-80
   enforcement of, 77, 90
Cognitive disabilities
   frames of reference, 111
   helped by occupational therapy, 7
   within psychological sphere, 63
Cognitive integration components; *see also*
      Appendix D
   within activity analysis, 219
   AOTA definitions of, 279
   within occupational performance mod-
      el, *113*
   of performance, 115-116
Cognitive psychology, and problem solving,
   157
Cognitive systems, coordinating, 39
Commission on Standards and Ethics,
   enforcing Code of Ethics, 75, 90
Communication
   complexity of human, 200-201
   computers used to aid, *11*
   as fundamental performance area, 114
   importance of comprehensive, 6
   tools for active listening, 207-208
   understanding verbal and nonverbal,
      205-206
   using correct medical terminology, 192
Community mental health centers, types
   of, 67
Community mobility, AOTA definition of,
   275-276
Compassion, and Moral Treatment, 19-20
Compensatory approach, to solution development, 164, *165*
Competence, maintaining high standards
   of, 77
Computers
   aiding patients with cerebral palsy, *11*
   augmentative communication devices,
      221, *223*
Concepts, definition of, 109
Conditional reasoning, strategy of, 236-237
Confidentiality, and trust, 205
Congenital disabilities, shown in photo-
   graphic essay, *10*
Consultants, role of, 253-254
Continuing education, 100-101
Continuous quality improvement, stan-
   dards of practice, 267
Continuum of care, providing comprehen-
   sive care, 59

Corporations
   offering employment, 59
   OSHA standards in, 179
Correctional facilities
   employment opportunities in, 68
   providing occupational therapy, 59
Costs
   affected by Medicare, 29
   incentives to reduce, 60
Critical thinking, in problem solving, 157-
   158
Cues, 235
Cultural aspects, affecting performance, 116

D

Davis, Carol, on steps to resolve ethical
      dilemmas, 79
Day treatment facilities, addressing social
      sphere, 66-67
Death, and dying, 201
"Deinstitutionalization" Plan, 29
Demographics
   employment trends, 69-70
   of occupational therapy practitioners, 54
   of settings, *61*
Denial, stage of loss, 201
Depression
   within psychological sphere of practice,
      63
   stage of loss, 201
Developmental growth
   assessing in twins, *11*
   photograph featuring disabilities in, *13*
Devices; *see* assistive devices
Diagnoses
   through clinical reasoning, 235
   using spheres of practice, 60, 62-67
Diagnostic-related groups (DRGs)
   fee organization of, 60
   and Medicare, *25,* 29
Dignity, in occupational therapy philosophy,
   41
Direct service functions, definition of, 123
Directions, terms referring to, 194-195, *196*
Discharges
   developing plans of, 131
   importance of plans, 168-169
   preparing summaries, 132
   standards of practice, 267
Disciplinary Action Information Exchange
      Network (DAIEN), publishing
      ethics offenders, 91
Disciplinary processes
   imposing sanctions, *91*
   policies and procedures, 90-91
Discontinuation, standards of, 267
Distal, as basic medical term, *195, 196*
Documentation
   importance of accurate, 169-171
   of treatment, 130
Domain of concern; *see also* Appendix D
   definition of, 112
   evolution of, 112-113
Dorsal, as basic medical term, *195, 196*